"Tapping into the analytic wisdom of their left brains and the intuitive wisdom of their right brains, the husband and wife team of Gregor and Maša Žvelc have co-created a profoundly humane, heartfelt, tender, and lovingly crafted masterpiece. Seamlessly interweaving theory and practice, *Integrative Psychotherapy* highlights the healing power of relationally focused treatments that privilege mindful awareness, compassion, acceptance, shared conscious presence, and co-regulation. Their holistic approach, at once inspired and inspiring, features the freshly revitalized, neurobiological concept of memory reconsolidation, which creates opportunity for rewiring the brain and updating mental schemas about self, others, and the world. Truly a gem of a book!!"

—**Martha Stark, MD,** faculty, Harvard Medical School, co-founder / co-director / faculty, Center for Psychoanalytic Studies, award-winning author of 8 books on psychoanalytic theory and practice, including *Relentless Hope: The Refusal to Grieve*

"*Integrative Psychotherapy* defines the most therapeutically astute utilization of mindfulness and compassion I've seen, because it goes beyond creating awareness of one's existing, limiting patterns to engage the brain's empirically confirmed process of transformational change through memory reconsolidation. The entire methodology is transdiagnostic and transtheoretical, so it is a broadly integrative framework with deep experiential process and active, respectful cultivation of the client's unique world of meaning."

—**Bruce Ecker,** LMFT, Coherence Psychology Institute co-director, co-creator of Coherence Therapy, and coauthor of *Unlocking the Emotional Brain: Eliminating Symptoms at Their Roots Using Memory Reconsolidation*

"Gregor and Maša Žvelc offer a thoughtful, finely layered account of the theory and practice of mindful, compassionate integrative psychotherapy. Numerous rich illustrations of therapeutic dialogue vividly demonstrate the 'science' and 'art' of integrative psychotherapy. They highlight how a sensitive, accepting, mindful and compassionate therapeutic relationship helps clients explore themselves more deeply towards integrating forgotten parts. This is an ideal textbook for students seeking a coherent and comprehensive, yet gentle, model of psychotherapeutic integration, while experienced therapists will value the knowledgeable and scholarly references to contemporary theory and research."

—**Dr Linda Finlay**, Integrative Psychotherapist in private practice, United Kingdom

Integrative Psychotherapy

Integrative psychotherapy is a groundbreaking book where the authors present mindfulness- and compassion-oriented integrative psychotherapy (MCIP) as an integration of relational psychotherapy with the practice and research of mindfulness and compassion.

The book elucidates an approach which is holistic and based on evidence-based processes of change related to the main dimensions of human experience. In this approach, mindfulness and compassion are viewed as meta-processes of change that are used within an attuned therapeutic relationship to create a powerful therapeutic model that provides transformation and growth. The authors offer an exciting perspective on intersubjective physiology and the mutual connection between the client's and therapist's autonomic nervous systems.

Comprised of creatively applied research, the book will have an international appeal amongst psychotherapists/counsellors from different psychotherapy traditions and also students with advanced/postgraduate levels of experience.

Gregor Žvelc, PhD, is an associate professor of clinical psychology at the University of Ljubljana. He is a Certified International Integrative Psychotherapy Trainer & Supervisor (CIIPTS) and Teaching and Supervising Transactional Analyst (TSTA). He is the co-founder and director of the Institute for Integrative Psychotherapy and Counselling, Ljubljana.

Maša Žvelc, PhD, is a Certified International Integrative Psychotherapy Trainer & Supervisor (CIIPTS). She is co-founder and co-director of the Institute for Integrative Psychotherapy and Counselling, Ljubljana, where she has a psychotherapy and supervision practice and leads training in integrative psychotherapy and supervision.

Advancing Theory in Therapy

Series Editor
Keith Tudor
Auckland University of Technology, New Zealand

About the Series
Most books covering individual therapeutic approaches are aimed at the trainee/student market.

This series, however, is concerned with advanced and advancing theory, offering the reader comparative and comparable coverage of a number of therapeutic approaches.

Aimed at professionals and postgraduates, *Advancing Theory in Therapy* will cover an impressive range of theories.

With full reference to case studies throughout, each book in the series will:

- present cutting edge research findings
- locate each theory and its application within its cultural context
- develop a critical view of theory and practice.

Books in this series:
Constructivist Psychotherapy
A Narrative Hermeneutic Approach
Gabriele Chiari, Maria Laura Nuzzo

Lacanian Psychoanalysis
Revolutions in Subjectivity
Ian Parker

Gestalt Therapy
Advances in Theory and Practice
Edited by Talia Bar-Yoseph Levine

Existential Therapy
Legacy, Vibrancy and Dialogue
Laura Barnett, Greg Madison

Integrative Psychotherapy
A Mindfulness- and Compassion-Oriented Approach
Gregor Žvelc, Maša Žvelc

For more information about this series, please visit: https://www.routledge.com/Advancing-Theory-in-Therapy/book-series/SE0646

Integrative Psychotherapy

A Mindfulness- and Compassion-Oriented
Approach

Gregor Žvelc and Maša Žvelc

Routledge
Taylor & Francis Group

LONDON AND NEW YORK

First published 2021
by Routledge
2 Park Square, Milton Park, Abingdon, Oxon OX14 4RN

and by Routledge
52 Vanderbilt Avenue, New York, NY 10017

Routledge is an imprint of the Taylor & Francis Group, an informa business

© 2021 Gregor Žvelc and Maša Žvelc

British Library Cataloguing in Publication Data
A catalogue record for this book is available from the British Library

Library of Congress Cataloging-in-Publication Data
A catalog record has been requested for this book

ISBN: 978-0-367-25906-8 (hbk)
ISBN: 978-0-367-25908-2 (pbk)
ISBN: 978-0-429-29048-0 (ebk)

Typeset in Baskerville
by Taylor & Francis Books

Contents

Figures and Table

Figures

Table

Series preface

This series focuses on advanced and advancing theory in psychotherapy. Its aims are: to present theory and practice within a specific theoretical orientation or approach at an advanced, postgraduate level; to advance theory by presenting and evaluating new ideas and their relation to the approach; to locate the orientation and its applications within cultural contexts both historically in terms of the origins of the approach, and contemporarily in terms of current debates about philosophy, theory, society and therapy; and, finally, to present and develop a critical view of theory and practice, especially in the context of debates about power, organisation and the increasing professionalisation of therapy.

When I initiated this series 20 years ago, I was keen to commission a volume on integrative psychotherapy but, for various reasons, one was not forthcoming and I put this particular project on the back burner. Now I'm glad I did and I'm even more glad that, subsequently, I met Gregor and Maša Žvelc, got to know them and their ideas, and asked them to contribute this particular volume to the series. Integrative psychotherapy is now an approach or modality in its own right, as reflected in the increased literature on the subject and the number of training programmes that take an integrative approach. At the same time, by advancing the concept of integration, integrative psychotherapy invites, even insists on a meta-perspective. The meta-perspective that the authors advance in this volume is that of a mindfulness- and compassion-oriented approach in which both mindfulness and compassion are viewed as meta-processes of change that are enhanced within the psychotherapeutic relationship. The book covers an astonishing range of ideas, including those about the self (observing/transcendent), consciousness (mindful and nondual), awareness (also nondual), change (based on evidence-based processes), growth and development (which includes the spiritual), and much more. The book is very well-organised: following an introduction to the field of integrative psychotherapy, the authors take the reader through a logical progression and unfolding of concepts and theories based on relational perspectives (on psychotherapy, the mind, and schemas) before outlining and illustrating the methods and interventions of their mindfulness- and compassion-oriented approach to integrative psychotherapy. In doing so, the authors provide a detailed account of a mindful and compassionate integrative clinical practice, which is both thoughtful and reflective, whilst also advancing the theory of integrative psychotherapy, and, thereby, fulfilling the brief of the series.

Keith Tudor

Abbreviations

ACT	Acceptance and Commitment Therapy
ANS	Autonomic Nervous System
EMDR	Eye Movement Desensitization and Reprocessing
FSC	Four States of Consciousness
MBCT	Mindfulness-Based Cognitive Therapy
MCIP	Mindfulness- and Compassion-Oriented Integrative Psychotherapy
PS	Physiological Synchrony
RNSS	Relational Needs Satisfaction Scale
SPA	Scale of Physiological Arousal

Acknowledgements

We feel sincere thankfulness for the many people who have supported us during the writing of this book. First of all, we are immensely grateful to our colleague and series editor, Keith Tudor. You have been an outstanding support and ongoing inspiration. We felt "held" during the process of writing.

We would also like to thank all our teachers and professional colleagues who inspired us and contributed to the development of ideas in this book.

We thank our teacher, Richard G. Erskine, for introducing us to integrative psychotherapy more than 20 years ago, for your continuing support and inspiration over the years.

We thank our teacher and colleague Ken Evans, who is sadly not with us any more, but his spirit lives with us in our workshops and integrative psychotherapy training.

Over the years, we have been influenced by a number of people whose workshops, training, and discussions have transformed our thinking and clinical practice. You are Steven Hayes, Roger Solomon, Ray Little, Leslie Greenberg, Diana Fosha, Joanna Hewitt Evans, Igor Krnetić, Mario Salvador, Eluned Gold, Biljana van Rijn, Bob Cooke, Anthony Jannetti, Branko Franzl, Daniel Siegel, and Bruce Ecker. The influence of each is present in our book.

We want to express sincere thanks to all the trainers at our Institute for Integrative Psychotherapy and Counselling, Ljubljana for ongoing support and exchange of ideas.

We would also like to thank colleagues at the International Integrative Psychotherapy Association (IIPA) and European Association for Integrative Psychotherapy (EAIP). These two professional organisations are our "professional" home.

We thank our friend, co-worker, and mindfulness teacher Melita Košak for ongoing support and for help with the development of mindfulness exercises. Your discussions and exchange of ideas have contributed immensely to the development of MCIP. Thanks for your trust in us during our years together at our institute.

We thank Anja Erjavec, who initiated qualitative research into mindfulness at our institute and helped us to develop our ideas and thinking about mindfulness. We also thank our colleague and mindfulness teacher Mateja Škorc for ongoing discussions regarding the integration of mindfulness in psychotherapy.

We thank all our trainees and supervisees for challenging our ideas, continual professional exchange, and also for believing in us and supporting us with the book. We grow and learn together!

We thank Jure Bon, Mihael Černetič, Matej Černigoj, and Tomáš Řiháček for a thorough reading of early chapters of this book and useful comments. Thanks also to Urban Kordeš, whose discussion about our early theories related to mindfulness helped to shape and ground our ideas.

We thank Leticia Slapnik Yebuah for her help with the design of the figures.

I (Gregor) thank Tau Malachi and Elder Gideon for introducing me to the gnostic nondual spiritual path and the importance of mindfulness and compassion.

Thanks to our friend, Robert Riley, who with his passion for the English language, helped to make our words sound good.

We thank each other, for mutual support, endless discussions, comments about the writing and endless patience, especially when one of us was upset.

We thank our parents for their support and love.

And last but not least we are immensely proud and grateful to our sons, Lan and Amadej, for giving us your support, curiosity, and encouragement during the writing of this book. We love you!

Gregor Žvelc and Maša Žvelc

Introduction

I dreamt that people from all over, from all religions and spiritual traditions, were gathering in the streets of my home town. They joined together in their prayer, meditation and contemplation.

This dream came to me (Maša) about a week before I was due to lead a round table discussion on the future of integrative psychotherapy at the European conference of integrative psychotherapy in 2015. Before I had this dream, I had been wondering what to say. The dream revealed to me the basic values of integrative psychotherapy: the attitude of togetherness, connectedness, openness, and respect towards each other. In my dream, we all felt that despite the differences, in our hearts we are all the same; we are all facing similar struggles and holding similar hopes. *I felt I belonged there.*

It was the spirit of integrative psychotherapy – learning from one another, sharing our knowledge and wisdom for the sake of the people. This spirit can be compared with the light of a candle: the flame of one candle may light many other candles so that the room becomes much brighter; and the flame of that first candle, which initially shared its light, does not vanish. It shines on with the rest of the lighted candles. And together, the light is stronger.

We have written this book over the course of one year and a half, but the journey of this book and our quest for integration started more than 20 years ago. At that time we were young psychologists, having experience in different psychotherapy schools: psychoanalytic psychotherapy, transactional analysis and cognitive-behavioural therapy. We were struggling with how to fit all this knowledge together. Then in 1999, we were introduced to relationally focused integrative psychotherapy by Richard G. Erskine in his workshop at the World Congress for Psychotherapy in Vienna. We were fascinated and touched by a gentle, deep, respectful, and compassionate approach to psychotherapy that valued and integrated different approaches. In the workshop, we witnessed the power of accepting awareness and compassion for transformation and growth. Relationally focused integrative psychotherapy gave us a new perspective with its focus on internal and external *contact*, which later become known as a major paradigm shift towards mindfulness and compassion. Instead of trying to change the client, this approach, through acceptance and valuing the client's phenomenology and their protective mechanisms, helps the client to go deeper into their world and integrate long-forgotten parts of self. Our journey towards integration had begun and is still continuing today.

We have been providing training in relationally focused integrative psychotherapy for the past 16 years. During this time, we have been in further professional training and workshops in different psychotherapy approaches including the developmental-integrative approach (Evans & Gilbert, 2005), acceptance and commitment therapy (ACT) (S. C. Hayes et al., 2012), emotion-focused therapy (EFT) (Greenberg & Watson, 2006), EMDR (F. Shapiro, 2001), relational transactional analysis (Hargaden & Sills, 2002), and accelerated experiential dynamic psychotherapy (AEDP) (Fosha, 2000b). We were also inspired by a number of authors who have written about trauma therapy (Levine, 1997; Ogden et al., 2006; Rothschild, 2000), the model of resolution of alliance ruptures (Safran & Muran, 2000) and polyvagal theory (Porges, 2011). On a personal level, we have been long-time practitioners of mindfulness, and have a long-standing interest in various spiritual traditions.

All these influences have transformed us and our work and have led to the development of mindfulness- and compassion-oriented integrative psychotherapy (MCIP). In this process we have further developed and integrated relationally focused integrative psychotherapy with practice, theories, and research in mindfulness and compassion. MCIP particularly integrates acceptance and commitment therapy (ACT) and knowledge from other third-wave behavioural approaches. The emergence of mindfulness- and compassion-oriented approaches has led to a paradigm shift in cognitive-behavioural approaches, and we think there is an increasing need to connect these ideas with other psychotherapy traditions. MCIP fulfils this need and provides integration of relationally focused integrative psychotherapy with mindfulness and compassion.

We have to emphasise that in our approach, mindfulness and compassion are viewed as meta-processes of change that are enhanced within the psychotherapeutic relationship. The primary task in MCIP is to invite the client to bring mindful awareness and compassion to their inner experience or parts of self. This promotes both greater psychological flexibility and transformation of dysfunctional schemas. Although we may teach clients some mindfulness exercises, this is not the primary focus in our approach. In MCIP, the qualities of mindfulness and compassion are at the heart of the therapeutic relationship.

In this book we provide a synthesis of knowledge, which advances the theory and practice of integrative psychotherapy. The book consists of three main parts: (1) Introduction to integrative psychotherapy, (2) Concepts and theories, and (3) Methods and interventions.

Part I introduces mindfulness- and compassion-oriented integrative psychotherapy (MCIP). In Chapter 1, "Development of mindfulness- and compassion-oriented integrative psychotherapy", we introduce psychotherapy integration and relationally focused integrative psychotherapy. We also describe the fundamental principles of MCIP.

In Chapter 2, "Evidence-based processes of change in integrative psychotherapy", we describe MCIP as a process-based therapy, which is founded on scientific research into the processes of change in psychotherapy. We present the *integrative model of processes of change* that describes evidence-based processes of change related to different dimensions of human experience: interpersonal, cognitive, affective, physiological, behavioural, spiritual, and systemic/contextual. Mindfulness and compassion are in the model presented as meta-processes of change that enhance all other described processes. We review the psychotherapy research studies related to each process of change. The model helps the therapist to track the client's experience from moment-to-moment and encourage the appropriate process of change. As Goldfried (1980) suggests, processes of change are at the level of abstraction between theory and interventions and so this chapter could have been included as a separate part of the book between Part II (concepts and theories) and Part III (methods and interventions). However, we decided to include this chapter in the first part of the book, as it is the basis for understanding the processes of change in all the subsequent chapters of the book.

Part II describes the fundamental theories and concepts of MCIP that are the basis for therapeutic methods and interventions. In Chapter 3, "Mindfulness and compassion in integrative psychotherapy", we differentiate between two main senses of self: the *personal sense of self*, which is related to our personal identity and self-narrative, and the *observing/transcendent self*. We describe the observing/transcendent self as awareness itself that is subjectively experienced as the experience of *being* and manifests in qualities of mindfulness, compassion, interconnection, and spirituality. We present the *diamond model of the observing self*, which describes the observing self and its relation to the main dimensions of human experience. The model describes four core processes of mindful awareness and compassion: present moment awareness, acceptance, decentred awareness, and compassion. We also introduce the model of *the triangle of relationship to internal experience* that describes three main relationships to internal experience: being merged with the experience, being distanced from the experience, and being a loving witness to our experience. The essential aim of MCIP is that the client during therapy activates the observing self and becomes a loving witness to their experience.

In Chapter 4, "Integrative psychotherapy as relational psychotherapy", we describe how MCIP as a relational form of psychotherapy views the client and therapist as a system of mutual influence. We present the integrative model of interpersonal relationship that helps us to understand our clients in terms of interpersonal functioning. One of the goals in MCIP is that clients develop the capacity for subject relations, which is seen in qualities of autonomy, connectedness, and mutuality. We emphasise the moments of *shared conscious presence* that can emerge when both the client and the therapist are in touch with the observing self and are fully present with each other.

In Chapter 5, "Relational mind and intersubjective physiology", we emphasise the significance of the intersubjective physiological field between the therapist and the client. We stress the importance of the therapist's physiological state during the therapy session. We discuss the importance of three pathways of the autonomic nervous system (ventral vagal, sympathetic, and dorsal vagal) and related autonomic states, based on Porges' polyvagal theory. We also review the research into interpersonal physiology and its importance for psychotherapy practice. We discuss the positive and negative aspects of physiological synchrony in the therapeutic relationship, the importance of therapist self-regulation and regulation of the client. We highlight the therapist's mindful awareness during therapy for the regulation of their own and the client's physiological states.*

In Chapter 6, "Relational schemas and memory reconsolidation", we describe the concept of relational schemas as a fundamental construct in MCIP that provides us with an understanding of the client's inner relational world and how this world impacts the relationship with others. We discuss how the change of dysfunctional schemas occurs through the process of memory reconsolidation and describe how mindfulness and compassion are crucial in this process. This chapter includes material from the article "Between self and others: Relational schemas as an integrating construct in psychotherapy", written by Gregor Žvelc and published in 2009 by the *Transactional Analysis Journal*. This earlier material has been re-worked and updated in the light of the contemporary theory of memory reconsolidation and our views regarding the importance of mindfulness and compassion for working with schemas.

In Chapter 7, "Beyond ordinary unhappiness: From personal to observing self", we discuss the differences between the two main senses of self: the personal sense of self and the observing/transcendent self. The personal sense of self is an expression of the self-narrative that is continually self-reinforcing and maintaining itself. We propose that all human beings suffer from *ordinary unhappiness*, which is the result of identification with our personal sense of self. Because of identification with the personal sense of self, people feel fundamentally separate from each other, live unconsciously according to their life-story, are preoccupied with themselves and experience loss of the present moment. We also present the *self-narrative-system*, which is a diagnostic and treatment planning tool that helps us to understand the client in terms of their self-narrative. The model shows how the person is living their internalised life-story and how they are continually reinforcing it in their life. We propose that activation of the observing self helps us to develop a mindful and compassionate relationship with our personal sense of self and overcome ordinary unhappiness. We further propose that a change of self-narrative paradoxically happens through mindful awareness and self-compassion.

In Chapter 8, "The multiplicity of mind, states of consciousness, and treatment planning", we present the model of the four states of consciousness (FSC). The model describes four different states of consciousness: restricted consciousness, Adult state of consciousness, mindful state of consciousness, and nondual awareness. The model helps us to understand the client in terms of their self-states and how activation of the client's mindful state of consciousness is crucial for the transformation of their personal sense of self. In the chapter, we also present the main phases of MCIP that are crucial for treatment planning.

In Part III, we present the practical methods and interventions of MCIP. In Chapter 9, "Methods of relational mindfulness and compassion", we present the *keyhole model of relational mindfulness and compassion*, which describes how mindfulness and compassion can be enhanced by the relational methods of inquiry, attunement, and involvement. The model provides integration of Richard Erskine's Keyhole model with mindfulness and compassion processes. We provide examples of interactions between the client and the therapist to illustrate how relational methods can enhance processes of the present moment, decentred awareness, acceptance, and compassion.

In addition to relational methods, mindfulness and compassion can be enhanced by different practices and exercises. In Chapter 10, "From mindful awareness and self-compassion to values-based living", we present different experiential exercises that are used in MCIP to help the client to bring mindfulness and compassion to their inner experience. We also present methods and interventions that help clients develop metacognitive awareness of schemas and self-states, and promote living according to values and meaning. Interventions are illustrated by examples of interactions between the client and the therapist.

In Chapter 11, "The therapist's mindful presence and physiological regulation in the therapeutic relationship", we highlight the importance of the therapist's mindful state of consciousness during the therapy session for effective psychotherapeutic work. We introduce the phrase "The therapist first", emphasising that the therapist should primarily bring their mindful attention onto themselves, starting with mindful awareness of their physiological state. This enables them to self-regulate, keep them within the window of tolerance and to stay present. We present different ways in which the therapist can regulate their own or their clients' hyper- or hypoarousal. A significant part of the chapter is the vignette of a psychotherapy session, where these methods of mindful awareness and physiological regulation are systematically and practically showed step by step.

In Chapter 12, "The transforming power of mindfulness: Mindful processing", we present a method of *mindful processing* that is used for processing disturbing experiences. In this mindful processing method, we intentionally invite the client to bring mindful awareness to their painful feelings, body sensations, or other experiences evoked by painful memories or dysfunctional schema, alternating between mindful awareness of experience and sharing their experience with the therapist. We present the seven phases of this method and describe how mindful processing promotes memory reconsolidation. The chapter includes some material from the article "Mindful processing in psychotherapy: Facilitating natural healing process within attuned therapeutic relationship", written by Gregor Žvelc and published in 2012 by the *International Journal of Integrative Psychotherapy*. In this chapter, these initial ideas are updated and developed into a comprehensive seven-phase method for the processing of disturbing experiences.

In Chapter 13, "Self compassion: The road to a loving and healing inner relationship", we present the method for processing unresolved and painful issues with the help of self-compassion. This method is illustrated through two vignettes of psychotherapy sessions that show the transforming power of self-compassion processing, which leads to memory reconsolidation and integration of the personal sense of self. The first vignette shows self-compassion processing connected to the situation of internal criticism, and the second vignette deals with bringing self-compassion to the client's past issues and "abandoned" Child self-state.

In writing this book, we have wholeheartedly adopted gender neutrality and consistently use singular "they" as a generic third-person singular pronoun. Although its use may at first sound unfamiliar, we think that it is not a coincidence that the Merriam-Webster dictionary chose the singular "they" as the word of the year for 2019. This reflects a major move in our society towards open-mindedness and inclusivity.

We hope that our book will be of service to all integrative psychotherapists as well as therapists of other approaches who are interested in the integration of mindfulness and compassion in their psychotherapy approach and value the importance of the therapeutic relationship. The book may also be of interest to any reader who is passionate about the transformative power of mindfulness and compassion.

Gregor Žvelc and Maša Žvelc

Part I

Introduction to integrative psychotherapy

1   Development of mindfulness- and compassion-oriented integrative psychotherapy

When students ask us what integrative psychotherapy is, we often tell them the ancient Indian parable of the "Blind Men and the Elephant". In this parable, some blind men wanted to know what an elephant is. Each of the blind men described the elephant in their own way, according to which part of the body they inspected. For one, who touched the trunk, the elephant was like a snake, for another whose hand touched the elephant's leg, it was like a tree-trunk. The blind man who touched the tail described it like a rope. Others described it as a wall, a spear, and a fan. Then, the blind men started to quarrel about the reality of the "elephant".

The field of psychotherapy is often similar to blind men who are quarrelling about the nature of truth. The history of psychotherapy is full of rivalries between psychotherapy approaches, where each approach wanted to prove that it possesses the truth and that it is better than another. Behavioural therapists criticised psychoanalysis, saying that it is unscientific. Conversely, psychoanalysts criticised behavioural therapy, saying that it produces only symptom relief. Humanistic schools were often called too optimistic, and humanistic schools thought that psychoanalysis and behavioural therapy were too deterministic.

Like a blind man, each psychotherapy approach often gives priority only to one or a few aspects of human experience. Some approaches focus on the cognitive dimension, others on emotions, some give priority to relationships, and others to values and meaning. However, as the parable suggests, all these dimensions are part of the whole and all are significant.

The parable of the "Blind Men and the Elephant" is often used to describe psychotherapy integration (Cooper, 2019; Walder, 1993). The psychotherapy integration movement emerged as an attempt to overcome the rigid boundaries and divisions of separate psychotherapy approaches, and to start an ongoing dialogue between different approaches and schools. Instead of defending and proving one's own view, different approaches to psychotherapy can learn from each other in an attempt to understand the greater reality and the whole of the human psyche.

Psychotherapy integration as a new paradigm in psychotherapy

The psychotherapy integration movement emerged as an expression of the need to overcome the limitation of a single approach to psychotherapy. Psychotherapists who had trained in a specific approach to psychotherapy started to look outside of their primary approach and began to learn from each other. Norcross and Alexander (2019) describe that "integration is characterised by dissatisfaction with single-school approaches and a concomitant desire to look across school boundaries to see what can be learned from other ways of conducting psychotherapy" (p. 4). Since 1980, integrative psychotherapies have significantly grown in different continents and countries (Gómez et al., 2019). In the 21st century, psychotherapy integration has become a "spirit of the time" or "zeitgeist" (Castonguay et al., 2015). Norcross and Alexander (2019) state that "approximately one quarter to one-half of contemporary American clinicians disavow an affiliation with a particular school of therapy and prefer instead the label of *integrative* or *eclectic*" (p. 13). To date, there are more than 460 published books on psychotherapy integration (Goldfried et al., 2019), and leading textbooks on psychotherapy often identify their theoretical orientation as integrative (Norcross & Alexander, 2019). We think that psychotherapy integration can be rightly called a new paradigm in psychotherapy which is gaining increasing acceptance in the field.

There are different pathways to psychotherapy integration: theoretical integration, common factors, assimilative integration, and technical eclecticism (Norcross & Alexander, 2019). Theoretical integration involves the synthesis of theories and methods of two or more approaches to psychotherapy in a new therapeutic approach. A common factors approach focuses on common ingredients and principles of change across different psychotherapy approaches with an attempt to "create more parsimonious and efficacious treatments based on those communalities" (Norcross & Alexander, 2019, p. 11). Assimilative integration involves grounding in one particular psychotherapy approach and selective integration of principles, views, and methods from other psychotherapy approaches. Technical eclecticism is the use of techniques from different therapeutic approaches without an overarching theoretical framework, but it is based on research evidence and clinical observation to select the techniques which work best for a specific problem or person.

The main characteristics of the integrative paradigm can be summarised by (a) dialogue and openness, (b) coexistence of different "truths" or "realities", (c) the importance of different dimensions of human experience, (d) the importance of tailoring the therapy to individual characteristics or needs of the client, and (e) the importance of psychotherapy research.

Dialogue and openness. The integrative paradigm is based on the spirit of open exploration of different psychotherapeutic approaches and transtheoretical dialogue. Integrative psychotherapists are open to different ideas and learning beyond any one particular approach. Fernández-Alvarez et al. (2016) describe how "in practice, psychotherapy integration characterises an ongoing rapprochement, convergence, and complementarity not only at the conceptual level, but also at the clinical and empirical level" (p. 820).

Coexistence of different "truths" or "realities". The integrative approach is focused not on finding one absolute truth, but on being open to the coexistence of multiple truths or realities. Sometimes these truths may be contradictory. Integrative psychotherapy embraces constructivist and postmodern perspectives. The "truth" that we are proposing in this book is also one of many truths based on our knowledge and life experience.

The importance of different dimensions of human experience. Psychotherapy integration is motivated by disillusionment with a single approach to psychotherapy (Norcross & Alexander, 2019), and an awareness that each psychotherapy approach has its domain of expertise that can be enhanced if integrated with other approaches. Integrative psychotherapists focus on various dimensions such as cognitive, affective, physiological, behavioural, interpersonal, socio-cultural, ecological, and spiritual. While wholeness may be ideal, our intention is to be holistic and not to exclude any of these dimensions.

Importance of tailoring the therapy to the individual characteristics or needs of the client. This principle is based on an awareness that no single approach to psychotherapy is always the most suitable for all clients in all situations. So, instead of wanting the client to adapt to a particular psychotherapy school and method, integrative psychotherapists are flexible in their approach and focused on the needs of individual clients in their specific context.

Psychotherapy research and psychotherapy integration

Clinical science has been dominated by the medical model, which emphasises randomised controlled trials to show the effectiveness of a particular psychotherapy approach. This has led to the development of many different psychotherapy packages and therapy manuals for a specific disorder, ignoring the reality of clinical practice that demands flexibility instead of conformity to a particular manual. Fraser (2018) describes several challenges to the medical model that have arisen over the past decade. Research findings show that adherence to a treatment protocol does not lead to better outcomes, and that therapists who are more flexible in their approach achieve the best outcomes (Wampold & Imel, 2015). Therapists also find it challenging to keep up with learning every new approach for a specific disorder and often find such approaches incompatible with their viewpoint (Fraser, 2018).

Meta-analytic studies of psychotherapy outcomes also challenge the classical medical model (Fraser, 2018). Wampold and Imel (2015) in their seminal book, *The Great Psychotherapy Debate*, conclude that "exemplary studies and methodologically sound meta-analyses unfailingly produced evidence that demonstrated that there were small, if not zero, differences among treatments" (p. 156). This is known in psychotherapy research as the "Dodo Bird Verdict", coming from the story of Alice in Wonderland in which the Dodo concludes: "Everyone has won and all must have prizes" (Luborsky et al., 1975). Based on research that there are few significant differences in outcomes between different psychotherapy approaches, psychotherapy researchers have focused on studying common factors and change processes that affect outcomes in different psychotherapy approaches. While there are numerous common factors, the most frequently proposed are the quality of the relationship and therapeutic alliance (Fraser, 2018), which consists of a therapeutic bond and agreement on goals and tasks of treatment. Norcross and Lambert (2018) describe how the therapeutic relationship is *evidence-based* and "makes substantial and consistent contributions to outcome independent of the type of treatment" (p. 303).

Whilst acknowledging the commonalities between treatments, "there are occasionally specific factors attributable to different treatments and different therapists" (Norcross & Alexander, 2019, p. 8). Both common factors and specific factors of change are important for the integrative practitioner. Norcross and Alexander (2019) write that "we integrate by combining fundamental similarities and useful differences between schools" (p. 8). In this way, we can embrace both factors that are common and also factors related to specific therapies.

In recent years, there has been an emergence of process-based therapies which are based on the transdiagnostic processes of change (Hofmann & Hayes, 2019). Instead of following specific therapy packages, the therapist encourages processes of change that have been found to be effective in psychotherapy research. Process-based therapies are congruent with the vision of the integrative paradigm. Instead of proving which therapy is more effective, they emphasise processes of change that can be found in different psychotherapy approaches and can be used with different clinical disorders. In Chapter 2, we provide a model of the processes of change that are used in our approach to psychotherapy integration.

What is integrative psychotherapy?

In line with Fernández-Alvarez et al. (2016), we think that it is important to distinguish the term *integrative psychotherapy* from the term *psychotherapy integration*. The term integrative psychotherapy refers to a specific approach based on psychotherapy integration, while the term psychotherapy integration refers to the broader framework and paradigm in psychotherapy. There are various integrative approaches such as accelerated experiential dynamic psychotherapy (Fosha, 2000b), integrative therapy (Petzold, 2002), emotion-focused therapy (Greenberg & Watson, 2006), cyclical psychodynamics (Wachtel, 2008; Wachtel & Gagnon, 2019), the transtheoretical approach (Prochaska & Diclemente, 2019), and many others.

Our approach to integrative psychotherapy is based on relationally focused integrative psychotherapy developed by Richard G. Erskine and his colleagues at the Institute for Integrative Psychotherapy (Erskine, 2015, 2019a; Erskine & Moursund, 1988; Erskine et al., 1999; Moursund & Erskine, 2004). The preliminary ideas of this approach were first presented in a series of lectures at the University of Illinois in 1972 (Erskine, 2015). Relationally focused integrative psychotherapy is based on principles of theoretical integration and the importance of common factors in psychotherapy, such as the therapeutic relationship. In this approach, the term integrative psychotherapy carries several layers of meaning. It refers to the integration: (a) of personality, (b) of psychotherapy approaches, and (c) within the psychotherapist.

Integration of personality

Relationally focused integrative psychotherapy aims at the integration of split-off parts of the personality and "making them part of the cohesive self" (Erskine, 2015, p. 1). Such integration promotes flexibility and enables people to "face each moment openly and freshly, without the protection of a preformed opinion, position, attitude, or expectation" (Erskine, 2015, p. 1). Relationally focused integrative psychotherapy also promotes the integration of the main dimensions of human experience: cognitive, affective, behavioural, and physiological "with an awareness of social and transpersonal aspects of the systems surrounding the person" (International Integrative Psychotherapy Association, 2020).

Figure 1.1 presents the model of the *self-in-relationship system* (Erskine & Trautmann, 1993/1997). This model presents four main dimensions of human functioning: affective, behavioural, cognitive, and physiological within a relational system (Erskine & Trautmann, 1993/1997). It also includes the spiritual dimension, which R. G. Erskine (personal communication, May 5, 2020) in his updated model puts in the centre of the diagram.

The cognitive dimension refers to thoughts, beliefs, and perceptions; the behavioural dimension refers to observed behaviour; the affective dimension to emotions; the physiological dimension to physical sensations and bodily processes; and the relational dimension to the relationship with other people and systems. The spiritual dimension refers to transcendental and existential aspects of our life and a deeper sense of purpose. All of these dimensions are viewed from a systems perspective, where the different dimensions influence and affect each other. Each dimension has an "interrelated effect on the other dimensions" (Erskine, 2015, p. 3). Based on a systems perspective, integrative psychotherapists try to understand "the function of a particular behavior, affect, belief, or body

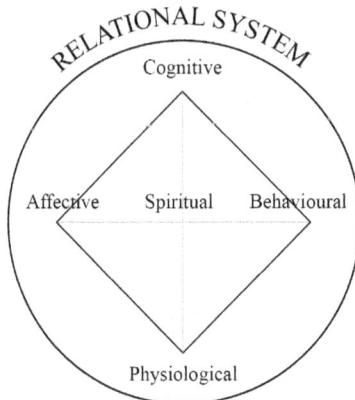

Figure 1.1 The self-in-relationship system
Note. Adapted from "The process of integrative psychotherapy" by R. G. Erskine and R. L. Trautmann, 1997, *Theories and methods of an integrative transactional analysis: A volume of selected articles* (p. 81), TA Press (Original work published 1993). Copyright 1993 by R. G. Erskine. Adapted with permission.

gesture on the human organism as a whole" (Erskine, 2015, p. 4). The client can be open or closed to contact in each of these dimensions. For example, some clients avoid emotions and are open to contact only on the cognitive dimension. Some clients are only open to contact on the behavioural dimension and have difficulties understanding the causes of their problems, and are also fearful of emotions. There are also clients who are overwhelmed with emotions. In integrative psychotherapy we assess in which dimension the client is open or closed to contact (Erskine, 2015). We make contact with our client first on the dimension where the client is open to contact and later on invite them to contact the dimensions where they are closed to contact. In this process, within an attuned psychotherapy relationship, we use the methods and interventions from the major psychotherapy traditions that target the phenomenological, behavioural, and relational levels of the client's functioning. One of the goals of integrative psychotherapy is that the client is in full contact with all dimensions.

Integration of psychotherapy approaches

Relationally focused integrative psychotherapy is the theoretical integration of aspects from different psychotherapy approaches. This is illustrated in the model of the self-in-relationship (Figure 1.1) that shows the dimensions of personality that are emphasised in different psychotherapy traditions. The cognitive approach to psychotherapy focuses on the question "Why?" (Erskine & Moursund, 1988). It assumes that change takes place through the client's understanding of their problems and conflicts – by insight. The behavioural approach to therapy focuses on the question "What?" (Erskine, 2015). It describes how our behaviour is shaped and maintained, and what changes are necessary to change dysfunctional behaviour. The goal is a reinforcement of new desired behaviour (Erskine & Moursund, 1988). "The affective approach to psychotherapy deals with the question 'How?' How does a person feel?" (Erskine, 2015, p. 3). The focus is on the client's phenomenological experience. The goal in this approach is awareness and expression of repressed emotions that "will produce an emotional closure and provide for a fuller range of affective experience" (Erskine, 2015, p. 3). The fourth dimension is the physiological dimension, where the focus is on working with the body. The fifth dimension is relational and refers to the relationship of the person with other people and larger systems, such as family, school, or the socio-cultural environment. In integrative psychotherapy the therapeutic relationship is one of the major factors of change and provides a context for work on all other dimensions. The sixth dimension is spiritual, where the focus is on finding meaning and purpose in life. This dimension is emphasised in different humanistic–existential psychotherapy approaches and transpersonal psychotherapy.

Erskine (2015) describes how "integrative psychotherapy takes into account many views of human functioning: psychodynamic, client-centered, behaviorist, family therapy, Gestalt therapy, neo-Reichian, object relations theories, psychoanalytic self-psychology, and transactional analysis" (p. 2). Each of these approaches provides important insights into the nature of the human being and "each is enhanced when selectively integrated with others" (Erskine, 2015, p. 2).

Integrative psychotherapy also integrates scientific research from different fields: neuroscience, psychotherapy research, and research from developmental psychology. Of particular importance are theories that describe the normal developmental process from infancy to old age, and how a person develops self-protective mechanisms based on interruptions in their healthy development. Object-relations theories, attachment theory, self-psychology, and Erikson's developmental theory, are important sources of knowledge that inform the integrative psychotherapist regarding ways of coping with interruptions to interpersonal contact.

Integration within a psychotherapist

The ultimate aim of the integrative psychotherapist is to develop their own personal integration of theories and methods, based on their characteristics and preferences. It also means a commitment by the practitioner for ongoing personal development, for internal integration and growth. In integrative psychotherapy the psychotherapist is not a detached professional who offers the client different techniques and homework assignments, but is someone who is fully present and involved in the relationship. The central assumption of integrative psychotherapy is that healing occurs through contact-in-relationship, where clients through contactful relationship with the therapist develop internal contact and integrate parts of their personality (Erskine et al., 1999). For this task, the personal integration of the therapist is of key importance.

There is no limit or end to this journey of integration, which is a process and not a goal. It is like walking to the east; such a journey never ends. There is always something further to integrate. So the aim of integrative psychotherapy is not to make another fixed and closed approach, but to be open to the continual process of assimilation and accommodation. Richard G. Erskine, our teacher, said: "You are not an integrative psychotherapist. You are becoming an integrative psychotherapist and that never ends" (R. G. Erskine, personal communication, June 10, 2000). This means being open to new research findings, new theories, and learning every day from our clients.

In this book, we present our particular integration based on relationally focused integrative psychotherapy.

Mindfulness- and compassion-oriented integrative psychotherapy (MCIP)

In this book, we present mindfulness- and compassion-oriented integrative psychotherapy (MCIP), which has been developed by the authors of this book over the past 12 years. MCIP has roots in Erskine's relationally focused integrative psychotherapy and aims to advance its theory and methods. Our model is an attempt to "integrate integrative psychotherapy." It provides further integration of Erskine's approach with mindfulness- and compassion-oriented approaches, practice, and research. MCIP integrates relationally focused integrative psychotherapy with the knowledge and practice of acceptance and commitment therapy (ACT) (S. C. Hayes et al., 1999, 2012) and is inspired by different mindfulness- and compassion-oriented approaches and theories (Desmond, 2016; P. Gilbert, 2010; Kabat-Zinn, 1990; Neff, 2003a; Segal et al., 2002; D. J. Siegel, 2007, 2018). MCIP is also influenced by the theory and research of memory reconsolidation (Ecker, 2015, 2018; Ecker et al., 2012; Lane et al., 2015) and Porges' polyvagal theory (Porges, 2011, 2017). The fundamental principle that holds all the various ideas and concepts together is the importance of the therapeutic relationship, and in MCIP, mindfulness and compassion are brought into the heart of the psychotherapeutic relationship. We do not see our approach as a final destination and hope that it will be further transformed and integrated.

Fundamental principles and characteristics of MCIP

Mindfulness- and compassion-oriented integrative psychotherapy is based on ten fundamental principles that underpin its theories and methods.

Intersubjectivity and focus on co-creation

MCIP is relational psychotherapy which is based on the fundamental principle that human beings are interconnected and influence one another. The client and psychotherapist are viewed as a system of mutual influence. They are both co-creating the intersubjective field (Stolorow, 1994) and influencing each other on both the conscious and unconscious levels. This fundamental principle is essential for understanding that all processes in psychotherapy are co-created by both the client and the therapist. In MCIP, we also pay special attention to physiological intersubjectivity, the mutual influence of the autonomic nervous system of both the client and therapist on each other.

The intersubjective approach also has important implications regarding the nature of "truth". In MCIP, the therapist's perspective is not more real than the client's and vice versa. The truth is co-created between the client and the therapist.

The phenomenological and experiential approach

MCIP is a phenomenological approach. The therapist is interested in the client's phenomenology, and together with the client explores their inner world. The fundamental principle of integrative psychotherapy is that every experience has its own meaning, logic, and is valuable. The therapist respects and is genuinely interested in the client's subjective world and invites the client to develop the same relationship with themselves. The phenomenological approach involves *bracketing*, which means giving in brackets the ideas and theories about the client

(Finlay, 2016). Such an attitude can provide real hearing, listening, and sensing of the client. In MCIP, therapists strive to be open for their clients' phenomenology, while at the same time being in contact with their inner world.

MCIP is an experiential approach to psychotherapy. The therapist helps the client to become aware of their experience and to experience their thoughts, emotions, and sensations in the here-and-now. The therapist is active in this approach in the sense of inviting the client to "experience", and not only to talk about their problems, and in leading the client to "root" their words into their body and emotional experience (Fosha, 2000b). The aim is that the client is in full contact with what they are thinking, feeling, and sensing.

Holism and the importance of all dimensions of human experience

MCIP is a holistic approach to psychotherapy and gives importance to all dimensions of human experience: cognitive, affective, physiological, behavioural, relational, and spiritual. All these dimensions influence each other and are part of the whole. The aim of the therapy is that the client comes into contact with and integrates all of these dimensions.

Process-based psychotherapy founded on the research validated processes of change

MCIP is based on empirically validated processes of change that have been established through psychotherapy research. These processes of change are related to the main dimensions of human experience and encompass both common and specific factors of psychotherapy. MCIP is process-oriented psychotherapy, which means that the therapist from moment-to-moment tracks the client's experience and encourages appropriate processes of change. In MCIP we give special importance to mindfulness and compassion processes as meta-processes of change and emphasise memory reconsolidation as the core mechanism of transformational change.

Mindful awareness and self-compassion as core processes of change

In MCIP, the therapist encourages the processes of mindful awareness and self-compassion within an attuned therapeutic relationship. The core change process in MCIP involves inviting clients to bring mindful awareness and self-compassion to their inner experience. Instead of focusing on changing the clients' thoughts, feelings, and sensations, we help them to change how they relate to the content of their mind. While describing mindfulness processes, Černetič (2005) says: "When a person stops trying to become different, he immediately becomes different in a profound, thorough way" (p. 78). This means that when clients develop a new accepting and compassionate relationship with themselves, at that very moment, they change. This principle is congruent with the paradoxical theory of change in gestalt therapy (Beisser, 1971). With mindful awareness and self-compassion, we relate in a profoundly different way to ourselves and promote transformation and change.

Importance of the relationship

MCIP is informed by attachment theory and other developmental theories that describe the importance of the need for relationships throughout our lives. Developmental theories provide us with an understanding about how the child's personality and the brain develop based on the early child–parent relationship. The therapist in MCIP uses developmental knowledge to understand clients from the perspective of their relationships, and how they developed protective patterns based on problematic interactions with significant others.

Congruent with these theories, the therapeutic relationship in MCIP is seen as both the foundation for change and also as one of the main healing agents. We strive to develop an attuned and secure therapeutic relationship based on the therapist's mindful presence, attunement, and compassion. The attuned therapeutic relationship also provides corrective relational experiences that promote the change in the client's relational schemas and memory reconsolidation.

Importance of the therapist's mindful presence and regulated therapy field

In MCIP we emphasise the importance of the therapist's mindful presence and awareness. Mindful awareness enables the therapist to track their own physiological states and regulate them when needed, while also leading the client to mindful awareness and regulation. Integration and growth are possible when we function within the window of tolerance (Ogden et al., 2006; D. J. Siegel, 1999, 2012) and therefore MCIP emphasises the importance of regulation for both the client and the therapist. The responsibility for regulation begins with the therapist. When the therapist's and the client's autonomic states are regulated, and their minds are within the window of tolerance, then the psychotherapy process can lead to integration, healing, and growth.

Trust in natural healing capacities and inner wisdom

MCIP is based on the assumption of an innate and natural self-healing capacity within each person and is congruent with the humanistic principle of organismic wisdom. In MCIP we propose that mindful awareness and self-compassion enhance this natural healing process in which the change occurs spontaneously as a result of the awareness and acceptance of internal experiences (G. Žvelc, 2012). Through mindful stillness, awareness, and acceptance, we create the conditions where our mind uses resources which are beyond the resources of everyday living and rational problem-solving. Mindful awareness and self-compassion awaken our inner wisdom, love, and the capacity for growth.

Ordinary unhappiness and the imperfect nature of the human condition

Our fundamental assumption is that we all experience "ordinary unhappiness" (Freud, 1895/2013) and are not perfect. We all experience both moments of happiness and sorrow, love and destruction, peace and anxiety, health and illness. Our view is inspired by S. C. Hayes and colleagues (2012), who criticise the assumption of healthy normality that is part of the traditional models of mental health. They propose an assumption of destructive normality, which is related to the negative effects of human language on mental health.

We propose that our ordinary unhappiness is related to phylogenetic and ontogenetic conditions and identification with our self-narrative, our personal sense of self. The assumption of ordinary unhappiness is connected to the fact that our life circumstances, phylogenetically and ontogenetically, are limited. Human beings from the beginning of their existence on Earth had to strive for and fight for survival and resources. Humans have fears of scarcity, of not having enough; and on the other hand, also fears of losing what they have. Fear, sorrow, and aggression exist in humans alongside compassion, altruism, love, and gratitude.

Apart from our life circumstances, our ordinary unhappiness is related to our identification with our self-narrative, our personal sense of self. When we are identified with our self-narrative, we are caught in constant processes of self-comparison and dissatisfaction with ourselves and striving to be better than we are. In MCIP we think that the suffering of human beings is partly connected to attempts to escape from ordinary unhappiness and attempts to improve our self-narrative. We have high ideals about how we should be: happy, without stress, in peace, not anxious, not depressed, not aggressive or angry, etc. However, these attempts can lead to constant dissatisfaction, comparison to others, self-criticism, and impossible expectations about being perfect. We propose that people's suffering would lessen if we could learn to see and accept our own and others' limitations, imperfections, and our common humanity. The profound realisation of this truth can liberate us from the inner critique, that we (or other people) should be different or better, and liberate us from the pressure to change. In this way we would also come to realise that we are all in the same boat – limited and experiencing ordinary unhappiness and suffering. Suffering (anxiety, stress, sorrow, aggression, illness) is an inevitable companion in our lives. We cannot change this fact by trying to fight it or by putting pressure on ourselves.

We think that our ordinary unhappiness and suffering can be lessened and transformed by acceptance and compassion related to our imperfect human condition, by stopping trying to change ourselves and by trusting that by such a surrender inner wisdom will emerge. Behind our personal sense of self, there is another sense of self – the *observing self*, which is related to *presence, being, mindful awareness, compassion,* and *transcendence*. This is a hidden potential within us, of which we are often not aware. Being centred within our observing self helps us to genuinely accept the imperfect nature of our personal sense of self and brings us closer to our inner purpose and meaning. By "pausing" with a loving presence, the greater our chances are that inner resources and wisdom will awaken that will help us to mindfully act according to our deepest values.

Importance of spirituality and living according to values and purpose

In MCIP, we give importance to the role of spirituality in human life, as well as the search for meaning and purpose. The therapist in MCIP is open to spiritual themes when they emerge in the course of psychotherapy, and views them as part of the universal striving to find meaning and a deeper sense of purpose. One of the goals in MCIP is to invite our clients to search for meaning in life, and to start to live life according to their deepest values and purpose.

2 Evidence-based processes of change in integrative psychotherapy

Mindfulness- and compassion-oriented integrative psychotherapy (MCIP) is based on evidence-based processes of change that have been found to be effective in psychotherapy research and lead to desirable treatment outcomes. In this chapter, we will describe the integrative model of evidence-based processes of change. The model provides process diagnostics, treatment planning, and a useful map for clinical interventions and strategies in MCIP.

Processes of change in psychotherapy

The focus on processes of change emerged with the work of Goldfried (1980), who proposed that different psychotherapeutic approaches may share common principles of change, which are at the level of abstraction between theory and therapeutic techniques. At the level of theories and therapeutic techniques, different psychotherapy orientations may differ; however, principles of change are common across different orientations. He proposed the following five main principles of change, which are common to different psychotherapeutic orientations: corrective emotional experience, feedback from the therapist that promotes new understanding, positive expectations that psychotherapy can be helpful, establishing a therapeutic alliance and promoting reality testing (Goldfried, 1980; Goldfried & Padawer, 1982).When Goldfried (1980) proposed focusing on the common processes of change instead of emphasising particular psychotherapy schools, the field was not ripe for such a major paradigm change. The field of clinical science has been dominated by the medical model, which tried to find a treatment that was effective for each particular clinical disorder. In contrast, researchers related to the psychotherapy integration movement have been increasingly studying different processes of change (Crits-Christoph et al., 2013; Greenberg, 2008; McAleavey et al., 2019; Norcross & Lambert, 2018).

In recent years, there has been an increasing focus on the processes of change and the emergence of process-based therapies (Fraser, 2018; Hofmann & Hayes, 2018, 2019). Hofmann and Hayes (2019) describe how process-based psychotherapy presents a new paradigm in clinical science compared to the medical illness model, which assumes that clinical disorders are treated with specific protocols. This new paradigm, instead of focusing on a particular treatment for a specific disorder, focuses on empirically validated transdiagnostic processes of change. Therapeutic processes are "underlying change mechanisms that lead to the attainment of a desirable treatment goal" (Hofmann & Hayes, 2019, p. 38). Hofmann and Hayes (2019) state that the main question of process-based therapy is: "What core biopsychosocial processes should be targeted with this client given this goal in this situation, and how can they most efficiently and effectively be changed?" (p. 38).

The integrative model of processes of change

Mindfulness- and compassion-oriented integrative psychotherapy (MCIP) is process-based psychotherapy. Therapists in MCIP track moment to moment their client's experience and encourage processes of change related to different dimensions of human experience. Figure 2.1 presents the integrative model of the processes of change. It sets out the processes of change related to the main dimensions of human experience: interpersonal, cognitive, affective, physiological, behavioural, spiritual, and systemic/contextual. The model also includes mindfulness and compassion processes that are meta-processes of change and are related to all of the main dimensions.

This model describes both problem areas as well as change processes that facilitate psychological health and well-being. In MCIP, we are focused on the individual client in their particular context. Case conceptualisation is developed based on the main problem areas and the central processes of change that need to be encouraged. We not only develop an overall case conceptualisation of a particular client but also pay attention to the client's immediate experience. We track the client's experience from moment-to-moment in terms of processes of change and facilitate the needed processes of change at a particular moment. Clients may need different interventions at different times (Cooper & McLeod, 2007), so the integrative psychotherapist is flexible in the use of interventions related to the processes of change.

Processes of change in the model encompass both common and specific factors of psychotherapy. While there are numerous processes of change to be found in psychotherapy research literature, we have included only the main processes that we think are crucial in MCIP. The processes related to the interpersonal, cognitive, affective, and physiological dimensions are congruent with Erskine's (2015) writings on integrative psychotherapy. Additionally, we have also included processes that are unique to our approach: mindfulness and compassion processes and processes related to the spiritual dimension.

The integrative model of processes of change is influenced by qualitative research on the client's experience of helpful aspects of integrative psychotherapy (Modic & Žvelc, 2015; Modic, 2019). Modic (2019) conducted interviews with 16 clients, who had been in integrative psychotherapy for at least one year. With the help of *The Client Change Interview* (Elliott et al., 2001), she researched helpful therapeutic factors and changes from the client's perspective. She developed a model of the client's experience of helpful therapeutic factors and changes.

MINDFULNESS AND COMPASSION	
PROBLEM AREAS	**META-PROCESSES OF CHANGE**
Preoccupation with past/future Fusion/Experiential merging Experiential avoidance Self-judgement, the judgement of others	Present moment awareness Decentred perspective Acceptance Self-compassion and compassion

DIMENSIONS OF HUMAN EXPERIENCE	
PROBLEM AREAS	**PROCESSES OF CHANGE**
INTERPERSONAL DIMENSION	
Maladaptive relational patterns, attachment issues, ruptures in alliance	Attunement Maintaining and repairing therapeutic alliance Corrective relational experience
COGNITIVE DIMENSION	
Lack of self-understanding Impaired mentalisation	Insight Mentalisation
AFFECTIVE DIMENSION	
Lack of awareness of emotions Avoidance of emotion Lack of expression of emotions Emotional dysregulation	Emotional awareness Acceptance of emotions Expression of emotion Emotion regulation
PHYSIOLOGICAL DIMENSION	
Problems in interoception Physiological dysregulation	Interoception Physiological regulation
BEHAVIOURAL DIMENSION	
Passivity and avoidance, impulsivity, lack of skills, behavioural inflexibility	Committed action
SPIRITUAL DIMENSION	
Lack of purpose and meaning of life Lack of contact with observing/transcendent self	Contact with values/meaning of life Contact with observing/transcendent self
SYSTEMIC/CONTEXTUAL DIMENSION	
Problems related to systems, such as family, school and work situation Problems related to the socio-cultural, political and ecological dimension	Changes related to external systems

Figure 2.1 Processes of change in integrative psychotherapy

Her model includes the following therapeutic processes: emotional processing, dual awareness, contact with painful content, acceptance and compassion for oneself, insight and understanding of oneself, the responsibility of the client for effective ongoing patterns of activity, and effecting changes outside the therapy sessions (Modic, 2019).

Mindfulness and compassion as meta-processes of change

Our approach to integrative psychotherapy gives primacy to mindfulness and compassion processes: *present moment awareness, acceptance, decentred perspective* and *compassion*. Mindful awareness and compassion promote change in each dimension of human experience. For example, mindful awareness promotes emotional processing (Sayers et al., 2015), affect regulation (Farb et al., 2012; A. M. Hayes & Feldman, 2004; Teper et al., 2013; Vago & Silbersweig, 2012), interoception (Farb et al., 2015), behavioural flexibility and values clarification (S. L. Shapiro et al., 2006). We understand mindfulness and compassion as meta-processes of change, which influence all other processes of change.

A large body of research shows that mindfulness and compassion are related to positive psychotherapy outcomes and have benefits for mental health. A meta-analysis of mindfulness-based therapies shows that mindfulness is effective for anxiety (Hofmann et al., 2010; Khoury et al., 2013), symptoms of depression (Goldberg et al., 2018; Hofmann et al., 2010; Khoury et al., 2013), and depression relapse (Goldberg et al., 2019; Kuyken et al., 2016). Mindfulness-based interventions were also found to be effective for patients with alcohol and drug use disorders (Cavicchioli et al., 2018), where large effects were related to the perceived craving, negative affectivity, and post-traumatic symptoms. Mindful meditation was also found to improve pain, depression symptoms, and quality of life in chronic pain patients (Hilton et al., 2017), and mental well-being in patients with multiple-sclerosis (Simpson et al., 2019). Meta-analyses of mindfulness-based interventions for mental-health workers show that mindfulness interventions improve well-being and reduce distress (Lomas et al., 2019; Spinelli et al., 2019). Present moment awareness, acceptance and decentred perspective/defusion are also extensively researched in acceptance and commitment therapy (ACT) (S. C. Hayes et al., 2012). These processes are crucial for psychological flexibility that is empirically linked to positive treatment outcomes (S. C. Hayes et al., 2012).

Compassion is also being increasingly researched. A meta-analysis of 14 studies shows that self-compassion is related to lower psychopathological symptoms with large effect size (MacBeth & Gumley, 2012). Compassion is the primary process in compassion-oriented approaches, such as compassion-focused therapy (P. Gilbert, 2010) and mindful self-compassion (Germer & Neff, 2013; Neff & Germer, 2013). M. Ferrari et al. (2019) have done a meta-analysis of 27 randomised controlled trials that investigated self-compassion interventions and psychosocial outcomes. They found that self-compassion interventions promote improvement in a range of clinical symptoms such as eating difficulties, rumination, self-criticism, depression, anxiety, and stress. Research also shows that self-compassion promotes well-being (M. Ferrari et al., 2019; Zessin et al., 2015) and that higher self-compassion is related to a lower level of shame (Sedighimornani et al., 2019). Modic (2019) found that mindfulness and self-compassion are important processes and outcomes in integrative psychotherapy. Mindfulness and compassion processes are elaborated in detail in Chapter 3.

Interpersonal dimension

Problems in the interpersonal dimension are related to attachment issues and maladaptive relationship patterns. They can manifest both in relationships outside of the therapy or within the therapeutic relationship itself as transference enactments or ruptures in the therapeutic alliance. MCIP is a relational form of psychotherapy where the therapeutic relationship is seen as the primary vehicle of change, which is congruent with numerous psychotherapy research studies that show that therapeutic relationship is consistently related to positive psychotherapy outcomes (Elliot et al., 2011; Norcross, 2010; Norcross & Lambert, 2018).

We emphasise three processes related to the therapeutic relationship: *attunement, maintaining and repairing the therapeutic alliance,* and *corrective relational experiences.* These are evidence-based processes that are consistently related to positive outcomes in psychotherapy. They were also found to be crucial helpful aspects of integrative psychotherapy in the qualitative research of Modic and G. Žvelc (2015).

There is some overlap between these three processes; however, because of their importance and significance in our approach, we list them separately. The first process is *therapeutic attunement,* which refers to the attunement of the therapist to the client's moment-to-moment experience. Erskine and Trautmann (1996) describe attunement as "a kinesthetic and emotional sensing of the other" that provides "reciprocal affect and/or resonating response" (p. 320). Attunement can be understood as a form of empathy that is frequently used in experiential therapies (Elliot et al., 2011). Meta-analytic studies of empathy show that empathy is related to positive treatment outcomes (Elliot et al., 2018; Norcross, 2010; Norcross & Wampold, 2018).

Attunement is closely related to the process of *maintaining and repairing the therapeutic alliance.* This refers to the agreement between client and therapist regarding goals of treatment, collaboration in tasks of the therapy and the presence of a positive emotional bond between client and therapist (Bordin, 1979). Therapeutic attunement facilitates the bond element of the alliance, with the therapeutic alliance being the common factor in psychotherapy that is consistently related to positive treatment outcomes (Crits-Christoph et al., 2013; Eubanks & Goldfried, 2019; Flückiger et al., 2018). Flückiger et al. (2018) have in a meta-analysis of 295 studies that covered more than 30,000 patients confirmed the importance of the robustness of the therapeutic alliance for a positive psychotherapy outcome. In integrative psychotherapy, the therapist consistently tracks the quality of the therapeutic alliance (M. Žvelc, 2008) and in the case of ruptures, the goal of the therapist is to facilitate their resolution (Safran & Muran, 2000). Research shows the importance of monitoring the alliance throughout the whole therapy and intervening when ruptures occur (Eubanks et al., 2018). There is growing empirical support regarding the importance of recognising and repairing ruptures in the alliance (Barber et al., 2013; Eubanks et al., 2018; Eubanks & Goldfried, 2019). A meta-analysis of research on repairing alliance ruptures shows that successful resolution of ruptures is moderately related to improved outcome (Eubanks et al., 2018).

Corrective relational experiences are the third primary process of change related to the therapeutic relationship. Alexander and French (1946/1980) observed that the therapeutic relationship can provide a corrective emotional experience. Such a corrective experience is at "the heart of change – it is the most essential of change principles" (Eubanks & Goldfried, 2019, p. 95). In integrative psychotherapy, the therapeutic relationship is not seen just as a prerequisite for other strategies and interventions, but as a central process of change. The therapist through the relational methods of integrative psychotherapy (inquiry, attunement, and involvement) (Erskine et al., 1999) offers a new relational experience, which is different from the old relational expectations of the client. This creates a juxtaposition experience (Erskine et al., 1999), which enables the client to reorganise their relational schemas based on new experiences with the therapist.

Corrective relational experiences could be defined as

> specific times in therapy when the client feels a distinct shift, such that she or he comes to understand or experience affectively the relationship with the therapist in a different and unexpected way, and is thereby transformed in some manner.
>
> (Knox et al., 2012, p. 191)

In addition to the relational methods of integrative psychotherapy, the therapist in MCIP may also use metacommunication and self-disclosure (Safran & Muran, 2000; M. Žvelc, 2008).

Mindful awareness and compassion are also crucial for a good therapeutic relationship and the related processes of change (Bruce et al., 2010; Horst et al., 2013). The mindful presence and compassion of the therapist may facilitate attunement, and strengthen the therapeutic alliance and may consequently provide new relational experiences. Geller and Greenberg (2012) describe how mindfulness promotes therapeutic presence, which enhances affect attunement and the therapeutic alliance. Geller et al. (2010) have found that clients' experiences of the therapeutic presence are related to their experience of positive change after the session and having a good therapeutic relationship. The development of the client's capacity for mindfulness and self-compassion can also be beneficial for interpersonal relatedness. Research shows that mindfulness is associated with relationship satisfaction (Kappen et al., 2018; McGill et al., 2016) and that higher self-compassion is related to more positive relationship behaviour, such as being more caring and supportive (Neff & Beretvas, 2013).

Cognitive dimension

Problems in the cognitive dimension are connected to problems in self-understanding and mentalisation. Fonagy and Target (2006) define mentalisation as "mental activity, namely, perceiving and interpreting human behaviour in terms of intentional mental states (e.g., needs, desires, feelings, beliefs, goals, purposes, and reasons)" (p. 544). The problems in this dimension can be found on a continuum that ranges from ordinary human experience to a pathology of mentalisation. We can say that we all experience a certain lack of understanding of ourselves since much of our experience is unconscious, but on the further end of the continuum there may be people who have serious deficits in their ability to understand self and others. These deficits may be seen, for example, in an inability to understand the subjective nature of internal states, in acting-out, psychosomatic problems, alexithymia, and problems in relationships.

The main processes of change in the cognitive dimension are related to *insight and mentalisation*. Clients in integrative psychotherapy report a better understanding of themselves as being both an important process during therapy as well as an important treatment outcome (Modic, 2019).

Insight is traditionally emphasized as a primary mechanism of change in psychodynamic approaches (Barber et al., 2013; Messer, 2013); however, most therapies promote some form of self-understanding (Castonguay & Hill, 2007). Insight refers to both the sudden inspiration of a new understanding (Aha! Experience) or to the "tendency to be able to achieve such understanding" (Gibbons et al., 2007, p. 144). Research shows that changes in insight during psychotherapy are related to the positive outcome of psychotherapy (Barber et al., 2013; Crits-Christoph et al., 2013; Høglend & Hagtvet, 2019). Mentalisation is a process of change, which has been increasingly studied in recent years. An improvement in mentalisation capacities has been strongly related to the decrease of symptoms over time in patients with borderline personality disorder (De Meulemeester et al., 2018).

In integrative psychotherapy, the main method for increasing insight and mentalisation is the method of inquiry, which is a sensitive exploration of the client's subjective experience (Erskine et al., 1999). Inquiry helps clients to understand the relational schemas and self-states that influence their experience. We may also use interventions that are typical for psychodynamic therapies, such as interpretation and confrontation. These interventions are used within a relational stance and are offered to the client as subjective ideas that can be rejected and not as objective facts. We may also use explanations of psychological processes and metaphors that may facilitate insight into subjective experiences.

We think that mindful awareness enhances the cognitive processes of insight and mentalisation. Various defence mechanisms are by definition connected with avoidance and non-acceptance of feared experience. With mindful awareness, we are promoting a new stance towards internal experience, which promotes relaxation of defence mechanisms and can lead to new insights. Mentalisation is also a process that is enhanced by mindful awareness and it shares some characteristics with mindfulness as both are concerned with awareness of our internal mental states. The main difference is that mentalisation is concerned with understanding the mental states of self and others and is not focused only on the present moment, but also on a reflection of our past and future (Choi-Kain & Gunderson, 2008). Wallin (2007) describes how mindful awareness can facilitate the essential aspects of mentalisation – "the recognition that mental states are only mental states, subjective rather than objective, fluid rather than fixed, something we have rather than something we are" (p. 165). The process of decentred perspective is in our opinion the primary process of mindfulness, which facilitates this shift in awareness.

Affective dimension

Problems in the affective dimension are related to problems in emotional processing that may manifest as a lack of awareness of emotions, avoidance of emotions, inability to express emotions, or emotional dysregulation. Both outcome and process research findings of psychotherapy agree that emotional processes are central for good psychotherapy outcomes (Elliot et al., 2013; Greenberg, 2008). In MCIP, we emphasise the following four core affective processes of change: emotional awareness, acceptance of emotions, expression of emotions, and emotional regulation. All four processes are empirically validated processes of change that are related to positive treatment outcomes (Crits-Christoph et al., 2013; Greenberg, 2008). While these processes may be important in all psychotherapies, they are especially emphasized in humanistic/experiential psychotherapy approaches, such as emotion-focused therapy (Greenberg & Watson, 2006), gestalt therapy (Perls et al., 1951), and accelerated experiential dynamic psychotherapy (Fosha, 2000b). In integrative psychotherapy, working with emotions is essential. Modic (2019) has in qualitative research found that clients describe awareness, acceptance, expression, and verbalisation of emotions as helpful aspects of their therapy. Better emotional processing was also found to be an important outcome.

Emotional awareness refers to awareness of the felt sense of emotion and putting the experience into words (Greenberg, 2008). "Emotional awareness is not thinking about feeling, it involves feeling the feeling in awareness" (Greenberg, 2008, p. 52). In integrative psychotherapy, awareness of emotions is accomplished by inquiring about the emotional experience and acknowledging the client's emotions (Erskine et al., 1999). A related process is the *acceptance of emotions* which helps to overcome emotional avoidance. Validation and normalisation of emotions help the client to accept and tolerate the emotional experience. Acceptance of emotion is consistently associated with positive mental health (Ford et al., 2018) and predicts experiencing less negative affect and depressive symptoms (Shallcross et al., 2010).

Expression of emotion is another crucial process in psychotherapy that is empirically related to change (Elliot et al., 2013). Lane et al. (2015), in their review of research literature, describe how emotional arousal appears to be an important process in all psychotherapies. In integrative psychotherapy, clients are invited to express and get in contact with repressed feelings (Erskine, 2015). However, Greenberg (2008) describes that emotional expression is not always useful. Research shows that productive processing is more critical than arousal alone (Greenberg et al., 2007). For productive processing of emotion, it is essential to have awareness and contact with emotion, agency, and emotional regulation (Greenberg et al., 2007).

Emotional regulation is another necessary process of working with emotions. Dysregulation of emotion may manifest in either numbing of emotions or being flooded with emotions. The goal is that the client functions in the optimal zone of arousal – the window of tolerance (D. J. Siegel, 1999). The optimal zone of arousal is related to a moderate level of emotional arousal, not so high as to be overwhelming and not so low as to be distanced from emotions (Lane et al., 2015). In integrative psychotherapy, the attuned therapeutic relationship provides an atmosphere of safety, acceptance, and validation that helps to regulate the client's emotion. Greenberg (2008) similarly describes the empirical evidence that the empathic relationship is crucial for emotional regulation. We may also use other techniques for emotional regulation, such as breathing, working with resources, and exercises related to mindfulness and compassion.

In integrative psychotherapy, we use the relational methods of inquiry, attunement and involvement (Erskine et al., 1999) to enhance the processes of emotional change. These methods invite the client to get in contact with their emotions, to reflect on them and express them. They are also essential for emotional regulation. We also use more active emotion-focused methods that have their origin in gestalt therapy, such as two chair work and the empty chair technique. These methods have been increasingly researched within emotion-focused therapy (Greenberg et al., 1993; Greenberg & Watson, 2006). We also use different methods for working with ego states, such as the psychotherapy of introjects and working with child ego states (Erskine, 2015). As research shows (Modic, 2019), integrative psychotherapists may also creatively use other empirically validated techniques for emotional processing, such as EMDR.

The development of mindful awareness and compassion promote and influence all of these emotional processes. Research shows that mindfulness promotes emotional processing (Sayers et al., 2015) and affect regulation (Farb et al., 2012; A. M. Hayes & Feldman, 2004; Hölzel et al., 2011; Teper et al., 2013; Vago & Silbersweig, 2012). Mindful awareness also promotes both awareness and acceptance of our emotions, which are the main mechanisms for the adaptive processing of emotions. Acceptance and a decentred perspective also help us to stay with our experience with openness and non-reactivity. This enables us to contain our experience, which results in the regulation of affects. Self-compassion enables us to develop kindness towards our pain and to experience common humanity, which is important for the acceptance and regulation of emotions (Hölzel et al., 2011).

Physiological dimension

The main problem area related to the physiological dimension is a lack of contact with the body associated with problems in interoception. Farb et al. (2015) define interoception as the "process of receiving, accessing, and appraising internal bodily signals" (p. 1). It refers to the ability to contact our body sensations and make sense of them. Many of our clients are cut off from their bodies and have difficulties in attending to and understanding the signals from their body, which may affect their well-being and adaptive behaviour. Many mental health problems are associated with problems in interoception such as affective disorders, addiction, eating disorders, chronic pain, dissociative disorders, post-traumatic stress disorder, and somatoform disorders (Farb et al., 2015).

Another problem area related to the physiological dimension is physiological dysregulation, which shows in chronic hyper- or hypo-arousal of the autonomic neural system. Porges (2011, 2017) in his polyvagal theory, describes the importance of regulating the autonomic neural system so that people can feel safe and stay within the social engagement system.

The main processes of change within the physiological dimension are enhancing *interoception and physiological regulation*. These processes of change have in recent years attracted increasing attention, especially in the field of trauma treatment and mindfulness (Dana, 2018; Farb et al., 2015; Levine, 2018; Ogden et al., 2006; Price & Hooven, 2018; Rothschild, 2000, 2017).

In MCIP, we invite the client to develop mindful awareness and acceptance of body sensations and body movements, which opens the way towards understanding the body's signals. In MCIP, we have developed a method called mindful processing (G. Žvelc, 2012) in which clients mindfully attend from moment to moment to their subjective experience, starting with body sensations. We also use various experiential experiments, where clients actively experiment with their body awareness and movements. In clients with a history of trauma, various action tendencies may have been inhibited, such as running away or defending (Levine, 1997, 2018). In the process of psychotherapy, they may complete incomplete movements that were inhibited because of unresolved trauma.

Physiological regulation is another process that is crucial in MCIP. If a client is in a dysregulated physiological state, the crucial task in therapy is to promote physiological regulation. Through therapy, we widen the client's window of tolerance (Ogden et al., 2006; D. J. Siegel, 1999), which helps the client to stay present with a whole range of body sensations, emotions, thoughts, and memories. The aim is for the client to activate their ventral vagal state, which is a resource of safeness (Porges, 2017).

In MCIP, the therapeutic relationship is the primary source of physiological regulation. If the therapist is present, in their own physiologically balanced state and attuned to the client, that will help to regulate the client's own physiological state. Another important process is that we help clients to regulate their physiology by inviting them into mindful awareness and self-compassion. Physiological regulation is promoted through different mindfulness exercises and self-help strategies, such as body scan, breathing, and mindful movement. As Hölzel and colleagues (2011) describe, mindfulness enhances awareness of internal body sensations, which may be an essential process for affect regulation. Clients are invited to use self-care strategies between sessions, which are related to the process of committed action described in the following section.

Behavioural dimension

Problems in the behavioural dimension are evidenced by passivity, impulsivity, lack of skills, and behavioural inflexibility. Some people, for example, avoid certain places and experiences and are not engaged actively in life. They may fear or experience shame in certain situations and because of that, they may avoid certain areas of life. Impulsivity is related to problems in controlling their behaviour, which may appear in problems with aggression, sexual promiscuity, or with alcohol. Some people may lack the specific skills that are necessary for a meaningful life. They may, for example, lack social skills, have problems in assertive behaviour, or they may lack self-regulation skills. Behavioural inflexibility refers to inflexible behaviour, which is manifested in repetitive malfunctioning patterns that are contrary to a client's values and wishes. For example, a client may end a relationship whenever it becomes too intimate.

Integrative psychotherapy research shows that taking responsibility for effective action and activities outside of the therapy sessions are important and helpful processes (Modic, 2019). They are related to the process of *committed action*, which is the primary psychotherapy process related to the behavioural dimension. Committed action is the central process of change in ACT (S. C. Hayes et al., 2012). It involves taking responsibility for our own life and engaging in behaviour that is true to our deepest wishes and longings (Luoma et al., 2007). In integrative psychotherapy, this process is accomplished by inviting the client to adopt new ways of behaving that are contrary to old script patterns, and that will evoke new responses from others that are inconsistent with dysfunctional relational patterns (Erskine, 2015). Such behaviour has to be true to the client's personal values and has to be meaningful. We may make contracts for behavioural change, from the tradition of transactional analysis (Berne, 1961, 1966), which share a similarity to the homework assignments in the behavioural tradition. However, we do not use the word "homework" as this often carries associations that are too closely reminiscent of a school setting. In contracts for behavioural change, clients make a commitment that they will engage in behaviour that is purposeful and meaningful for them. Committed action may involve learning new skills that the client lacks, either in psychotherapy or outside of the therapy setting. It may involve the deliberate practice of certain behaviour. Within the process of committed action, different techniques from the behavioural tradition may be used that are empirically related to successful psychotherapy outcomes, such as behavioural activation, exposure, and skills training/experimentation (S. C. Hayes & Hofmann, 2018).

Mindful awareness and compassion are also crucial for change in the behavioural dimension. Behavioural change often includes engaging in a new way of behaving that may evoke unpleasant emotions. Mindfulness and self-compassion can help clients to stay with and contain their emotions while engaging in a new desired behaviour. Both processes promote psychological flexibility (S. C. Hayes et al., 2012). Mindful awareness may help us to develop a decentred awareness of our maladaptive schemas and to choose behaviour that is congruent with our values. Similarly, S. L. Shapiro et al. (2006) propose that mindful awareness facilitates both exposure to feared stimuli and cognitive, emotional, and behavioural flexibility. Research shows that mindfulness reduces rumination (Jain et al., 2007) and promotes greater engagement and attention to the task (Norris et al., 2018).

Spiritual dimension

The spiritual dimension is in our approach to integrative psychotherapy related to our innermost meaning and purpose in life and experience of transcendence. It is often referred to as the transpersonal dimension. Spirituality means different things for different people. Some may find a sense of higher purpose in life in engagement in different spiritual or religious traditions while others may experience this in contact with nature or in selfless service to other human beings. The spiritual dimension may also have for some people a negative connotation because it can remind them of a particular church or religion. In our approach, the spiritual dimension is related to anything that transcends our limited personal sense of self and gives meaning and direction to our lives. This dimension is crucial in humanistic–existential approaches such as logotherapy (Frankl, 1946/1992, 1969/1994; Yalom, 2001), Jungian analytic psychology (Jung, 1951/2010), and transpersonal psychotherapy (Assagioli, 1965/1993; Grof, 1988).

The problem area related to the spiritual dimension is the lack of meaning and purpose in life. Some clients have difficulties in finding meaning and values that would give a direction to their life, experiencing life as empty and meaningless. The focus on meaning is central both to various humanistic and existential psychotherapy traditions and also to the third-wave behavioural approaches such as ACT.

The primary psychotherapy change process related to the spiritual dimension is *contact with values*. Values give meaning and purpose in life and guide our lives (Luoma et al., 2007). In MCIP, we invite the clients to search for meaning and purpose in their lives and to find values that are true to their deepest longings and wishes. True values are not something that were uncritically introjected from significant others but are an expression of our innermost being. Mindful awareness may be crucial for coming into contact with values and discovering our meaning and purpose in life (S. L. Shapiro et al., 2006). Brown and Ryan (2003), for example, have in research found that individuals who are acting mindfully are more congruent with their values.

The second process of change, related to the spiritual dimension, is *contact with an observing/transcendent self*. Contacting the observing self is a core meta-process of change, which influences other processes of change. This is also congruent with a new conceptualisation of psychological flexibility in ACT, which gives primacy to the observing, perspective-taking self (S. C. Hayes et al., 2019). The authors present a Chinese version of the ACT hexagon in which the perspective-taking self influences all other flexibility processes. They describe how "the perspective-taking self empowers an experiencing self, as well as greater acceptance, defusion, and contact with the present moment – the four 'mindfulness' processes in psychological flexibility" (S. C. Hayes et al., 2019, p. 35). The observing self has in recent years attracted research interest from a number of different fields, including neuroscience (Josipovic, 2010, 2014) and contextual behavioural science (McHughs & Stewart, 2012; McHughs et al., 2019).

The observing self is often referred to as the no-thing self, pure consciousness, or the essential/spiritual self. Hölzel and colleagues (2011) describe how mindfulness leads to a shift in perspective on the self, which we conceptualise as a shift from a personal sense of self to the observing/transcendent self, which is awareness itself and is the context of all of our experiences (see Chapter 3). In MCIP, the client is invited to reflect on the source of mindful awareness itself, which may result in an awareness of the transcendent self. Becoming aware of the transcendent self may manifest in spiritual experiences and a sense of transcendence. It may manifest in the experience of timelessness, inner peace, interconnectedness with other people, compassion, and acceptance (S. C. Hayes et al., 2012).

Mindfulness practices have been used for centuries in different wisdom traditions such as Buddhism, mystical Christianity, the Kabbalah, and Sufism. While in Western psychology the aim of mindfulness practice is usually better mental health, in wisdom traditions this was not the primary aim. Their primary aim was spiritual development and enlightenment and not an enhancement of the personal self. Mindfulness and compassion may spontaneously awaken interest in spirituality. Research shows that practitioners of mindfulness have a variety of spiritual and mystical experiences (Vieten et al., 2018). It is important that as psychotherapists we are open to the spiritual dimension, as some clients will bring spiritual issues into the psychotherapy session. This is congruent with McAleavey and colleagues (2019), who in their list of empirically based principles of change include the importance of accommodating the client's need for spiritually oriented psychotherapy.

Systemic/contextual dimension

The individual does not exist in isolation but in a matrix of larger systems, including such as the culture, family, school and work environments, the rules and the laws of the state, and other socio-cultural factors. We are all influenced by these socio-cultural contexts and also our relationship with nature.

Influence of external systems

Sometimes the main problem arising in the course of therapy is related to a context that is external to the individual. For example, a client's problems may be a symptom of the pathology of the whole family. Parents' drinking problems and constant fights may be a leading cause of anxiety and stress in children. Problems may also be related to the negative influences of peers or relationships with teachers and sports mentors. For example, the pandemic in 2020 and each country's response to it through the imposition of emergency laws and regulations (such as individual isolation, education at home with the closure of schools, working from home with the closure of businesses or unemployment etc.) affected the whole population. In integrative psychotherapy, we are sensitive to these contexts and their influence on both groups and the individual. If the main problem is in the external system, interventions focused on changes in the system may be indicated, such as family/couple therapy, working with the school/teachers, or working with the individual with an awareness of systemic issues.

Socio-cultural context

People's lives are embedded in a broader socio-cultural context that includes issues such as age, religion, political affiliation, gender, sexual orientation, class, status, race, and ethnicity (Evans & Gilbert, 2005). The socio-cultural context influences our being in the world, both consciously and unconsciously. It is important that therapists reflect on their own socio-cultural background and develop a decentred perspective towards their assumptions, which stem from their culture. In this way, they can better understand their clients who may come from a different socio-cultural background, instead of looking at them with the limited vision of their own worldview. The integrative psychotherapist may "transcend culture by honoring the unique world view and values of the client and consequently allow cultural issues to influence the process and direction of the therapeutic work" (Evans & Gilbert, 2005, p. 59). Every client should be understood within their frame of reference and their socio-cultural context (Evans & Gilbert, 2005).

Ecological dimension: relationship to nature

Ken Evans at the Eighth European Conference of Integrative Psychotherapy, said: "Don't forget the sheep." With these words, he expressed the importance of the ecological dimension in psychotherapy. Various authors have emphasised the importance of the ecological dimension in psychotherapy (Buzzell & Chalquist, 2009; Evans & Gilbert, 2005; Rust, 2008; Totton, 2011). Evans and Gilbert (2005) described how the ecological dimension – meaning our relationship with the natural world – is often neglected by psychotherapists. They describe how the current paradigm of Western psychology "is that of development where growth is seen as 'more', and self is largely understood as 'customer'" (Evans & Gilbert, 2005, p. 59). This paradigm is focused more on self-realisation and the predominance of human needs, above all else. They propose that it is vital to raise ecological consciousness among psychotherapists, which means that the personal and professional values of each psychotherapist should include concerns for the preservation of all life forms on earth and not just humans (Evans & Gilbert, 2005). Mindfulness and compassion processes may be central in this shift towards ecological consciousness. Schutte and Malouff (2018) have in their meta-analysis of 12 research samples found a significant correlation between mindfulness and connectedness to nature. Greater awareness, acceptance, and compassion may naturally awaken greater compassion towards nature and all life forms on the planet.

Processes of change in clinical practice

During this journey through the different dimensions, we have described the main processes of change that are research-based and have been found to be effective in psychotherapy. The model of processes of change helps us to conceptualise the client's problems in terms of the main dimensions and change processes. All these processes of change are interconnected and influence each other. Change in one dimension can facilitate change in other dimensions. The fundamental assumption is that it is beneficial to work on different dimensions, to facilitate change within the whole system.

In integrative psychotherapy, we determine the main problems in each dimension and the main processes that need to be enhanced with each client. We then tailor the treatment according to each client, instead of rigidly trying to fit the client into our particular therapeutic schema. While overall case conceptualisation may act as a guide for the course of the therapy, the therapist also tries to identify processes that are important to address in the moment-to-moment process of therapy. The main questions are which process at which point in psychotherapy would be most beneficial to enhance. The integrative psychotherapist is therefore flexible and willing to decentre from their own ideas and theories in order to be present and available for the client. In determining which process is important to address, we follow Erskine's (2015) guidelines on attending to where the client is open or closed to contact. At the beginning of the therapy we will focus on dimensions where the client is open to contact, to facilitate trust and safety. Later we will invite the client into areas that are more difficult and painful. At different moments in therapy, a client may show openings at dimensions where they are usually closed to contact.

The process of therapy, according to the integrative model of processes of change, can be summarized in the following way:

1   Identifying problem areas related to each dimension.
2   Identifying in which dimension is the client open or closed to contact.
3   Identifying the process of change that would be most beneficial to enhance taking into account the client's readiness and willingness to work in that dimension.
4   Tailoring methods and interventions to facilitate the selected process of change.
5   Monitoring the impact of our interventions and change in the overall system.

Part II

Concepts and theories

3 Mindfulness and compassion in integrative psychotherapy

In this chapter, we integrate current ideas from the science and practice of mindfulness and compassion with concepts of integrative psychotherapy. We present two new models that can be used for the understanding of mindfulness and compassion in psychotherapy: the *diamond model of the observing self* and the *triangle of relationship to experience*.

In the literature, we find many different understandings and definitions of the term mindfulness. Mindfulness is described as a state of present-centred awareness, as a personality trait, meditation practice, or an intervention (Vago & Silbersweig, 2012). Kabat-Zinn (1994) describes mindfulness as "paying attention in a particular way: on purpose, in the present moment and nonjudgmentally" (p. 4). In mindfulness- and compassion-oriented integrative psychotherapy (MCIP), we view mindfulness primarily as a process of accepting awareness of the present moment. This process can be developed by different means in both our everyday lives as well as in psychotherapy. Bishop and colleagues (2004) proposed two main components of mindfulness: (a) sustained attention to the present moment; and (b) a specific quality of attention characterised by acceptance, openness, and curiosity to experience. Congruent with this definition, Cardaciotto et al. (2008) conceptualise mindfulness as "the tendency to be highly aware of one's internal and external experiences in the context of an accepting, nonjudgmental stance toward those experiences" (p. 205). The first component of mindfulness refers to continual awareness of the present moment, instead of focusing on the past or future. The second component describes a nonjudgemental stance towards experience that manifests in "acceptance, openness, and even compassion towards one's experience" (Cardaciotto et al., 2008, p. 205). Such a stance towards private events enables a person to be with their experience without judgment, interpretation, or attempts to change it. D. J. Siegel (2007) similarly describes this mindful stance towards internal experience with the acronym COAL: Curiosity, Openness, Acceptance, and Love.

Awareness alone does not necessarily lead to a state of mindfulness (Černetič, 2005, 2017). Some clients are very aware of their anxiety; however, they are fighting with it and trying to get rid of it, which can lead to an increase in anxiety. So awareness has to be coupled with acceptance and openness to experience to be qualified as mindful awareness (Černetič, 2017). Acceptance is often confused with passivity or resignation, but in mindful awareness, we are fully present with our internal experience without preoccupation or avoidance (Cardaciotto et al., 2008). This results in increased contact with internal experience.

In addition to mindfulness, the process of compassion has in recent years attracted increasing clinical and research interest (Germer & Neff, 2013; P. Gilbert 2009, 2010; Neff, 2003a; Neff & Germer, 2013). P. Gilbert (2009) defines compassion as "basic kindness, with deep awareness of the suffering of oneself and of other living things, coupled with the wish and effort to relieve it" (p. xiii). Tirch et al. (2014) similarly describe compassion as involving three main characteristics: "mindful attention to and mindful awareness of suffering, an understanding and felt sense of suffering and its causes, and motivation to remain open to suffering with the intention or wish to relieve it" (p. 8).

In our approach to integrative psychotherapy, mindfulness and compassion are viewed as core psychotherapy processes that can be enhanced by different methods and techniques within the attuned therapeutic relationship. The therapist's mindful presence and compassion are the basis for helping the client towards mindful awareness and compassion. There is a growing body of research showing the benefits of mindful awareness and compassion from both psychology, psychotherapy research, and neuroscience (Cavicchioli et al., 2018; Farb et al., 2012; Farb et al., 2007; M. Ferrari et al., 2019; Goldberg et al., 2018; MacBeth & Gumley, 2012; Teper & Inzlicht, 2013; Teper, et al., 2013). Mindful awareness and compassion are evidence-based processes that can be enhanced in psychotherapy.

Mindfulness and compassion as core processes in integrative psychotherapy

Martin (1997) proposed that mindfulness is a common factor in different psychotherapies. Similarly, Dunn et al. (2013) propose that mindfulness is a transtheoretical clinical process. In MCIP, this process is viewed as an essential element in the process of change.

Germer (2005) described three different ways of integrating mindfulness into psychotherapy that is collectively referred to as mindfulness-oriented psychotherapy. Therapists may (1) personally practise mindfulness which helps them to bring the quality of a mindful presence in relation to their clients; (2) use a theoretical frame of reference, which is informed by mindfulness research, mindfulness practice, or Buddhist psychology; (3) teach clients how to develop mindfulness practice.

In MCIP, although we use all three ways of integrating mindfulness into psychotherapy work, we give priority to the mindful presence of the therapist and the theoretical frame of reference, which is based on mindfulness research and contemplative wisdom traditions. While a therapist may invite the client to learn mindfulness meditation and occasionally teach some technique, this is not the primary focus in our approach.

MCIP has strong roots in humanistic psychotherapy and is relational psychotherapy, which sees client and therapist as an intersubjective system of mutual influence. From this perspective, mindfulness and compassion are not seen primarily as techniques to be learned, but as processes that are enhanced within an attuned psychotherapeutic relationship. In this way, our approach differs from mindfulness-based approaches such as MBCT (Segal et al., 2002), where the primary intervention is teaching the clients the techniques of mindfulness meditation.

The concept of contact and mindful awareness

As we describe in Chapter 1, MCIP is based on Erskine's relationally focused integrative psychotherapy. G. Žvelc (2009a, 2012) proposed that Erskine's relationally focused integrative psychotherapy already uses mindfulness in its approach, even though the word "mindfulness" is not explicitly mentioned in his writings on integrative psychotherapy. The main theories and methods of relationally focused integrative psychotherapy are "based upon the philosophy of an accepting awareness within an attuned therapeutic relationship" (G. Žvelc, 2012, p. 44). The main relational methods of integrative psychotherapy are inquiry, attunement, and involvement (Erskine et al., 1999). G. Žvelc (2012) suggests that these methods "invite the client into state of awareness and acceptance of his/her internal experience, which is the main mechanism of mindfulness ... [They] invite the client in contact with self and others and promote the integration of dissociated states of self" (p. 44).

Relationally focused integrative psychotherapy is also a compassion-oriented approach, even though the process of compassion is not fully elaborated on in writings about integrative psychotherapy. The relational methods of inquiry, attunement, and involvement are compassion-based methods that provide a compassionate response to the client's suffering (Erskine, 2019c).

In previous writings and presentations, we have argued that the concept of contact is closely related to the contemporary construct of mindfulness (G. Žvelc, 2009a; G. Žvelc et al., 2011). We think that humanistic and existential therapy approaches were using mindfulness processes in psychotherapy for a long time before mindfulness became popularised within the cognitive-behavioural tradition. However, this process was not conceptualised as mindfulness but was understood by different names, such as *contact* in gestalt therapy. Mindful awareness is a process of accepting awareness of internal and external stimuli. Similarly, contact can be both internal and external. Internal contact refers to full awareness of our internal experience, while external contact refers to awareness of external events (Erskine & Trautmann, 1996). Erskine (1993) describes that "with full internal and external contact, experiences are continually integrated" (p. 185).

The concept of contact comes into relationally focused integrative psychotherapy from gestalt therapy (Perls et al., 1951). As with gestalt therapy, Erskine et al. (1999) describe contact as a process:

> Contact is really a verb, not a noun; it is dynamic rather than static. It is similar to a flashlight beam playing over the contents of a darkened room, lighting up first this object and then that one. It is not a random movement,

though; in full and healthy contact, there is a shuttling between internal and external events, with neither overbalancing the other. We move from awareness of self to awareness of our environment and especially of other people in that environment.[1]

As contact is a primary mechanism of change in integrative psychotherapy, integrative psychotherapy is in its essence a mindfulness-oriented approach. The central concept of integrative psychotherapy is that of restoring the client's full contact with themselves and others, which could equally be described as mindful awareness. Congruent with this, G. Žvelc et al. (2011) proposed the following revised definition of contact, which is congruent with mindfulness: "We would redefine contact as full, accepting awareness of internal experiences and external events" (p. 246). It is important to note that such awareness does not mean inactivity or passivity in the face of external events that are not acceptable (domestic violence, racism, etc.). Quite the opposite is true since greater internal and external contact results in us not denying the reality of the situation and leads to taking appropriate action.

The observing/transcendent self

In this section, we present the concept of the observing self, which is one of the core concepts in MCIP. The concept of self has a long history in psychology, starting with William James' (1890/2007) conceptualisation of self as a subject and self as an object. The development of mindfulness approaches in psychotherapy and neuroscience mindfulness research has brought a new perspective to our understanding of the sense of self. Lutz et al. (2006) describe how both neuroscience and Buddhist models of self distinguish between "a minimal subjective sense of 'I-ness' in experience, or ipseity, and a narrative or autobiographical self" (p. 524). Farb et al. (2007) have found neurological support for two fundamentally distinct forms of self-awareness: narrative self-reference and the self in the present moment. In MCIP, we similarly differentiate between two different senses of self: the *personal sense of self* and the *observing self*. The personal sense of self is connected to our personal identity and our corresponding self-narrative that has been developed and constructed based on our life experiences. It is our "usual sense of self" – what we take ourselves to be. However, beyond the personal sense of self, there is another experience of self – the observing self (Deikman, 1982; S. C. Hayes et al., 1999).

The observing self is awareness itself that is subjectively experienced as a simple experience of *being* and conscious *presence*. It is the "transparent center, that which is aware" (Deikman, 1982, p. 94) and is distinct from the contents of awareness, such as thoughts, emotions, or body sensations. Deikman (1982) has proposed that Western psychology has missed this differentiation between awareness and contents of awareness and has usually described the self as content or structure. He describes the reality of the observing self with the proposition: "I am aware; therefore, I am" (p. 94). From this perspective, observing self could also be described as "*the self-as-awareness*". It is our essential sense of self that is awareness itself. We experience the world through our awareness; however, awareness itself cannot be observed, it can only be experienced (Deikman, 1982, 1996), and it has transcendental qualities (Deikman, 1982).

This description of the observing self is congruent with the experiences of meditators from different wisdom traditions (Deikman, 1982). D. J. Siegel (2007) describes how in mindfulness meditation there is a different quality of self: "As the immersion in mindfulness unfolds, bare awareness of the ipseity of one's experience emerges – the sense of a grounded self beneath the layers of constructed identity" (pp. 243–244). D. J. Siegel (2007) describes such an experience as a "sense of the essential nature of the mind" (p. 99), which "implies an invariant quality, a grounded essence of our being that is not just a function of the transient contexts that come and go in our lives" (D. J. Siegel, 2007, p. 99). Although both Assagioli (1965/1993) and Deikman (1982) had described the observing self, it was not an accepted part of mainstream psychotherapy. It was seen as part of some mystical and spiritual traditions, a concept that could not be proved by scientific means. With the development of mindfulness approaches, the concept of the observing self has in recent years been gaining increasing empirical support and interest. Contextual behaviour science, which is the basis of acceptance and commitment therapy, is providing empirical support for the use of the observing self in psychotherapy (S. C. Hayes et al., 2012; McHughs & Stewart, 2012; McHughs et al., 2019). S. C. Hayes (1984) has written a seminal article *Making sense of spirituality*, which was the first description of the observing self in contextual behavioural science. In ACT literature, this sense of self is also described as the *self-as-context* or *transcendent self* (S. C. Hayes et al., 2012). The transcendent self is "an aspect of self that metaphorically cannot be looked at but instead must be looked from" (S. C. Hayes et al., 2012, p. 85). It is a perspective through which we observe all our experiences. It is a stable sense of self, a stable perspective of I/HERE/NOW (Villate et al., 2012). As the observing self has transcendental qualities, we will refer to the observing self also as *transcendent self*.

Qualities of the observing/transcendent self

The observing/transcendent self is a crucial aspect of ourselves that is at the heart of psychological health and healing. In MCIP, we invite the client to come into contact with this sense of self, which brings with it qualities that promote well-being and psychological growth. The qualities of the observing self are: mindful awareness and presence, transcendence and spirituality, interconnection, compassion, stable perspective, and a container of experience.

Mindful awareness and presence

The *observing self* manifests as mindful awareness – an accepting nonjudgmental awareness of our experience. In addition to present moment awareness and acceptance, an important quality of mindful awareness is its decentred perspective

(Safran & Segal, 1990), which enables us to differentiate between ourselves and our experience. When we are in contact with the observing self, we become aware of the continually changing contents within our consciousness. We may be aware of our thoughts, emotions, physical sensations, or external environment.

Mindful awareness is also experienced as a *conscious presence* or *being*. It is related to a *being mode* of mind (Segal et al., 2002), which is characterised by "'accepting' and 'allowing' what is, without any immediate pressure to change it" (p. 73). It is related to the immediate experience of the present moment. In contrast, our everyday *personal sense of self* is related to a doing mode, which is goal-oriented and motivated "to reduce the gap between how things are and how we would like them to be" (p. 73). This mode of mind could also be described as a problem-solving mode of mind (S. C. Hayes et al., 2012).

Transcendence and spirituality

The observing self has transcendental qualities. This aspect of self has been described in different spiritual traditions and is "at the heart of human spirituality" (S. C. Hayes et al., 2012, p. 184). It can only be experienced and not grasped as an object, and so it is often referred to as the *no-thing* self and *pure awareness* (S. C. Hayes et al., 1999; S. C. Hayes et al., 2012). In mindfulness meditation, we observe and pay attention to our internal experiences as well as external stimuli. We can ask ourselves, who is the one who is aware? Who is aware of thoughts, emotions, sensations, and the external world? Such inquiry compels us to become aware of awareness itself. When the focus of our awareness becomes the observing self, we may touch the transcendental dimension of the human psyche.

Metaphorically, the transcendent self is like the sense of looking from behind our eyes (Villate et al., 2012). We cannot look back and see our own perspective. If we try to do that, we will do it again from our own perspective. This sense of self cannot be described in the way we describe any other objects – it is no-thing and at the same time everything (S. C. Hayes, 1984). It has qualities of spaciousness and timelessness (S. C. Hayes et al., 1999). These qualities are an essential part of different spiritual traditions, which describe spirituality with terms such as nothing/everything or infinite (S. C. Hayes, 1984; S. C. Hayes et al., 2012). We could describe it as our essential, spiritual self.

Interconnection and compassion

With our personal sense of self, we experience ourselves as inherently separated from other human beings; the transcendent self, in contrast, is inherently interconnected with others (S. C. Hayes, 2019; S. C. Hayes et al., 2012; Villate et al., 2012). If we are in contact with the observing self, we can also experience the other person as a conscious human being. In this sense we can experience interconnection and a sense of shared consciousness (S. C. Hayes et al., 2012). Villate et al. (2012) describe how contact with a transcendent sense of self is the basis for compassion, connection, and pro-sociality. The observing/transcendent self is also crucial for self-compassion. When we are in contact with the observing/transcendent self, we have an open and accepting relationship with ourselves, which is the basis for self-compassion.

Stable perspective

The observing self is always present as a stable perspective from which we can observe all experiences. While the contents of awareness are continually changing, the I as the fulcrum of perspective does not change (Deikman, 1982; S. C. Hayes, 1984). It provides a stable and changeless perspective over time; we have been our self as a perspective throughout our whole life. In this sense, the transcendental sense of self is a stable sense of self. It is something in our life which is always present although we are often not aware of it.

Container of experience

The transcendent self is a context in which our every experience is viewed, yet it is different from all experiences. It is a container of all that we perceive and experience (S. C. Hayes et al., 2012). This aspect of a transcendental sense of self is crucial in psychotherapy. Even if clients are experiencing painful emotions or thoughts, there is an aspect of them that is not touched by this experience. This helps them to adopt a witnessing mode of relationship to their experience (Žvelc, 2009a).

As we have already described, the observing self is intrinsically connected to the quality of mindful awareness and compassion. In MCIP, we encourage clients to contact the observing self and to bring mindful awareness and compassion into their lives and into their psychotherapy process. In the following sections, we will describe two new models that provide us with an understanding of mindfulness and compassion processes in psychotherapy: *the diamond model of the observing self* and *the triangle of relationship to experience*.

The diamond model of the observing self

One of the core models in integrative psychotherapy is the self-in-relationship system (Erskine & Trautmann, 1993/1997), which is often referred to as the diamond model (see Figure 1.1, Chapter 1). In this model, we see the interrelationships between different dimensions: cognitive, affective, physiological, behavioural, relational, and spiritual. In integrative psychotherapy, we pay close attention to all these dimensions of human experience and are interested in where a client is open or closed to contact. With different psychotherapy methods, we are then able to help the client to achieve full internal and external contact.

Figure 3.1 represents our integration of the self-in-relationship system with the concept of the observing self and mindful awareness. We call it the *diamond model of the observing self*.

The model was inspired by D. J. Siegel's (2007, 2018) visual metaphor of the *wheel of awareness* that represents mindful awareness. In his illustration, the central hub of the wheel describes the experience of being aware, while the rim represents the objects of awareness (D. J. Siegel, 2018, p. 108). This illustration was an inspiration for the graphical presentation of the diamond model of the observing self, where the observing self is in the centre of the self-in-relationship model.

The observing self in the figure is symbolically represented as the sun with its rays (illustrated by arrows) "shining" towards different dimensions: cognitive, affective, physiological, behavioural, and relational. The sun is a metaphor for the observing self, which is often in spiritual traditions described as the light of awareness or spiritual sun. The innermost circle represents the observing self and different rays the process of mindful awareness of different contents of experience, which are represented by the square and the circle. In Figure 3.1, there is also an arrow pointing back at the observing self, which symbolically represents

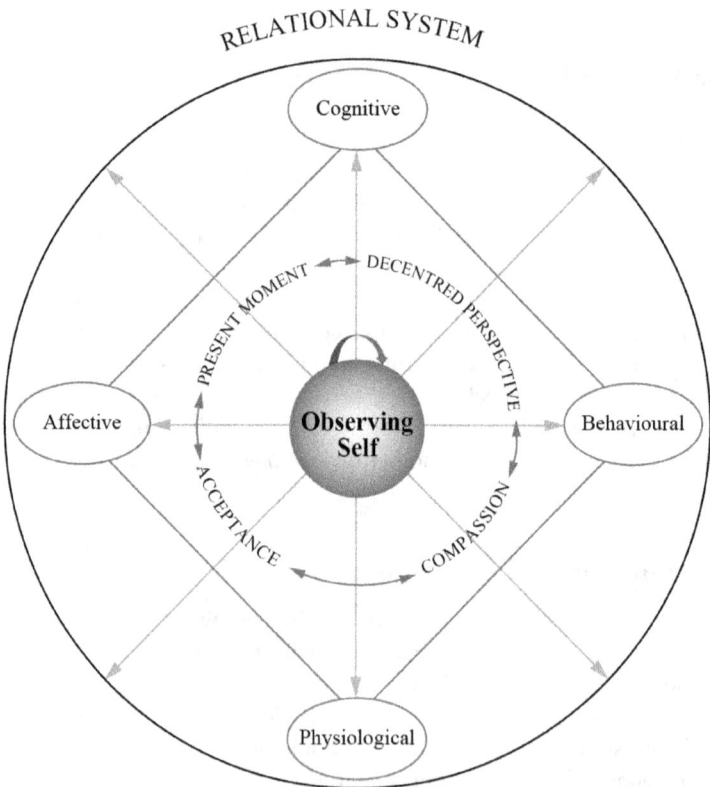

Figure 3.1 The diamond model of the observing self
Note. Adapted from "The process of integrative psychotherapy" by R. G. Erskine and R. L. Trautmann, 1997, *Theories and methods of an integrative transactional analysis: A volume of selected articles* (p. 81), TA Press (Original work published 1993). Copyright 1993 by R. G. Erskine. Adapted with permission.

awareness of awareness itself. This drawing is inspired by D. J. Siegel's (2018) illustration of the wheel of awareness (p. 108), where the spoke of attention turns back into the hub, which illustrates the awareness of awareness.

Figure 3.1 symbolically shows the mindful awareness of both internal and external experiences. In integrative psychotherapy terminology, this is described as internal and external contact (Erskine, 2015). Internal contact refers to awareness of our thoughts, emotions, body, and behaviour and is in the figure portrayed by rays pointing to dimensions in the square. Rays pointing to the circle portray our external contact – our contact with other people or the environment.

The observing self in the centre refers to the sense *I am aware*, while rays pointing to different dimensions describe the content of our experiences that we are currently aware of. While the observing self is constant and stable, the contents of our awareness are continually changing. The rays, "shining" from the observing self, represent four key processes of mindful awareness and compassion: present moment, decentred perspective, acceptance, and compassion. These processes are illustrated within a circle that shows how all these processes are related to each dimension. In the next section, we describe each of these core processes in more detail.

Processes of mindful awareness and compassion

As we describe in previous sections, the observing self manifests in qualities of mindful awareness and compassion. Mindful awareness has certain qualities that distinguish it from the "ordinary" form of awareness, which is related to the personal sense of self. While the ordinary awareness of the personal sense of self is often judgemental and oriented towards past and future, mindful awareness has the following qualities: an awareness of the present moment, acceptance, and a decentred perspective. These qualities are the main processes of mindful awareness that are enhanced in mindfulness- and compassion-oriented integrative psychotherapy. They are key processes of mindfulness in ACT (S. C. Hayes et al., 2012) and other third-generation behavioural approaches such as MBCT (Segal et al., 2002). In addition to the processes of mindful awareness, the observing/transcendent self also has qualities of self-compassion and compassion to others (S. C. Hayes et al., 2012).

Present moment awareness

Mindful awareness is always in the here and now. We are continually aware of what is happening in the present moment. We are, for example, aware of our thoughts, emotions, body sensations. I may notice that I feel tense in my chest, at the next moment I am aware that I have a thought "what is this tension about", then I experience sadness, then I hear a loud noise from the kitchen … The contents of our mind represented by the rectangle and circle are continually changing; there is always something new emerging in the present moment (see Figure 3.1). In this way, we are aware of the stream of our own consciousness, of the different contents of our mind that are in constant flux. The diamond model of the observing self differentiates between awareness itself and the contents of awareness. While awareness itself is constant, the contents of awareness are continually changing.

According to the diamond model of the *observing self*, we may be unaware of specific thoughts, emotions, body movements/sensations, or our current behaviour. For example, being unaware of our emotions may result in an inability to describe and understand them. A lack of awareness may also manifest in relation to other people and the external environment. Client Andrea, for example, described how she is often not present with her husband. While talking with him, she is often disconnected and feels numb. She also described how she is often on autopilot and not being aware of her environment, such as a beautiful landscape, when she is outside walking in nature.

Problems in the present moment awareness may manifest in a preoccupation with the past/future in experiences like rumination, regrets about past, re-experiencing traumatic memories, constant worry, and anxiety. The corresponding process of change is present moment awareness. In MCIP, we bring the client into contact with the present moment with a variety of different psychotherapeutic methods. The diamond model of the observing self helps us to distinguish which aspects of inner experience the client is not aware of and need to be attended to.

Acceptance

Mindful awareness has the quality of being accepting and open to all our experiences. This means that we do not try to avoid or deny experience but remain open and in full contact with it. In this process, our experiences are allowed and accepted. We relate to our experiences without attachment or aversion. Acceptance is a crucial process of mindfulness, which helps us to "embrace one's immediate experience in a nonjudgmental way and without struggle" (S. C. Hayes et al., 2012, p. 77). This is also related to the concept of "letting go" (Kabat-Zinn, 1990). We are not trying to cling to a particular experience, and neither are we trying to move away from it. Acceptance is related to nonjudgment. We are not judging the experience as bad or good. The observing self is in itself nonjudgmental and could be described as pure awareness of what is happening in the present moment.

The lack of acceptance of internal experience manifests in the avoidance of emotions, physical sensations, and thoughts. The client may be aware of internal experiences (e.g. his emotions) but is in a constant struggle to control them and avoid being present with them. Such a process could be described as experiential avoidance (S. C. Hayes et al., 2012), which "occurs when a person is unwilling to remain in contact with particular private experiences" (p. 72).

Experiential avoidance is often a key factor in drug abuse, eating disorders, and any other problems that are based on attempts to control unpleasant internal experience. In the process of integrative psychotherapy, we invite our clients to embrace and accept their experiences.

Decentred perspective

Mindful awareness is decentred regarding the contents of our experience. We are fully present with our thoughts, emotions, and physical sensations, without being merged with them. There is a clear differentiation between the I, who is aware, and the content of my experience. For example: if we have negative cognition such as "I don't deserve to live" we can just observe this thought without identifying with it. It is just thought and not myself. Decentring is crucial also for the acceptance of our experiences.

Safran and Segal (1990) describe decentring as "a process through which one is able to step outside of one's immediate experience, thereby changing the very nature of that experience" (p. 117). Bishop et al. (2004) describe how mindfulness invites the person to become aware of thoughts and emotions and to "relate to them in a wider, decentered perspective as transient mental events rather than as reflections of the self or as necessarily accurate reflections on reality" (p. 236).

Decentred perspective is a crucial process of mindful awareness (Segal et al., 2002; S. L. Shapiro et al., 2006). Deikman (1982) describes a similar process as *deautomatization*, which is the "undoing of the automatic processes that control perception and cognition" (p. 137). In acceptance and commitment therapy, a similar concept is *defusion*, which rather than changing thoughts and emotions, helps clients to change the context in which thoughts and emotions occur (Luoma et al., 2007). Cognitive defusion, for example, helps clients to look *at* their thoughts, rather than *from* their thoughts (S. C. Hayes & Spencer, 2005).

Decentred perspective is also related to the description of S. L. Shapiro et al. (2006) of *re-perceiving*, which they describe as a meta-mechanism of mindfulness:

> Through the process of mindfulness, one is able to disidentify from the contents of consciousness (i.e., one's thoughts) and view his or her moment-by-moment experience with greater clarity and objectivity. We term this process reperceiving as it involves a fundamental shift in perspective. Rather than being immersed in the drama of our personal narrative or life story, we are able to stand back and simply witness it.[2]

When clients are merged with the content of their experience, we may use different interventions to facilitate a decentred perspective. This perspective enhances the ability to observe and stand back from the contents of our consciousness such as thoughts, emotions, or physical sensations. Contact with the observing self naturally promotes the experience of differentiation between awareness and the contents of awareness. Such a decentred perspective helps clients to contain painful private experiences. For example, the client may be invited to observe painful thoughts and emotions as passing events in the mind.

Compassion

Contact with the *observing self* leads to both self-compassion and compassion towards others. The mindful processes of present moment awareness, acceptance, and decentred perspective are crucial for compassion. With mindful awareness, we bring acceptance and love to all our experiences, both pleasant and unpleasant. Compared to mindful processes, compassion is directed towards painful experiences and to the person who suffers, whether ourselves or others. It also involves an active intention to relieve the suffering. The process of self-compassion refers to developing kindness and love towards our pain, suffering, and inadequacies.

Self-compassion involves:

> being touched by and open to one's own suffering, not avoiding it or disconnecting from it, generating the desire to alleviate one's suffering, and to heal oneself with kindness. Self-compassion also involves offering nonjudgmental understanding to one's pain, inadequacies, and failures, so that one's experience is seen as part of the larger human experience.
>
> (Neff, 2003b, p. 87)[3]

This definition implies three main components of self-compassion: self-kindness, common humanity, and mindfulness (Neff, 2003a, 2011). It means being kind to ourselves, when we are experiencing pain, understanding that our pain, suffering, and imperfection are part of being human and bringing accepting awareness to our painful experiences. A lack of self-compassion may manifest in self-judgement and self-criticism, and it may be the key issue behind different problems such as shame, low self-esteem, depression, and social anxiety.

In MCIP, through the compassionate presence of the therapist and different psychotherapeutic methods we invite the client to be self-compassionate. Although the compassionate therapeutic relationship is the main factor in developing this, we also use different interventions that invite the client to enhance self-compassion. Self-compassion is intimately connected to compassion for others and so, developing self-compassion often gives birth to compassion for other human beings. Sometimes the reverse is also true; compassion for others may facilitate compassion towards ourselves.

The observing/transcendent self and nondual awareness

In Figure 3.1 we can see that rays from the observing self are pointing out towards different dimensions and that there is also an arrow pointing back at the observing self. These describe two different aspects of awareness that are related to the observing self:

- Mindful awareness of internal and external stimuli.
- Nondual awareness.

When our attention is focused on the contents of our mind or the outside environment, we are experiencing the observing self as continual awareness of the present-moment – mindful awareness. In the model, this is portrayed by rays pointing out towards different dimensions. However, when mindful awareness is turned inwards, to awareness itself, this can manifest in the experience of transcendence and *nondual awareness* (Josipovic, 2019). In Figure 3.1, this is portrayed as an arrow pointing from the observing self back towards itself. This drawing represents awareness of awareness itself. D. J. Siegel (2018) describes how awareness of awareness itself often leads to experiences of "love, joy, and a wide-open, timeless expanse" (p. 116).

The diamond model of the observing self is the core model in our integrative approach. It can be used for assessing and enhancing mindfulness processes in relation to each personality dimension. The therapist can track from moment-to-moment the client's mindful awareness in relation to specific dimensions of the personality. The model helps in understanding:

- A client's lack of contact with a particular dimension.
- The mindful processes that need to be encouraged in order to promote mindful awareness of a particular dimension.

The triangle of relationship to experience

G. Žvelc (2009a) has described three main relationships with phenomenological experience, which are useful to consider in the psychotherapy process:

1 Being merged with the experience.
2 Being distanced from the experience.
3 Being witness to our experience.

Based on these ideas, we have developed a model of the triangle of relationship to experience, which can be used as a process for tracking clients' mindful awareness from moment-to-moment (Figure 3.2). While the diamond model of the observing self describes processes of mindful awareness and compassion related to

Loving witness
(high awareness, acceptance and decentred perspective)

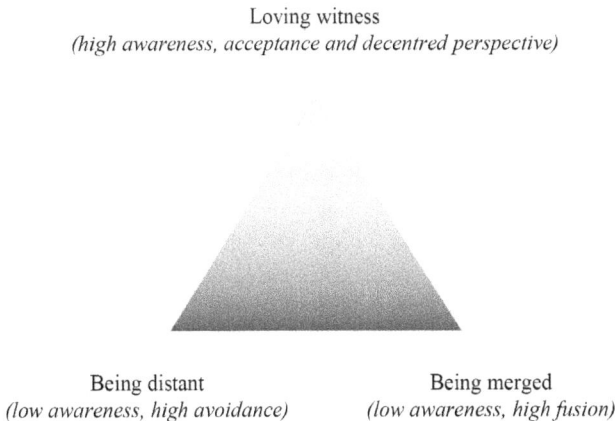

Being distant   Being merged
(low awareness, high avoidance)   *(low awareness, high fusion)*

Figure 3.2 The triangle of relationship to internal experience

different dimensions of the human being, the triangle of experience helps us to assess the client's relationship to their experiences and intervene accordingly.

Figure 3.2 describes three main relationships to internal experience in the form of a triangle. Each relationship is connected to different expressions of mindful processes: present moment awareness, acceptance, and decentred perspective. Being *merged* with our experience and being *distant* are bipolar opposites. The right side of the continuum describes merging with our experience, while the left side describes avoidance of our experience. Both poles of the continuum are characterised by low present-centred awareness and manifest in lack of contact. When being distant, we are not aware of certain aspects of our experience that we are avoiding. Being merged with our experience is also connected with low awareness, as in this state we are not aware of other stimuli beyond the contents that we are merged with. The upper point of the triangle is related to high present moment awareness, acceptance, and decentred perspective. This relationship to internal experience is described as being a *loving witness* to our experience and is characteristic of the observing self and related to mindful awareness. In the following sections, we will describe these three relationships to experience in more detail.

Being merged with the experience

When we are merged with our experience, we are so identified with it that we cannot make space between ourselves and the experience. We *are* our experience and this creates difficulty with decentring from the contents of our awareness. S. C. Hayes et al. (2012) describe this state as fusion. It could also be described in terms of low awareness of the present moment, as awareness is fixed on some specific content of awareness. When we are merged with our experience, we have difficulty perceiving any other present experiences except the content we are merged with.

We think that many disorders described by DSM-V could be described in these terms of merging with the contents of awareness. This merging could be either with thoughts, emotions, or body sensations. For example, clients with post-traumatic stress disorder may be completely overwhelmed by their emotional experiences such as fear or terror and related painful physical sensations. Another example is with clients experiencing depression, who may be completely identified with the belief that they are not worthy of living, and it would be better if they die. In cases of obsessive-compulsive disorder, clients overidentify with intrusive thoughts, which they react to, even if they are logically not reasonable. While these may be extreme cases of merging with the experience, all of us in our everyday life often experience fusion with our beliefs, emotions, and physical sensation. Merging can be found on the continuum from the decentred perspective of mindful awareness to extreme cases of merging, which can be the main characteristics of psychopathological states.

Being distanced from the experience

When we are being distanced from internal experience, we are not aware of our thoughts, emotions, and sensations (Žvelc et al., 2011). Clients may, for example, say that they are numb and do not feel anything, or that they do not have any memories from their childhood or the previous session. Besides non-awareness, this mode is also connected to the process of avoidance of internal experience. The process of avoidance is an essential part of different defence mechanisms as described by psychoanalytic theory (McWilliams, 2011). For example, the defence mechanism of repression is one of the major defence mechanisms, which results in non-awareness of different contents of our awareness. At the lower end of the left side of the continuum (see Figure 3.2), we find the defence of dissociation, which results in avoidance not only of particular contents of awareness but of entire self-states. While repression involves active defence and deals with unpleasant experiences, dissociation is an automatic response to an unbearable traumatic experience (Howell, 2011).

The triangle of experience describes the continuum of distance, from full contact with experience (characterised by witnessing) to extreme distance characterised by dissociation. If being distant from experience becomes chronic, this may be part of different problems that clients come to therapy with. Clients with a schizoid personality disorder or dissociative disorders may experience extreme distance from the internal experience.

Being distanced from internal experience is also part of our everyday human experience. We are often not fully present with our experience, especially with experiences that are difficult to bear. When we experience difficult or painful emotions, thoughts or body sensation, we may tend to push them out of awareness with different defence mechanisms. We may also use different strategies to run from our experience, such as overeating, overworking, and in extreme cases also self-destructive behaviour such as cutting.

Being a loving witness to our experience

This relationship to internal experience is a characteristic of the observing self and related to mindful awareness. It can be described as a way of being with our experience with present moment awareness, acceptance, and decentred perspective. This helps us to be with our experience without identifying with it. A person can fully feel their body sensations and emotions and at the same time witness them. Being a loving witness to our experience could be described as full contact with our experience, where there is a clear differentiation between the observing self and the content of experience. A person can observe their thoughts, emotions, physical sensations, and behaviour as they occur from moment-to-moment without avoiding them or becoming merged with them. In this type of relationship, we are present with our experience with love and acceptance. The loving witness is not detached as a cold observer, which may be connected to the "being distanced" mode. The loving witness is "loving" in the sense of embracing experiences and accepting them unconditionally, whether they are pleasant or unpleasant.

The triangle of relationship to internal experience is a useful model when working with our clients. We can track from moment-to-moment how clients relate to their experience. The main dimensions of the triangle should be understood on a continuum and not as either/or experiences. Sometimes clients are moving towards one end of the triangle, and in another moment, they can be more on another end. Although sometimes clients are chronically more on one side of the triangle, even in that situation we can observe small changes and movements to other sides.

Being witness to our experience is a crucial mechanism of change in MCIP. We invite our clients to become a loving witness to their experience. We invite them to become mindful of their experience with the help of the main mindfulness processes: awareness of the present moment, acceptance and decentred perspective. These processes are used moment by moment. When clients are merged with their experience, decentring from their experience will be the primary process of change. We may also encourage the process of present moment awareness and invite clients to become aware of broader stimuli in the present moment and not just the contents they are merged with. We may, for example, be working with a woman client, who is merged with the thought "I will die of anxiety". Decentred perspective will help her to distance herself from her thought and observe it with curiosity and acceptance. The process of present moment awareness will also help her to develop a wider field of awareness and to become aware that there are also other contents of awareness present (for example the warm look of the therapist, calm sensations in her feet, or the thought "there is still hope for me").

When the client is moving towards the "being distanced" pole of experience, our general strategy is to increase the process of acceptance and present moment awareness. For example, client Peter was avoiding his experiences of sadness following the breakup with his girlfriend. He was telling his story without any emotional tone and was trying to find different reasons and excuses for a problematic relationship. He was moving towards the pole of distance regarding his own experience. The therapist gently invited him back into the present moment: "*You talked about the breakup with your girlfriend. Gently notice, what are you feeling in your body right now.*" Such interventions helped him to become fully present with his sadness and to complete the mourning process related to the loss of his girlfriend.

The clinical use of the diamond model of the observing self and the triangle of relationship to experience are described in detail in Part III of the book.

Notes

1 From *Beyond empathy: A therapy of contact-in-relationship* (p. 5), by R. G. Erskine, J. P. Moursund, and R. L. Trautmann, 1999, Brunner/Mazel. Copyright 1999 by Taylor & Francis. Reprinted with permission of the publisher (Taylor & Francis Ltd, www.tandfonline.com).
2 From "Mechanisms of mindfulness," by S. L. Shapiro, L. E. Carlson, J. A. Astin, and B. Freedman, 2006, *Journal of Clinical Psychology*, *62*(3), p. 377 (https://doi.org/10.1002/jclp.20237). Copyright © 2006 by Wiley Periodicals, Inc. Reprinted with permission.
3 From "Self-Compassion: An alternative conceptualization of a healthy attitude toward oneself," by K. Neff, 2003, *Self and Identity*, 2, p. 87 (https://doi.org/10.1080/15298860390129863). Copyright 2003 by Taylor & Francis. Reprinted with permission of the publisher (Taylor & Francis Ltd, www.tandfonline.com).

4 Integrative psychotherapy as relational psychotherapy

Integrative psychotherapy is a relational form of psychotherapy (Erskine et al., 1999; Erskine, 2015; Moursund & Erskine, 2004). The client and the therapist are viewed as a system of mutual influence. They influence each other on both conscious and unconscious levels and create a system of reciprocal influence – the *intersubjective field* (Stolorow, 1994). We view all phenomena that occur in psychotherapy from the perspective of this co-creation and mutual influence. We pay attention to the client's intrapsychic world, the therapeutic relationship, and the therapist's subjective experience.

There are two different modes of working with clients within the intersubjective field: "1. the intrapsychic mode (internal relationship of the client with himself); and 2. the relationship mode (the relationship between client and therapist)" (G. Žvelc, 2014, p. 168). Both modes are essential, and the focus is sometimes more on intrapsychic relating and sometimes more on the relationship between the client and the therapist. In MCIP, mindfulness and compassion are crucial in both modes of relating.

In the *relationship mode*, the main emphasis is on the client–therapist relationship. The mindful presence and compassion of the therapist is crucial for attunement and developing interpersonal contact. D. J. Siegel (2007) describes this mode as an interpersonal attunement. In the *intrapsychic mode*, the focus is on the relationship between the observing self of the client and their inner world. We invite clients to connect with the observing self, which helps them to bring mindful awareness and compassion towards their inner world. The goal is the development of a client's new way of relating to self, which is based on self-compassion and mindful awareness. This new internal relationship is in stark contrast to the internal criticism or self-judgment that many people experience. D. J. Siegel (2007) describes such an internal relationship as intrapersonal attunement. It results in increased internal contact (Erskine, 2015; Erskine & Moursund, 1988). In this mode there is less emphasis on the relationship between the client and the therapist although it remains essential for the client. The therapist provides an atmosphere of safety, compassion, and presence, while the client relates to their inner world.

In both modes of relating the therapist is aware of the co-creation of relationship and pays attention to their client's experience, their own personal experience, and the intersubjective field. Mindfulness in a relationship can be described as "relational mindfulness" (Falb & Pargament, 2012; Surrey, 2005). Surrey (2005) states that in a relational approach to mindfulness, the therapist maintains a tripartite awareness of self, the other person, and the flow of the relationship. In MCIP, therapists from moment-to-moment mindfully track their changes in thoughts, emotions, and body sensations. They are almost simultaneously aware also of the client's experience and the quality of the intersubjective field, which is from moment-to-moment co-created by both the client and the therapist.

The process that flows between the intrapsychic and relational aspects of therapeutic work is interdependent and circular (Žvelc & Žvelc, 2011). When clients feel safe, accepted, and have trust in the therapist, they can risk the next step in the exploration of their inner world. Experiencing the mindful presence and compassion of the therapist helps them to bring mindfulness and compassion to their own inner experience. The experience of a safe therapeutic relationship also helps clients to verbalise and communicate their experience to the therapist. However, if the therapeutic relationship is not perceived as safe and trusting, clients will have difficulty in exploring their inner world.

The dynamic of the psychotherapeutic relationship is also dependent on the therapist's intrapsychic relationship and their ability for internal contact. The therapist's mindful awareness of their inner experience and self-compassion will manifest in both nonverbal reactions and the quality of interventions and will have an impact on the client. As the client and the therapist form an intersubjective system, the client–therapist relationship will also influence the therapist's internal contact and their interventions.

In integrative psychotherapy we monitor the quality of the therapeutic relationship and therapeutic alliance throughout the psychotherapy process. In the event of ruptures of the alliance, it is important to focus on the psychotherapy relationship and initiate the repair of the alliance (Eubanks et al., 2018; Safran & Muran, 2000; M. Žvelc, 2008). Maintaining and repairing the working alliance are seen as a continual process in psychotherapy and not a one-off event.

Developmental theories in integrative psychotherapy

Integrative psychotherapy is based on the fundamental philosophical assumption that people are relational beings that exist within a matrix of relationships. Evans and Gilbert (2005) describe this assumption with the proposition: "You are therefore I am" (p. 15). Contact with others is the primary motivation of human beings, and disruption or the lack of interpersonal contact may be related to the development of different psychological disturbances, both in childhood as well as later in life (Erskine, 1997; Erskine et al., 1999).

Integrative psychotherapy is informed by relational developmental theories that describe the development of a child's personality through relationships with significant others (Erskine, 2019a, 2019b). Object relations theory, self-psychology, and other developmental theories, such as attachment theory provide us with an understanding of early child development and possible disruptions in healthy human development (G. Žvelc, 2011; Žvelc & Žvelc, 2006). They help us to understand the client through the eyes of early relationships (M. Žvelc, 2011).

Object relations theory

Object relations theories have described how the structure of the personality is developed through interaction between the child and significant other people – objects (Fairbairn, 1941/1986; Fairbairn, 1943/1986; Guntrip, 1968/1993; Winnicot, 1953/1986, 1960/1986). Personality structure develops through the internalisation of the relationship with significant others. The pioneer of object relations, Fairbairn (1941/1986) wrote that the child's primary need is that parents love him and that parents accept his love. Because the need for relationship is the primary human need, the child will do everything to maintain the relationship – even if the price is a loss of self. Fairbairn (1943/1986) describes how children internalise negative experiences with objects, to maintain the illusion of a good relationship with their caregivers, taking onto themselves the "badness" of the caregivers in order to maintain the relationship with "good" external objects. Because of failures in relationship, the child's ego becomes fragmented into different self-object units which results in the development of various psychopathologies (Fairbairn, 1943/1986).

Object relations theorists have further described important insights into the nature of early relationships and their representation in the internal world. Winnicot (1960/1986), for example, has described the importance of the *good-enough* mother for the child's adequate development of self. Because of inadequate relational experiences, the child may develop a split between their *true* and *false* self. The child may start to submit to parental demands and expectations and may lose contact with their true self.

Self-psychology

Self-psychology developed by Heinz Kohut focuses on the importance of relationships for maintaining a cohesive self (Kohut, 1977). Children need the optimal empathic environment for the satisfaction of basic psychological needs. There are three primary self-object needs of the child: the need for merging, the need for idealisation and the need for twinship (Kohut, 1984). Adequate parental attunement to these needs is crucial for the development of the child's cohesive self.

Attachment theory

Integrative psychotherapy is also based on attachment theory. The child's need for attachment is the basic human need which motivates the infant to seek proximity with caregivers (Bowlby, 1969). The need for attachment is evolutionary-based and is crucial for the survival and protection of the child from danger. Ainsworth et al. (1978) have described how the child forms different patterns of attachment to the primary caregiver. They describe secure attachment and two insecure attachment types (avoidant and anxious-ambivalent). Children with secure attachment feel that they can rely on their parents for meeting their emotional needs. They experience their parents as a secure base from which they can explore the world and return for safety when they are feeling distressed. Children with avoidant attachment avoid emotional contact with their parents and deny their attachment needs, while children with anxious-ambivalent attachment show a pattern of preoccupation and ambivalence towards their parents. Main and Solomon (1990) have also described disorganised attachment, which arises in children who lived with parents who were highly unpredictable and is related to a disorganised pattern of behaviour towards the primary caregiver. These attachment patterns have been confirmed in numerous researches and provide the scientific basis for the understanding of relational processes in integrative psychotherapy.

Research shows that early attachment between the child and the parent is crucial for the development of the brain (Cozolino, 2002; Schore, 1994, 2001; D. J. Siegel, 1999). Schore (1994, 2001, 2003) describes the importance of affect regulation and attunement in the early relationship for the development of secure attachment and optimal brain development. An adequately attuned mother regulates the child's autonomic nervous system and modulates states of non-optimal high or low arousal. Attunement and regulation are crucial for a sense of connection, safety, and development of secure attachment. They enable the child to develop the capacity for self-regulation and internal contact. Secure attachment manifests in positive working models of self and others. Children with secure attachment feel that they are worthy of love and that they can rely on other people for safety and comfort. Secure attachment is related to numerous health benefits, such as greater resilience (Rasmussen et al., 2019). Secure attachment is also related to the ability of mentalisation and affect regulation (Fonagy et al., 2004). The lack of interpersonal contact, chronic misattunement, or abuse, negatively impact on the development of the brain and lead to insecure or disorganised attachment patterns (Schore, 2001, 2003).

Attachment research shows that attachment is a life-long process and that there exists a relative continuity of attachment patterns throughout our life (Wallin, 2007). Research shows that attachment patterns are transmitted across generations (Benoit & Parker, 1994; Cassibba et al., 2017; Fonagy et al., 1991; Hautamäki et al., 2010). Cassibba et al. (2017) have for example found empirical support for attachment transmission from grandmother to mother to adult offspring. However, attachment patterns can be changed during life (Chopik et al., 2019). A new trusting and accepting relationship with the therapist can lead to the development of secure attachment (Wallin, 2007). This is congruent with research that shows an increase in attachment security after psychotherapy (Strauß et al., 2018; Taylor et al., 2015).

The integrative model of interpersonal relationships

Based on object relations theory, self-psychology and attachment theory, G. Žvelc (2010a, 2011) developed the integrative model of interpersonal relationships. This model describes three basic bipolar dimensions of interpersonal relationships, which refer to three main developmental lines: (1) Autonomy – Dependence, (2) Connectedness – Alienation, and (3) Mutuality – Self-absorption (G. Žvelc, 2011).

Autonomy – Dependence refers to the process of separation and individuation, moving from complete dependence to the development of independence and autonomy. Individuals who have developed autonomy can differentiate between self and others and have developed the capacity for being alone. Dependence, on the other hand, manifests in symbiotic relationships, dependency, and increased separation anxiety. This developmental process has been described by a number of different object relations theorists (Fairbairn, 1941/1986; Fairbairn, 1943/1986; Kernberg, 1976; Mahler et al., 1975; Winnicot, 1960/1986).

The dimension Connectedness – Alienation describes the individual's ability to connect and be close to others. It can manifest either in intimate and close relationships or at the other pole of the continuum in feelings of alienation and isolation from others. This dimension describes the developmental process related to the development of intimate attachment to other people (Bowlby, 1969; Stern, 1998/2018).

The third dimension, Mutuality – Self-absorption, describes the individual's capacity for mutuality in relationships. It describes the developmental task of intersubjectivity, which is crucial for empathy and reciprocity in relationships (Aron, 1996, 2000; Benjamin, 1995; Stern, 2004). Individuals with high mutuality can establish reciprocal relationships in which another person is seen as a subject with their own desires and interests. At the other pole of this dimension we find individuals with high self-absorption manifesting in grandiosity, omnipotence, and egocentric relationships.

G. Žvelc (2010a, 2011) describes two main types of relationships, which are related to these interpersonal dimensions: subject and object relationships. In the *subject relationship*, the individual experiences other people as subjects with their own internal world. They are capable of recognising and acknowledging the subjectivity of another person and able to establish mutual relationships based on respect and reciprocity. The subject relationship is related to the healthy poles of the main dimensions of interpersonal relationships: autonomy, connectedness, and mutuality. Subject relationships are congruent with Martin Buber's (Buber, 1999) description of the I–Thou relationship, which involves mutuality, contact, and seeing the other person without preconceptions. At the other end of the continuum, we find the *object relationship*, which describes a relationship in which other people are viewed as objects for the satisfaction of the first person's needs. Other people are not seen as separate but as an extension of self. There is no reciprocity, and another person is seen only according to whether they can satisfy the first person's needs. Object relationships are related to the negative poles of the main dimensions of interpersonal relationships: dependence, alienation, and self-absorption. They are congruent with Buber's description of the I–It relationship, which is characterised by a lack of reciprocity and relating to another person as the object (Buber, 1999).

While healthy relationships involve a balance between the object and subject relationships, problems in relationships are related to the inability to establish subject relationships. Such individuals relate to other people as objects and have difficulties in forming intimate, reciprocal, and autonomous relationships. The subject relationship is, on another hand, crucial for genuine interpersonal contact. In such a relationship, we can "mutually recognize each other and can be intimately connected and autonomous at the same time" (G. Žvelc, 2010a, p. 501).

Subject relationships are related to the development of intersubjectivity, which is a developmental stage characterised by the capacity to recognise the other person as a separate centre of subjectivity with whom an individual can share their subjective experience (Stern, 1998/2018). Benjamin (1995) similarly proposes that developing the ability to recognise the mother as a separate subject with her own subjective world is the fundamental developmental achievement.

This integrative model provides a non-pathological understanding of different relationship difficulties. Instead of seeing the client, for example, as "narcissistic", we may understand the client's struggles with an increased dimension of self-absorption and alienation. The model also has an important implication for understanding the attachment patterns in psychotherapy (G. Žvelc, 2010b). Rather than seeing the attachment patterns as distinct and fixed types, we see them on a continuum ranging from "normal" expression to problematic. Secure attachment is found in the "healthy" poles of these interpersonal dimensions and is related to the capacity for autonomy, connection, and mutuality (G. Žvelc, 2010b). Insecure attachment, on the other hand, is related to the "unhealthy" poles of these dimensions. Avoidant attachment manifests in increased alienation, whereas preoccupied attachment is found in increased dependency (G. Žvelc, 2010b). Our thinking is congruent with Erskine (2009), who also described a dimensional approach to understanding attachment. He proposed that attachment issues could be understood on the continuum between attachment style, attachment pattern, and attachment disorder.

Developing the capacity for subject relationships

In our approach to integrative psychotherapy, the integrative model of interpersonal relationships is the basis for understanding relational processes. The three main relational dimensions can be understood as personality traits. We each have our own general expression of these dimensions, which manifest most of our life, and as therapists, we can understand each client based on them. For example, with a client who may be showing increased alienation and self-absorption in their life, the goal would be the development of a sense of connectedness and mutuality. The three primary dimensions can also be viewed as processes. At any given moment, we may experience a different movement towards the other pole of a continuum, with altered contexts and changing relationships causing us to express different poles of a dimension. In a relationship, we may in some moments feel a sense of deep connection; whereas, after an interpersonal conflict, we may become withdrawn and alienated from the other person. This similarly occurs in a psychotherapeutic relationship. For example, the client Martin, was very withdrawn during most conversations, but when the therapist asked him about his music career, he opened up and started to look the therapist in the eyes. The therapist had an immediate experience of aliveness and connection.

These relational processes are co-created in the psychotherapy relationship. All three dimensions can be viewed as a property of the relational field between the therapist and the client. For example, when the client is moving towards the pole of dependency, we may ask ourselves, "where am I on this continuum?" The answer may show that we are both creating this "sense of dependency" in the therapy room. The therapist, for instance, may be fearing that the client is going to end the therapy, and this may cause the client to appear more dependent. The client's fears of separation may, in turn, influence the therapist into discouraging the client from autonomy. So rather than seeing these dimensions only in the client, we are attentive to the emerging relatedness between the therapist and the client.

Some clients may have difficulties in establishing subject relationships, manifesting extreme expressions of the negative poles of these relational dimensions. For example, the client Andrea displayed an extreme expression of the dependence dimension. She could not tolerate being alone and experienced extreme anxiety when she was separated even for only brief moments from her partner. Another client, Steve, manifested an extreme expression of self-absorption. He was very egocentric in his relationships, "using" other people for his own personal benefit, and was incapable of feeling empathy for other people. Developing the capacity for subject relationships may be for such clients an important goal in psychotherapy. The new relational experiences with the therapist, mindful awareness, compassion, and mentalisation are the main processes of change that promote the development of subject relationships.

The relationship with the therapist is the main area in which clients encounter new relational experiences that encourage them towards subject relationships. In this process, the therapist's capacity for subject relationship is crucial. The therapist needs to embody qualities of connectedness, autonomy, and mutuality, differentiating between self and the client. The therapist must be open to connecting with and relating to the client as a person with their individual subjectivity. We think that this relational stance of the therapist is the basis for the client's development of subject relations. As the child develops through a relationship with a significant other, so the client may move towards subject relations with the help of a new relationship with the therapist.

Attunement to relational needs

Inquiry, attunement, and involvement are the main relational methods of integrative psychotherapy (Erskine et al., 1999). They are crucial for the development of the therapeutic relationship that may gradually help the client to develop a sense of connection, autonomy, and mutuality. The therapist in integrative psychotherapy is attuned, present, and involved in the relationship, being attentive to different relational needs that emerge in the relationship with the client. Erskine et al. (1999) have described eight primary relational needs that manifest in the psychotherapy relationship and also in everyday life: (1) Security, (2) Valuing, (3) Acceptance by a stable, strong, and protective other person, (4) Mutuality, (5) Self-definition, (6) Making an impact, (7) Having the other initiate, and (8) Need to express love. These needs are not only the needs of childhood but are important throughout our whole life and they can only be satisfied in a responsive human relationship. Lack of satisfaction of relational needs may result in loneliness and may gradually lead to loss of hope, anger, and depression (Erskine, 2015).

Žvelc et al. (2020) have empirically validated the construct of relational needs with the help of factor analysis. In their research, they found that Erskine's (2015) descriptions of relational needs are empirically related to five main dimensions of relational needs: (1) The need for authenticity, (2) Support and protection, (3) Having an impact, (4) Shared experience, and (5) The initiative from others.

The *need for authenticity* refers to the need for being oneself (authentic) in relationship with others. Satisfying this need is experienced when being with others as we truly are (Žvelc et al., 2020). The *need for support and protection* is related to Erskine's (2015) need for acceptance by a stable, dependable, and protective other person. When this need is met, the person feels that they can rely on a stable, strong, and dependable other person. The *need to have an impact* is the need to influence another person so that the other person is affected in some desired way (Erskine, 2015). The *need for shared experience* is the need to be in the "presence of someone who is similar, who understands because he or she has had a like experience, and whose shared experience is confirming" (Erskine, 2015, p. 50). The *need for the initiative from others* is the need for other people to initiate an exchange and make contact (Erskine et al., 1999).

The therapist attunes to these needs in the psychotherapeutic relationship and adopts a relational style congruent with the emerging relational needs of the client (Moursund & Erskine, 2004; Erskine, 2015). For example, when the client's main need is for shared experience, the therapist may selectively share with the client a particular aspect of their experience. If the main need is for a stable and dependable other person, the therapist may provide the experience of stability and strength. The self-disclosing of personal experience may not be an optimal intervention in this case. However, Žvelc et al. (2020) describe that in psychotherapy, we cannot satisfy the client's archaic relational needs; the psychotherapist may "validate and normalize these needs, which may initiate a grieving process for the unsatisfied relational needs of the past" (p. 3).

Žvelc et al. (2020) have developed the "Relational needs satisfaction scale (RNSS)", which measures the satisfaction of five main relational needs and can be used for the assessment of the client's relational needs and evaluation of psychotherapy from the perspective of relational functioning. The scale has satisfactory reliability and adequate construct and convergent validity (Žvelc et al., 2020). Research shows that higher satisfaction of relational needs is related to secure attachment, self-compassion, greater well-being and better overall satisfaction with life (Žvelc et al., 2020). RNSS is translated into several languages. The factor structure of the scale has also been confirmed in a Czech sample (Pourová et al., 2020).

As therapists we are only human, and cannot expect to be perfectly attuned, and indeed this is not our task. As the mother is only a good enough mother (Winnicot, 1960/1986), so also the therapist is only a good enough therapist. This means that the therapist will inevitably make mistakes and will occasionally be non-attuned or mis-attuned to the client (Guistolise, 1996; M. Žvelc, 2008). Although mistakes may lead to ruptures in the therapeutic alliance (Safran & Muran, 2000; M. Žvelc, 2008), if the therapist is actively engaged with ruptures in the relationship, they may become fertile ground for making changes in the psychotherapy. In MCIP, the therapist from moment-to-moment mindfully tracks the quality of the relationship. If ruptures in the relationship occur, then the therapist may engage in a rupture resolution process (Safran & Muran, 2000) through the use of *metacommunication*, which involves communicating about what is implicitly happening between the client and the therapist. It is an "attempt to bring ongoing awareness to the emergent patient–therapist interactive process" (Safran & Kraus, 2014, p. 382). Safran and Muran (2000) describe it as *mindfulness in action* as the therapist invites the client to collaboratively explore what is happening at the present moment in the relationship. Working with ruptures can invite the client to see the therapist as a subject – with their own desires, virtues, and mistakes. If a repair is possible in the relationship, this may lead to an increasing recognition of another person having their own mind. The client may also experience how differences and conflict can be tolerated and eventually resolved. In this way the client gets a new model of how differences and connection can coexist, which is the basis of mutual subject relationships.

Moments of meeting and subject–subject relations

Stern (2004) has described how in psychotherapy *moments of meeting* may occur that are crucial for change. These moments can be described as *subject–subject* relating between the client and therapist. In *subject–subject* relations, both client and therapist experience a deep sense of mutual connection, which involves recognition of each other as a separate subject. These are moments of authentic contact between two persons and may be one of the crucial processes of change.

Buber (1999) described such moments as the I–Thou relationship, which involves mutuality and seeing the other person without preconception. In such moments of real meeting, both therapist and client can be changed by the other (Evans & Gilbert, 2005; M. Gilbert & Orlans, 2011). Such moments cannot be planned and appear spontaneously when both participants are open and authentic. Evans and Gilbert (2005) describe that "such human contact at its most poignant moment can be a meeting of souls" (p. 131).

M. Gilbert and Orlans (2011) describe how it is important that the therapist maintains the I–Thou relational stance, even if the client is not yet ready for an authentic encounter. As Evans and Gilbert (2005) have described, the process of therapy may move through different phases, from an I–It relationship to I–It/I–

Thou before moving eventually to the I–Thou relationship. The development of subject relations is for some clients a gradual process of change, from relating to the therapist as an object, to gradually seeing the therapist as a subject. The developmental process between client and therapist mirrors the developmental process that occurs in early relationships. The child first relates to a significant other person as an object before later in the course of development, coming to view the significant other person as a subject (Benjamin, 1995). Some clients never had a good enough object relationship and did not safely attach to the parent. For such clients, the first goal may be the establishment of a good enough object relationship with the therapist before being able to recognise the therapist as a subject.

Shared conscious presence and transcendent relational field

Contact with the observing self, mindful awareness, and compassion may contribute to the development of the subject–subject relationship and moments of meeting. When both the client and the therapist are in contact with the observing/transcendent self and embody mindful presence, this may manifest in a new quality in their relationship. The client and therapist may recognise each other beyond the personal self and may experience the state of *shared conscious presence*. They may experience how consciousness itself is what we all share (S. C. Hayes et al., 2012). Such moments of recognition have a spiritual quality and may manifest in experiences of *nondual awareness*, which is experienced as a sense of interconnection, boundless awareness, and compassion (Josipovic, 2016, 2019). Schuman (2017) similarly describes that at the moment when the client and the therapist are fully present with one another, there may emerge a *transcendent relational field*, which has a quality of transpersonal awareness. In such moments "boundaries between self and other are temporarily relaxed, yielding an interpersonal experience of belonging, connectedness, and deep intimacy unbounded by the sense of separate self" (p. 79). The transcendent relational field is experienced as a "space in which we are connected" (Schuman, 2017, p. 79). It is felt like a shared state of consciousness (Schuman, 2017). We propose that such experiences of oneness and connection are not experiences of merging that are often related to a problematic symbiotic relationship. Such spiritual experiences include the awareness that in terms of a personal self, we are different and separate, but at the level of the observing/transcendent self we are all interconnected and "one". Contact with the observing/transcendent self may enable clients to develop a decentred perspective in relationship to themselves and other people. This process may help them come to understand that although other people have their own subjective worlds it is consciousness itself that we all share. This leap in understanding may help the client to develop a greater sense of connection and compassion to "all sentient beings".

5 Relational mind and intersubjective physiology

As people we sense other human emotions and body states and react to them. This process happens automatically. We can sense someone's emotional and physiological states, even when the other person is not aware of them or does not want to show them. For instance, although someone is not expressing fear or is perhaps repressing it and not feeling it, the other person may still sense some fear within themselves or some stiffness in their body. A baby has a happy expression in their eyes because their mother is happy. If somebody's heartbeat accelerates or cortisol level rises, the other person's heartbeat will also accelerate, and their cortisol levels may also rise. Our physiological states are contagious. We are living together in the same intersubjective physiological field.

We are mutually connected, and we communicate on many levels. Our brains, minds, and bodies are related. This continuous co-creative dialogue with others can be described as the intersubjective matrix (Stern, 2004). In addition to verbal and also visible nonverbal communication, there is, underneath, running mostly out of awareness a process of physiological interaction. The autonomic nervous systems of two or more people interact and influence each other (Palumbo et al., 2017; Porges, 2011, 2017).

When you introduce yourself to new people, do you remember their names? People, while they present themselves and shake hands, often cannot recall the name of the person being introduced. Why is that? It is because their mind is at that moment occupied with another task: their autonomic nervous system is scanning to check if the other person represents safety or threat. Porges (2011, 2017) calls this automatic, subconscious process for determining risk or safety in the environment, *neuroception*. It is an interpretative process which "leads to a 'neural' decision" (Porges, 2017, p. 102) as to whether there is a danger or not, mostly through the subconscious "interpretation of facial expressivity, intonation, and gestures" (Porges, 2017, p. 102). This automatic subconscious "scanning of safety" also happens in the therapeutic relationship. The client through the process of neuroception senses the physiological state of the therapist and vice versa.

The fundamental method of integrative psychotherapy is co-creating a therapeutic relationship, in which clients feel safe enough to explore their internal world and integrate the split parts of themselves (Erskine, 2019a; Moursund & Erskine, 2004; Žvelc & Žvelc, 2011; M. Žvelc, 2011). This secure base, which underpins the therapeutic relationship, enables a client "to take the risk of feeling what he is not supposed to feel and knowing what he is not supposed to know" (Wallin, 2007, p. 3). Thus the key question for the therapists is how we, as therapists can help create a good therapeutic relationship. There are a number of different ways in which to create, repair, and maintain an effective therapeutic alliance. The methods of inquiry, attunement, and involvement (Erskine, 2015; Erskine et al., 1999) and metacommunication (Safran & Muran, 2000) can be beneficial. However, they are only useful if the therapist is in their regulated, optimal arousal zone of the autonomic state.

In this chapter, we emphasise the importance of *the interaction of the therapist's and the client's physiologies* and propose that the *therapist's autonomic nervous state profoundly influences the therapeutic work*. For effective psychotherapeutic work, we stress the importance of the therapist's regulated autonomic nervous system (ANS), which allows the therapist to function inside the window of tolerance (D. J. Siegel, 1999). In terms of the polyvagal theory (Porges, 2017), activation of the ventral vagal nervous circuit of the therapist is needed so that they can interact in the therapy with their social engagement system (Dana, 2018).

Polyvagal theory and autonomic states in psychotherapy

The polyvagal theory describes three hierarchical states of the autonomic nervous system (ANS), which reflect activation of the following pathways: "the ventral vagal circuit, supporting social engagement behaviours, the sympathetic nervous system, supporting mobilised defensive (flight/fight) behaviours and the dorsal vagal circuit, supporting immobilised defensive behaviours" (Porges, 2017, p. 7). The social engagement system, mobilised defensive behaviour, and immobilised defensive behaviour correspond to the three different states of activation: the optimal arousal, hyperarousal, and hypoarousal zone (Ogden et al., 2006). The ventral vagal and dorsal vagal circuits are two branches of the parasympathetic nervous system (Porges, 2011, 2017). As in polyvagal theory, we use the terms autonomic states and physiological states interchangeably.

Ventral vagal circuit and social engagement

When we feel safe, the social engagement system is activated through the ventral vagal nervous circuit (Porges, 2011, 2017). We are in the optimal arousal zone (Ogden et al., 2006) and function within the window of tolerance (D. J. Siegel, 1999). The ventral vagal state is the neurobiological foundation for health, growth and restoration (Dana, 2018; Porges, 2011). In this state we can feel calm, grounded, happy, or meditative (Dana, 2018). We can be engaged, active, interested, passionate, and joyful (Dana, 2018). Our heart rate slows, our eyes soften, our voice and our face are soft and kind, and we move to reach out to the other (Dana, 2018; Porges, 2017). Clients and therapists in this state are open to connection and are ready to engage (Dana, 2018). The therapist's ventral vagal state communicates to the client's ANS that it is safe here. This facilitates the psychotherapeutic alliance, the collaborative bond between the therapist and the client (Bordin, 1979). In this state cortical functioning is maintained, and the different processes on cognitive, emotional, and body levels can be integrated (Ogden et al., 2006). Here "hope arises and change happens" (Dana, 2018, p. 27). Dana (2018, p. 26) calls ventral vagus the "compassion" nerve, since it supports compassionate connections and self-compassion.

The activation of ventral vagal state in both the therapist and the client is crucial for psychotherapy work. It supports the therapeutic alliance, connection, mentalisation, awareness, compassion, and integration. The therapist in the ventral vagal state has the potential to influence the client positively, to regulate the client's physiology and offer to the client safety and connection (Dana, 2018; Geller, 2018). Teaching clients to inhibit their defensive system in a safe environment and to activate their defensive system in a risky situation is a crucial goal of therapy. We propose that the ability to activate the ventral vagal state is the biological foundation for a satisfying and fulfilling life as well as for a harmonious society.

Sympathetic nervous system and mobilisation

Mobilisation and immobilisation are defensive states; they are activated when a threat is perceived. In the mobilised state of ANS, the sympathetic nervous system is activated. The sympathetic nervous system enables alertness, energy, and movements. It mobilises energy to prepare the person for the intense muscular action of either fight or flight, to protect or defend (Porges, 2011). The mobilised state is indicated by increased heart rate, fast breathing in the upper chest, dilated pupils, wide eyes, eyelids tense or raised, sweating, and other increased body sensations (Levine, 2018; Porges, 2011; Rothschild, 2017). The client may talk irrepressibly, be restless or very tense and stiff; they may be overwhelmed with fear, rage, or terror. Social engagement is not possible in this state, contact with self and with the therapist is limited. When overwhelmed by this state, we become emotionally flooded, reactive, impulsive, hypervigilant, and our cognitive processes are disorganised (Ogden et al., 2006).

Dorsal vagal circuit and immobilisation

The other defensive system, which is usually activated when mobilisation behaviours are not sufficient, is immobilisation, caused by the dorsal vagus (Porges, 2011, 2017). In this state, shutdown and collapse are experienced, protecting the person from physical and psychological pain (Dana, 2018). In this zone sensations are relatively absent, emotions are numbed, cognitive processing is disabled, and body movements are reduced (Ogden et al., 2006). Clients look frozen as if being not there, even appearing spaced out. They can dissociate. They lack vitality, have a flat or frozen face, are pale, their heart rate is slowed or unstable, switching between fast and slow (Dana, 2018). They may gaze out of the window or into space, have vacant eyes, collapsed posture, and loss of speech (Dana, 2018).

Introspectively, it feels like a sense of being alone, lost, and in despair and unreachable (Dana, 2018). It also manifests in feelings of shame.

In both systems, mobilisation and immobilisation, the ability to accurately read the cues from the environment is affected, and that can lead to faulty neuroception (Porges, 2017). Faulty neuroception means that a person perceives a threat, when there is no danger, or does not recognise a threat, where there is.

Autonomic dysregulation syndrome

The survival reactions induced by mobilisation and immobilisation are designed to be temporary, and turn off when the threat is over. Prolonged ongoing mobilisation or immobilisation can become toxic and affects the individual's health (Dana, 2018; Levine, 1997, 2018). It leads to what is called *autonomic dysregulation syndrome* (Levine, 2018), which is a stress-related disorder of regulation. Autonomic dysregulation syndrome appears in symptoms such as body tension and pain, chronic fatigue, episodes of dizziness, and digestive problems (Levine, 2018). It can be connected, but not exclusively, to certain cardiac arrhythmias, low or high blood pressure, a specific type of asthma, fibromyalgia, and migraines (Levine, 2018). We suggest that empathic distress and burnout could also be listed as symptoms of autonomic dysregulation syndrome. We find the term useful because it is an umbrella concept which covers different physical problems with the same origin – the lack of sufficient autonomic regulation. We agree with Levine (2018) that "opportunity for treatment lies in interventions that re-establish organismic self-regulation" (p. 22). Many of our clients and supervisees have signs of autonomic dysregulation syndrome. For the clients, and for the therapist as well, it is crucial that they learn to be aware of their autonomic states and recognise when regulation is needed and learn to apply fundamental strategies for self-care.

Coupling of the autonomic states

The sympathetic nervous system and dorsal vagal circuit can be coupled with the activation of the ventral vagal circuit and social engagement system (Porges, 2017). In this case, we can go to mobilisation or immobilisation behaviour without defence, still feeling safe. The coupling of the social engagement system with the sympathetic nervous system enables us to engage in stimulative activities. It is observed in play, performance, sports, and problem-solving tasks (Dana, 2018; Ogden, 2018; Porges, 2017). The coupling of the social engagement system with the dorsal vagal circuit enables us to enjoy low-arousal activities. It is observed during intimacy, deep relaxation, and safe stillness (Dana, 2018; Ogden, 2018; Porges, 2017).

This potential for coupling autonomic states means there are different ANS arousal states with different qualities. Arousal of the sympathetic branch, as well as dorsal vagal activation, do not necessarily reflect the threat; they can have many faces. Rothschild (2017) for example presents six degrees of ANS arousal. The possibility of coupling the sympathetic and dorsal vagal activation with activation of the ventral vagal circuit has significant meaning in therapy. It suggests that we may proceed with the therapy when the client's sympathetic system is aroused but coupled with the ventral vagal activation, which enables social engagement and connection with the therapist. For example, we may encourage our client to express anger towards their father in the therapy. The client's ANS mobilises. At the same time, they feel safe in the therapeutic relationship (feeling that the therapist understands and supports them); and so their social engagement system is also active, and the client is open to connection with the therapist. In this case, the therapy is useful. We may compare this coupling of the activation of autonomic states with what is termed "dual awareness", which is crucial for processing trauma (F. Shapiro, 2018).

The importance of the therapist's autonomic states

At the root of most problems there are emotional problems, and concomitant with that, impairment in self-regulation. At the beginning of therapy clients often have a narrow window of tolerance and they can quickly become dysregulated. In the course of therapy we work on widening this window of tolerance by helping clients to activate their social engagement system. We help them to recognise when they are approaching dysregulated states, then we co-regulate them and finally help our clients to regulate them for themselves. To be able to do this, we as therapists have to offer the clients our balanced, ventral vagal presence (Dana, 2018; Geller & Porges, 2014). If the therapist is in the ventral vagal autonomic state, they may have a "positive" influence on the client's ANS. The therapist, whose physiological state is inside the window of tolerance, conveys safety to the client and helps to regulate the client's autonomic states. This leads to a safe therapeutic relationship that enables effective psychotherapy. For the therapist to be able to maintain or return to a regulated, ventral vagal autonomic state, we propose an essential strategy: *continuous mindful awareness of one's own physiological states during the session.* This is congruent with research findings showing that mindfulness and interoceptive awareness promotes self-regulation (Farb et al., 2012; Goldin & Gross, 2010; A. M. Hayes & Feldman, 2004; Price & Hooven, 2018; Taren, et al. 2013; Teper et al., 2013; Vago & Silbersweig, 2012).

Intersubjective physiology research: Measuring physiological synchrony

Interaction between the physiological systems of two or more people is a significant mechanism which is indicative of our implicit connectedness. Sensing the heartbeat of another person is not just a poetic metaphor, it is a scientifically proved process, called *physiological synchrony.*

Physiological synchrony is a process that occurs when "physiological activity between two or more people is associated or interdependent" (Palumbo et al., 2017, p. 1). Palumbo et al. (2017) carried out a systematic review of 61 research articles on physiological synchrony (PS) where different measurements of PS had been used: cardiovascular (heart rate, heart rate variability), respiratory (respiratory rate, respiration volume time), or skin measurement (skin conductance, skin temperature) (Palumbo et al., 2017). Their review shows that "social processes also operate at the physiological level" (Palumbo et al., 2017, p. 29). Research proves the existence of PS within the mother–child dyad, family triads, couples, team members, as well as the client–therapist relationship and others. For example, this is seen in the synchronisation of the heartbeat and breathing of a mother and her child and in the skin conductance response of the therapist in association with the client. Research also informs us about the connection between people's hormonal levels. For instance, the cortisol levels among partners correlate positively (Saxbe & Repetti, 2010), as well as the cortisol levels of fathers, mothers, and their adolescent children (Saxbe et al., 2014). There is some evidence that PS is higher between people who are more psychologically close to each other, but there are some findings where PS is also found among strangers (Palumbo et al. 2017). Some studies suggest that PS is most noticeable during active interactions (Suveg et al., 2016).

There are two different processes of physiological synchrony. For *morphostatic synchrony* "behavioural interactions tend to upregulate and downregulate physiology to promote regulation" (Helm, et al., 2014, p. 523). This usually occurs when persons are within the range from mildly negative affective states to fairly positive. This process is also called co-regulation. In contrast, *morphogenic synchrony*, which happens mostly in moments of high stress or risk situations, "upregulates or downregulates physiology and leads to dysregulation" (Helm et al., 2014, p. 523). For example, if two partners are yelling and shouting at each other this affects them both physiologically and they both get more and more upset. Morphostatic physiological synchrony between mothers and children or partners is associated with higher relationship satisfaction (Helm et al., 2014; Suveg et al., 2016), whereas morphogenic synchrony is connected to conflict and negative interactions (Levenson & Gottman, 1983; Saxbe & Repetti, 2010; Suveg et al., 2016).

A systematic review of physiological synchrony research shows that there is often someone in the interaction who "leads" the physiology of the other, resulting in the other person synchronising to the physiology of the leader (Palumbo et al., 2017). Within dyads of mother and infant, for instance, it is the mother who has the role of the leader with the child following the mother's physiological patterns. If the mother's physiology is calm and regulated, the mother calms and regulates the baby, and this is a prerequisite for secure attachment. If the mother's autonomic state is dysregulated, this negatively affects the child's physiology and mental health (Gerhardt, 2004; Schore, 1994; Van Den Bergh et al., 2008; Weinstock, 2005). Psychotherapy research has confirmed the existence of physiological synchrony between therapists and clients, both in individual as well as in couple therapy (Bar-Kalifa et al., 2019; Karvonen et al., 2016; Päivinen et al., 2016; Palmieri et al., 2018; Tschacher & Meier, 2019). Physiological synchrony in therapy was assessed by measuring heart rate, heart rate variability, electrodermal activity, skin conductance, or respiration. The research confirms the connection between PS and a good therapeutic alliance (Bar-Kalifa et al., 2019; Tschacher &

Meier, 2019) and empathy (Marci & Orr, 2006; Marci et al., 2007; Messina et al., 2013; Robinson et al., 1982). Tschacher and Meier (2019) found that clients rated progress in the therapy as higher in the sessions where the "client's heart rate acceleration met therapist's heart rate deceleration" (p. 13). This can be interpreted as the therapist down-regulating the client's physiology. Palmieri et al. (2018) found that therapists in the experimental situation in which they felt secure were more likely to take the lead role in physiological synchrony.

Emotional contagion and mimicry

The processes of physiological synchrony are probably connected to emotional resonance (D. J. Siegel, 2007) and emotional contagion (Hatfield et al., 2014). The primary mechanism underlying emotional contagion is mimicry, the "unconscious or automatic imitation of speech and movements, gestures, facial expressions and eye gaze" (Prochazkova & Kret, 2017, p. 99). The existence of mimicry between people is scientifically proven (Prochazkova & Kret, 2017). The ability to feel the emotions of another involves our sensory and motor neural pathways. Someone may observe the muscle movements of another person, including micro-movements. Through the process of automatic mimicry, they perform the same movements and through sensing this, there is emotional resonance. Findings suggest that "people are generally not consciously aware of subtle changes in a partner's facial characteristics and do not voluntarily react to them" (Prochazkova & Kret, 2017, p. 103). One piece of research interestingly shows that partners can track moment-to-moment changes in their partners' faces and respond with congruent facial expressions, even when these changes cannot be noticed by the eye (Dimberg et al., 2000). Through the process of evolution we are wired to imitate others, sense them, and through that understand the other's mind (P. F. Ferrari & Gallese, 2007; Iacoboni, 2009). This enables empathy, connection, and compassion (Iacoboni, 2009) as well as the ability to predict another's intentions, which is crucial for self-protection. The neurobiological mechanism, which may explain these phenomena of intersubjectivity, is the functioning of mirror neurons (P. F. Ferrari & Galesse, 2007; Stern, 2004).

Mirror neurons and intersubjectivity

According to P. F. Ferrari and Gallese (2007), mirror neurons and other mirror-related mechanisms constitute the neural basis of embodied simulation, the core mechanism of intersubjectivity. Di Pellegrino et al. (1992) while studying the premotor cortex in monkeys, unintentionally discovered that some premotor neuron activation, when for instance the monkey observed the movement of the experimenter taking food from a box, coincided with the neuron activation when the monkey did that same movement. Later on, these neurons, which discharge in both situations, when the monkey does the action and when it observes another individual doing a similar action, came to be called mirror neurons (Rizzolatti et al., 1999).

Our mirror neuron system perceives the states of others and alters our emotional and body states "to match those we are seeing in the other person" (D. J. Siegel, 2007, p. 167). For example, this means that similar neurons will fire when a person cries or when she sees or hears another person crying or even when she perceives someone else who is about to cry. Mirror neurons enable the perceiving and inferring of the intentions of others which is crucial for "mind-reading" (P. F. Ferrari & Gallese, 2007). However, inferring the intentions of others is not direct knowledge of what others feel or will do. We interpret the action of the other and infer the intention through our own bodily sensory-motor knowledge, which is dependent on our representations of the world (P. F. Ferrari & Gallese, 2007). This means that the same act (like someone lifting a hand) could trigger different "reading" of the underlying intention by different individuals, depending on their past experiences, which are encoded in their implicit relational schemas.

Clinical applications of intersubjective physiology research

Intersubjective physiological research findings have crucial implications for psychotherapy. They provide empirical support for the importance of physiological processes within the therapeutic relationship and give us insights into the theory of psychotherapy methods. We emphasise the following research findings that are of key importance for understanding the intersubjective nature of the therapeutic relationship:

- The physiological states of the therapist and the client are interconnected; they tend to synchronise.
- The therapist responds to the client's physiology and the client to the therapist's.
- The process of physiological synchrony enables the therapist to feel and understand the client's states. It is a crucial process behind empathy and attunement.
- There are two kinds of physiological synchrony: the morphostatic, which enables co-regulation; and morphogenic, which leads to dysregulation.
- There is someone in the relationship who leads the physiology of the other. In psychotherapy, the therapist should take the role of the "leader", who leads the dysregulated therapy field towards regulation.

The critical questions are these: how much physiological synchronisation is needed in psychotherapy (Kleinbub, 2017), what kind of synchronisation, and when?

Research into morphostatic and morphogenic synchrony (Helm et al., 2014) suggests that only morphostatic physiological synchrony between therapist and client, which leads to co-regulation, may have a positive effect on the alliance and other therapeutic processes.

We think that the effect of physiological synchrony (PS) in the therapy is mediated by the autonomic states of the therapist and the client. If the therapist and the client are within the optimal physiological arousal zone, in the ventral vagal state, then PS leads to a good therapeutic bond, feelings of connection, and understanding. On the other hand, if either the therapist or client is in the dys-regulated autonomic state, then synchronisation, if it is not recognised and stop-ped, is counterproductive.

We can conclude that physiological synchrony is needed in the psychother-apeutic relationship, as it enables empathy, attunement, and feelings of connec-tion. However, high physiological synchrony can reflect weak differentiation and may not lead to change and development. For instance, if the client is anxious and in a mobilised autonomic state, the therapist's autonomic state will through synchronisation also become aroused and mobilised. Through this process, the therapist can "feel" what the client is feeling. The danger is that if the therapist remains synchronised with this dysregulation, both therapist and client will stay anxious and mobilised, and the therapy would not be helpful. It is the therapist's responsibility to "see" that they are locked in the dysregulation field and that it then becomes necessary to *interrupt the process of synchronisation*. In other words, the therapist interrupts the morphogenic synchrony by activating the ventral vagal pathways and through this process of self-regulation returns to the window of tolerance. By being in the optimal arousal zone, the therapist will then be able to co-regulate the client through the process of morphostatic synchronisation. The role of the therapist is to "lead" the client's physiological state in the direction of a regulated autonomic state.

The therapist interrupts the relational dysregulation with *mindful awareness* of their present physiological state. This helps the therapist to differentiate between themself and their client and to re-establish their own safe internal space. From this place of safety, they can take the "lead" and bring the client to a safe and regulated state of physiology and mind.

From our supervision practice, we have learned that therapists are often not aware of their dysregulated autonomic states during therapy. In such cases, the therapy ends up going in circles and often leads to ruptures in the alliance. Therapists also report experiencing pain and other physiological disturbances after therapy sessions such as anxiety, headaches, or sleeplessness. A therapist's prolonged dysregulation can ultimately lead to empathic distress (Klimecki & Singer, 2012) and symptoms of burnout (Rothschild, 2006). Because of this, we emphasise the importance of the therapist's mindful awareness of physiological states during the therapy sessions, which helps to regulate defensive states.

According to the research findings on intersubjective physiology and from our own therapy and supervision practice, we conclude that the *therapist's autonomic state is the fundamental factor in psychotherapy*. It affects how we as therapists "are" in the therapy. How we are in psychotherapy influences "what we say and do" (Geller & Greenberg, 2012; Geller, 2018; Ogden, 2018). This is congruent with the authors who propose that the therapist's presence is crucial in the psy-chotherapy process (Erskine, 2015; Geller & Greenberg, 2012; Geller & Porges, 2014). Activation of the ventral vagal state enables the therapist to be fully pre-sent in psychotherapy (Geller, 2018; Geller & Porges, 2014). The therapist's therapeutically effective presence is grounded in awareness and acceptance; it is a mindful presence. This mindful presence related to the ventral vagal state is, therefore, crucial for all other tasks in psychotherapy.

Therapist's mindful presence and self-regulation in psychotherapy

Even though the psychotherapeutic literature does acknowledge the importance of the psychotherapist's physiological states (Dana, 2018; Geller, 2018; Geller & Greenberg, 2012; Geller & Porges, 2014; Ogden, 2018; Rothschild, 2017; D. J. Siegel, 2007), we think that in general it is still not sufficiently emphasised. The therapist's physiological state influences their emotions, cognitions, behavioural responses, and also the client's physiological state (Porges, 2017). This raises the critical question: how can the therapist achieve a regulated physiological state, which will facilitate the client's optimal development and growth? Based on the research findings that mindfulness and interoceptive awareness promotes regulation (Goldin & Gross, 2010; A. M. Hayes & Feldman, 2004; Price & Hooven, 2018; Taren et al., 2013) and on our clinical experience, we propose that this is possible when the therapist is from moment-to-moment mindfully aware of their own physiological states. We suggest that mindful awareness activates ventral vagal regulation. Through mindful awareness the therapist decentres from dysregulated states, observes them in a nonjudgmental and accepting way, and by that self-regulates. Reminding and teaching therapists how to be mindfully aware within each therapy session of their physiological states and to self-regulate is the fundamental task of training and supervision.

Activation of the social engagement system enables the therapist to engage with the client effectively (Dana, 2018; Ogden, 2018). The ANS of the therapist is then in an optimal arousal zone, within the window of tolerance (Ogden et al., 2006; D. J. Siegel, 1999). Therapists within the window of tolerance can think clearly (Rothschild, 2017), can use metacognitive functions, like reflection and mentalisation, and can interact with their client in an adequate way (D. J. Siegel, 1999). If the therapist is not within the window of tolerance, their thinking, emotional processes, and behaviour can become rigid or chaotic, and probably will not be adaptive to the challenges of psychotherapy (D. J. Siegel, 1999). If therapists can modulate their arousal, they will be able to regulate their clients and to adapt to other challenges in psychotherapy as well. For the therapists, it is essential to feel, to be mindful of and to regulate their sensations and emotions. This enables them to use their "calm, centred social engagement capacity to track and guide the client from the hyperaroused (sympathetic) state towards internal regulation and the neuroception of safety" (Levine, 2018, p. 18). The therapist who is mindfully tracking their own physiological states during each therapy session and regulates them when needed also provides self-care for their own well-being and prevention of empathic distress and burnout.

To enable clients to feel safe in therapy, we as therapists want to provide cues of safety for them. This is possible only if we feel safe ourselves. That means that our ANS is not in the defence state and that our social engagement system is activated. Only therapists in the ventral vagal state can send their clients' ANS these cues of safety. Clients' feelings of safety are a prerequisite to all techniques we do in therapy and often, especially with traumatised clients, this is the crucial goal of therapy. "Cues of safety are the efficient and profound antidote for trauma" (Porges, 2018, p. 61). The therapist in the ventral vagal state has the potential to automatically, without conscious engagement, through the process of physiological synchrony, calm down a client's physiology. This is the passive, implicit way of regulating another, called *co-regulation* (Helm et al., 2014; Porges, 2017).

Physiological regulation in the psychotherapeutic relationship

Physiological regulation is a complex neural activity (Porges, 2011). We define it as a process of modulating the physiological arousal states of a person, bringing them to an optimal arousal zone. In situations where there is no actual danger, physiological regulation is the ability to come out of the defensive autonomic states to the window of tolerance and activation of the social engagement system. It is the ability to lower ANS arousal, if the person is in a mobilised state, and to heighten the activation if the person is in an immobilised state. When a person is in a mobilised state, led by the sympathetic system, the vagal brake is needed (Dana, 2018). When a person is in an immobilised state, led by the dorsal vagus, then a person can return to ventral vagal regulation through sympathetic activation (Dana, 2018; Porges, 2011). For the regulation of both defensive states, the aim is to activate in the client feelings of safety. Physiological regulation is also crucial for emotional regulation, where the intensity and duration of emotions are being modulated (Fonagy et al., 2004; Greenberg, 2008; Greenberg & Paivio, 1997).

Self-regulation is the ability of a person to modulate their ANS system on their own. Co-regulation or relational regulation is when one person helps to regulate the other person. One person can regulate the other in either an implicit, passive way or active way (Porges, 2017).

We all experience dysregulated states. The therapist during the course of a therapy session may swing between regulated states, states which are approaching dysregulation, and dysregulated states. As therapists we do become hyper- or hypoaroused. It is essential that, with mindful observation of our physiological states and self-regulation, we prevent ourselves from becoming highly dysregulated and come back to an optimal autonomic state.

In the therapy process, some clients may suffer from dysregulated states more or less regularly, while other clients come to defensive states only when approaching painful or traumatic memories or when they perceive misattunement in the therapeutic relationship. With mindful awareness of their own states and mindful observation and inquiry about the autonomic states of their client, therapists can, through recognising the signs, evaluate the client's arousal zone. They can then use this knowledge as a *map for their actions* in the psychotherapy.

The therapist from their regulated state helps to regulate the client in two main ways:

1   Relational implicit regulation. The therapist within the therapeutic relationship automatically co-regulates a client with the help of their own mindful, compassionate, regulated ventral vagal state.
2   Active/explicit regulation. In this process, the therapist actively invites the client to self-regulate. In MCIP this is done in one of two ways: by enhancing mindful awareness and self-compassion, or by using other strategies. In the first case, the therapist encourages connection with the client's observing self, which enables mindful awareness and self-compassion and through that the self-regulation process. In the second case, the therapist may teach the client other strategies and techniques of self-regulation.

Relational implicit regulation in the therapeutic relationship

People, as well as other mammals, can all regulate each other's physiological states (Helm et al., 2014; Porges, 2017; Reeck et al., 2016). A person develops the ability to self-regulate through the process of co-regulation (Porges, 2017; Schore, 1994, 2019). We call this process relational regulation. If we look at this developmentally, it is through the process of regulation by their mother or significant other that a child develops the ability to self-regulate (Gerhardt, 2004; Schore, 1994; D. J. Siegel, 1999). Imagine that a baby boy is upset. His mother takes him into her arms, gently swings him, lovingly looks at him, and gently talks to him. The baby's physiological state calms down. With this regulation from his mother, his prefrontal lobe develops and connections between the prefrontal lobe and subcortical areas are built (Gerhardt, 2004). The child can be regulated by the other only if the other is in the optimal arousal zone, thereby providing safety.

In therapy, we can effectively use this co-creative process when the therapist is in the ventral vagal state, which enables them to be present. A therapist with their mindful presence offers cues of safety and relationally regulates the client (Geller & Porges, 2014). The client's physiology resonates with the therapist's calm and grounded presence (Geller, 2018). Through the look of their eyes, a kind and gentle facial expression, soft voice, open body posture and breathing, the therapist conveys safety to the client and influences the client's physiological state (Geller & Porges, 2014). The client may, through the process of neuroception (Porges, 2017) and physiological synchrony, sense the safe and calm cues of the therapist's neural system and in turn feel safer and more relaxed. This is the implicit way of regulation. Although the process may look simple, therapists can quickly become dysregulated when working with destabilised clients (Rothschild, 2006). It is essential to train therapists how to be mindfully present, how to mindfully detect their dysregulated states, how to self-regulate, and how to respond to clients' dysregulated states.

Active regulation of the client in the therapeutic relationship

A therapist can also use the *active* way of regulating clients to bring them to the ventral vagal state. Implicit relational regulation is the foundation for active regulation. Active regulation requires conscious voluntary behaviour for changing physiological states (Porges, 2018). When clients get stuck in defensive autonomic states, we lead them into activating a mindful and self–compassionate state. We first educate clients about the meaning and the signs of their autonomic states (Dana, 2018; Rothschild, 2000). We explain to them that their dysregulated symptoms are survival strategies from the past, which were adaptive in stressful or traumatic situations and helped them physically and psychologically to survive. We lead them to self-acceptance of their protective strategies and self-compassion. Through mindful awareness of their body sensations, we teach them to detect which autonomic state they are in. Awareness of ANS states, naming them and assessing their intensity, decentres the clients from their experience and gives them a sense of control and safety. Through this process, they understand what is happening inside of them. In this way, their unpleasant, scary and "crazy" sensations become meaningful.

When the clients' arousal is rising, and they are approaching a dysregulated state or have already become dysregulated, it is essential to slow down the therapy process and initiate the process of self-regulation (Rothschild, 2000). We make a contract with our clients that when we perceive that they are in dysregulated states, we will ask them to make a mindful pause. For instance, we may ask them to stop talking for a while and to observe their physiological state mindfully. It is important to make such a contract in advance so that clients are not surprised when they are being "stopped". Also, they can be asked to give us a sign when they notice their dysregulated state. It is essential that when the client is in a dysregulated state, we nonjudgmentally initiate the process of mindful awareness and self-compassion, and in this way help the clients to self-regulate.

When clients start to observe and verbalise their internal processes from the position of the loving witness, this begins the mindful regulation process. By mindful awareness of breathing, body sensations, emotions, and thoughts, the client's physiological arousal can be regulated. It is also essential to be mindfully aware of what the body would like to do (like breathing more deeply, moving, shaking, jumping …) and to follow these tendencies. The therapist helps the client with an accepting attitude and interventions like: *"Whatever you feel, it's OK. The body is telling you an important story. Gently embrace whatever you are noticing."* The therapist is validating the client's experiences by communicating that they are important (Moursund & Erskine, 2004). In this way, we are developing acceptance of inner states. Acceptance counteracts the intention of experiential avoidance. Promoting self-compassion is also essential for the self-regulation process. Self-compassion counteracts self-rejection and self-criticism, awakens an accepting and loving inner relationship towards ourselves and by this returns safety to our psychophysiological system. Mindfulness and self-compassion activate ventral vagal regulation and help the client to feel safe again.

We may also use other resources to help a client to access their ventral vagal state: breathing with longer exhalation, soothing objects, photographs of pets and nature, imagining a safe place, situations of connection, of awe (Dana, 2018) and use of sound (Erbida Golob & Žvelc, 2015). The therapist can also propose that the client gently touches themselves. We have found that it can be very beneficial if the client puts their hand on their chest in a kind and loving way.

We suggest not to "leave" the client, or ourselves, in a dysregulated state, because if we did, both the client and the therapist would be unable to think clearly and would not be able to "integrate and make sense of what is happening" (Rothschild, 2017, p. 32). And furthermore, the body would continue to suffer. We may need to activate vagal brake many times during the therapy session (Dana, 2018; Rothschild, 2000, 2017) meaning that we "pause" and make time and space for mindful awareness, self-compassion, and regulation.

6 Relational schemas and memory reconsolidation[1]

The construct of schemas can serve as a common language for discussing and understanding psychotherapy. Relational schemas are the fundamental theoretical construct of MCIP that provides us with an understanding of the inner relational world of the client and how this world impacts relating to others.

Relational schemas are schemas of an individual's subjective experience of a relationship. They are "generalizations of repeated experiences of being with others and thus represent prototypes of relational events" (G. Žvelc, 2010c, p. 8). Relational schemas refer to the cognitive, affective, physiological, and behavioural aspects of an individual's subjective experience of relationship. They affect the way we establish interpersonal relationships and how we relate to ourselves. Relational schemas are usually developed in early childhood and are revised and reshaped throughout life.

The notion of relational schemas has previously been used by Baldwin (1992) and Safran (1990). According to Baldwin et al. (2003), a relational schema contains "an image of self (e.g., as inadequate), an image of other (e.g., as critical), and a script for a pattern of interaction between self and other (e.g., if I make a mistake, he will reject me)" (p. 153). Similarly, Safran (1990) describes relationship schemas as structures of relationships between oneself and significant others. The term "relational schemas" stresses the interrelatedness of how we experience ourselves and other people. As Stern (1998/2018) pointed out, a child develops representations of interactions, and not of separate experiences of self and others. This process is based on the subjective experience of the self in relation to other people. Stern (1995) uses the term "schemas-of-being-with" (p. 93) to describe such representations of a relationship.

Relational schemas are structures that have developed based on various relational experiences. They reduce vagueness and unpredictability, enhance our sense of security, and determine how we experience and perceive other people and ourselves in relationships with them. To structure and organise our experience of the world is a basic human need with a biological and evolutionary function (Berne, 1966; Erskine, 1997). The formation of relational schemas enables us to predict the behaviour of others quickly. In certain situations, fast responses and assessments of the emotional states of other people are crucial.

Affect regulation and development of a sense of self

The basic need of all children is for contact with other people because they cannot survive on their own. Children need a constant and stable other person who will look after their needs and regulate their experience in an appropriate way. Parents do this from birth onwards (Bowlby, 1969; Schore, 1994; D. J. Siegel, 1999; Stern, 1998/2018). If a young daughter is frightened, for example, the mother holds her and calms her down. If she is sleepy, the mother puts her to sleep. Parents not only regulate unpleasant experiences but also induce positive ones. Thus, in the presence of a significant other, a child can experience much greater satisfaction than he could if playing alone. One of the main tasks of parenting a young child is the regulation of unpleasant emotional states and the creation of positive ones (Horowitz, 1998; Schore, 1994; Stern, 1998/2018). A baby is thus in a relationship with the "other," who regulates his or her experience of self. Parents can also regulate which emotion a child will experience and, very importantly, its somatic state. In all these interactions, there occurs a significant change in the child's neurophysiological state. A child has different types of experiences in relationships with others and, when these are repeated, they form a relational schema of such relationships. By forming relational schemas, children develop the ability to regulate their own experience. For example, children learn to calm down, put themselves to sleep, regulate their anger and hunger, and so on. Activation of relational schemas enables children to experience self-regulation. When, for instance, a child is frightened, a schema is activated that provides the experience of comfort. Such schemas are adaptive and crucial for the development of a child's personality.

Let us imagine that a boy is playing with a puppet, and then his mother joins him, takes the puppet in her hands, and plays with him. This gives the boy much more pleasure than if he was playing alone. When such interactions are repeated, the moment will come when he will play with the puppet and experience a similar state to the one he previously experienced while playing together with his mother. We can say that the repeated interaction between the mother and the child led to the formation of a relational schema. This schema involves experiencing the self ("happy") in interaction with another ("causing happiness"). When a child comes into contact with the puppet, the schema is activated, and the child experiences similar happiness as if he or she were playing with mother. The puppet thus serves as a stimulus that activates the relational schema.

Nonverbal and verbal relational schemas

Stern (1998/2018) states that a child forms generalised representations of a relationship with a significant other very early. This happens before the development of speech and refers to the representation of a child's nonverbal experience. In relational schemas theory, we have termed such schemas "*nonverbal relational schemas*". They refer to behavioural, affective, and physical experiences of the self and other people. These schemas are coded in implicit memory, which is related to those parts of the brain that do not require conscious processing in order to store and recall (D. J. Siegel, 1999). Implicit memory is the earliest type of memory; it is already present at birth. When a person draws on implicit memory, they are not aware of the act of remembering. Explicit memory on the other hand requires awareness for both storing and recall. A person will in this case be aware that they are remembering something. When implicit memory is activated, behaviour, emotions, and images are activated. Nonverbal implicit schemas lead us to interpret current stimuli, behave accordingly, and experience certain emotions and images without being aware of the influence of previous experience on the reality of the moment.

With the development of speech, the schemas begin to involve language and the verbalisation of nonverbal experience. Adequate attunement to the child enables parents to find the right names for the child's experiences. Attributing meaning to nonverbal experience is not always precise; it depends on the parents' attunement to the child and the appropriate naming of the child's experience. To illustrate this, imagine a young boy who is experiencing fear. His mother perceives this and holds him in her arms while naming her child's response as fear, and the child is comforted. In this way, the child may develop a verbal description of the experience: "I am afraid, but I can rely on my mother." But parents may misinterpret their child's experience. In such a case, the mother might not recognise and verbalise the child's fear but rather be annoyed with the child for being "cranky", leaving her child without the appropriate words to describe their nonverbal experience.

Some relational schemas integrate both nonverbal and verbal schemas, although some schemas stay with us only in nonverbal form. When such implicit schemas are activated, we may experience specific feelings and body sensations towards ourselves or other people without being aware that we are experiencing memories from the past. The person may feel that they are experiencing something familiar, but is not aware of what that may be. This is related to Bollas's (1987) concept of the "unthought known".

Relational schemas networks and self-narrative

Relational schemas exist at different levels of generalisation. They can be quite specific and refer to specific themes and relationships, such as relational schemas of a person's relationship with their mother, father, or both parents. On the other hand, relational schemas can also be more generalised, for instance, those of a relationship with men or women in general, or authority figures. In this case, a relational schema is a network of interconnected specific schemas.

For example, in his childhood, the client Eric was frequently humiliated by his father, who was verbally abusive and overly demanding. The experiences with his father were generalised as a relational schema of a relationship with an abusive father. In addition to this relationship with his father, Eric also had similar experiences with his grandfather and his piano teacher. These experiences were connected with the schema of the relationship with the father. In this way, a network of relational schemas was formed (experiencing shame when exposed to criticism from other men). This schema was often activated in Eric's relationships with men, through which he experienced a good deal of shame leading him to avoid social contacts, especially with other men.

Networks of relational schemas at the highest level form an overarching relational schema – our *self-narrative*. The terms self-narrative refers to our narrative identity, which gives coherence and integration to our experiences. McAdams and McLean (2013) describe how narrative identity is "a person's internalized and evolving life story, integrating the reconstructed past and imagined future to provide life with some degree of unity and purpose" (p. 1). The self-narrative functions as the central organiser of our experience and integrates different relational schemas, both verbal and nonverbal. Experiences and relational schemas which are in accordance with the self-narrative will interconnect, while experiences which depart from it will be denied or stored separately. Although the term "narrative" is usually used for verbal stories, in line with Lichtenberg (2017) we understand the narrative as being broader, encompassing both nonverbal and verbal domains.

Activation of schemas and self-states

Erskine et al. (1999) describe that "the expectations for the future are often echoes of the past" (p. 167). Activation of schemas determines how we will perceive another person and how we will behave towards them. Schemas enable prediction and quick orientation in contacts with other people. In Chapter 5, we describe how with *neuroception* we continually evaluate other people and situations in terms of safety, risk, or danger (Porges, 2017). We think that neuroception is dependent on relational schemas that provide templates for activation of the autonomic nervous system based on previous relational experiences.

Activated relational schemas reawaken the primary relational experience. The context of a relationship affects which schemas and which elements of a schema will be activated within a relationship. A schema can be activated by an actual event that is associated with a schema, or it can be set off via memory or imagination. In other words, schemas can be activated through certain external or internal stimuli. In the case of an internal stimulus, an association, a certain thought, feeling, or sensation can trigger the activation of a schema. Any element of a schema – word, image, action, smell – can activate another. For example, the smell of a certain perfume can activate the schema of a relationship with our mother, or a stomach ache can activate the schema of being with a worried father, who was frightened of illness.

Relational schemas cannot be observed directly, but their activation can be seen in different patterns of subjective experience and behaviour; in the *self-states*. The term self-state refers to patterns of emotion, thinking, behaviour, and physiological reactions. Activated relational schemas are manifested either in the emotional attitude toward other people (or events) or intrapsychically in the form of internal dialogue between different self-states. To illustrate this, we will continue with Eric's story.

As we said, Eric's father was very strict, severely criticising his son's every mistake and verbally abusing him. These experiences became generalised as a relational schema. An event that is associatively linked to this schema can activate the schema and cause Eric to experience a certain self-state. In this case, Eric criticised himself for every small mistake he made, and, in doing so, he internally re-experienced shame and humiliation. Each mistake served as a stimuli for the activation of the relational schema. It triggered Eric to humiliate himself and further strengthen the schema. Based on a relational schema, Eric also anticipated criticism from other people, even if they had a positive attitude towards him. Even in the case of minor criticism from his colleagues at work, he felt humiliated, ashamed, and as if something was wrong with him.

Relational schemas can be *adaptive* or *dysfunctional*. Adaptive schemas are open to change and adaptive concerning the current situation. In Eric's case they were dysfunctional, as they were not adaptive to the current situation, were causing high stress, they were rigid and were not open to change. We propose that there are two fundamental types of disturbances in the development of relational schemas. The first is a lack of adaptive relational schemas, and the second is the development of dysfunctional relational schemas.

A lack of adaptive relational schemas

Relational schemas play an important function in the development of personality. They enable self-regulation and the development of a sense of self. However, such schemas only develop when a child has a good-enough parent who is attuned to the child's needs. When parents do not provide adequate attunement and regulation of the child's internal emotional states, such children will not develop relational schemas that would later enable them to regulate their own experience (e.g., calming or amplifying positive emotion). In an emotional sense, they are left on their own, which means they may experience intense emotional states that they cannot adequately regulate. Later in life, such individuals may have major problems regulating their own emotions, sometimes being swept away by strong feelings, without being able to regulate them. In terms of the polyvagal theory (Porges, 2017), we propose that such a lack of adaptive relational schemas may be related to insufficient vagal brake.

Development of dysfunctional schemas

Experiencing deprivation and/or trauma leads to defensive processes in a child. These defensive processes arise through a child's creative adaptation to absent or inadequate contact with parents. The child adapts to the situation to avoid the pain and at the same time to maintain the relationship with significant others. A child may deny certain facts and dissociate from emotional states. Body sensations and emotions may become separated from verbal meanings and images. The child may also become withdrawn and afraid of significant others. Based on repeated similar experiences, the child forms a relational schema of such an interaction. We refer to such a schema as a *dysfunctional relational schema*. It is a generalisation of the subjective experience of an inadequate relationship or lack of contact with a significant other. Dysfunctional schemas resist change and accommodation and can lead to a dysfunctional relationship with self and others. In childhood, such schemas are entirely adaptive, enabling the child to survive in a dysfunctional environment. However, for the adult they are dysfunctional, as they are remnants of past experiences that have not been updated with new information. Dysfunctional relational schemas distort the perception of current situations and lead us to behave and feel in a way that is not adaptive in relation to the present. Such schemas may lead to *faulty neuroception* (Porges, 2017) and can activate either the sympathetic or dorsal vagal parasympathetic system leading to behavioural strategies of mobilisation or immobilisation. The person can, for example, feel very threatened in relation to benign stimuli. The sweet smile of another person can be interpreted as dangerous, based on the relational schema of being with an unpredictable mother, who could change her mood very quickly from extreme kindness to rage.

Dysfunctional schemas have a defensive function and protect the person from both external and internal danger, even if the "real" danger is a long time past. They prevent the person from experiencing certain elements of subjective experience (emotions, body sensations, memories) and behaviours. Only those experiences that are coherent with the schema are allowed, while others are denied or dissociated. Dysfunctional schemas resist accommodation because they fulfil the important function of protection from painful and distressing subjective experience. In this way, a person does not have to face unpleasant memories and emotional states. Based on a dysfunctional schema, the person can feel "numb" and "empty" with their loved ones, which was an important strategy in the past – to avoid feeling the pain related to rejecting and "cold" parents. However, such schemas represent a source of dissatisfaction in adult life and often lead to clinical problems. They are "fixed structures that prevent the person from experiencing the freshness and uniqueness of the moment" (G. Žvelc, 2010c, p. 9). They interrupt intrapsychic and external contact (Erskine et al., 1999) and prevent the person from being spontaneous, aware, and intimate (Berne, 1967). To understand the process more clearly, let us look at a clinical case.

Peter spent his childhood with a verbally and physically abusive mother who was addicted to alcohol. In response to constant humiliation as a child, Peter dissociated many feelings. Anger and sadness were not allowed in his relationship with his mother along with any signs of rebellion. He also experienced extreme shame and became obedient and adaptable. Peter concluded that he was not safe and that he was a bad person. All this enabled him to survive the kind of relationship he had with his mother. If as a child Peter had rebelled and expressed his anger, he would have experienced even greater abuse from his mother. Thus, his reaction was his best attempt at adapting to the situation. Because such experiences were repeated many times, he formed a relational schema of the relationship with his mother, which included feelings of not being safe, shame, extreme adaptability, and the belief that he was a bad person. The schema also included experiencing other people as dangerous and abusive. Later in life, Peter had major problems with feeling unsafe in relationships. He did not trust his girlfriend and expected that she would sooner or later hurt him and abandon him. He also felt like he did not deserve her. At the slightest criticism from her he experienced shame and tried to please her. He had difficulty expressing anger and sadness; he could not stand up for himself and felt inadequate in his relationship with her. The dysfunctional relational schema of being with an abusive mother was being almost continually activated in his intimate relationship.

Relational schemas and change in psychotherapy

Dysfunctional relational schemas and lack of adaptive schemas are often the sources of the client's symptoms. In MCIP, we address with different methods and interventions dysfunctional schemas and promote the development of new adaptive schemas. There are three main psychotherapeutic tasks related to relational schemas: (1) Developing decentred awareness of relational schemas and psychological flexibility, (2) Change of dysfunctional relational schemas and memory reconsolidation, and (3) Developing new adaptive schemas.

Developing decentred awareness of relational schemas and psychological flexibility

In MCIP we emphasise the development of a new relationship with the schemas, which is based on mindful awareness and compassion. Through mindfulness processes and compassion, an individual can develop a new relationship towards their schemas that is based on the present moment, acceptance, decentred awareness, and compassion. Such new relationship enables a person to be freed from the grasp of dysfunctional schemas and enables them to live life fully according to their values. This process is in acceptance and commitment therapy (ACT) described as psychological flexibility. S. C. Hayes et al. (2012) define psychological flexibility as: "contacting the present moment as a conscious human being, fully and without needless defense – as it is and not as what it says it is – and persisting with or changing a behavior in the service of chosen values" (pp. 96–97). Through mindfulness and compassion processes, clients are invited to be fully present with their experience and to develop a decentred perspective towards their schemas. Decentred awareness of relational schemas enables the person to become aware of how their relational schemas are influencing their lives. Based on greater mindfulness and compassion they may start living life according to their values and meaning, even if relational schemas are activated. In this way, the clients come to feel greater internal freedom, as they are no longer merged with their schemas. The client Lana, for example, became aware of her schema, which was behind her avoidance of going to university to study mathematics: "I am not capable and others are better than me." Even though she had excellent marks in secondary school, she lacked the courage to go further. Decentred awareness related to the schemas helped her to go on to pursue her studies. In Chapter 10 we describe various methods and interventions that help the clients to develop decentred awareness of relational schemas. Decentred awareness of relational schemas is also the first step related to the task of changing dysfunctional schemas through the process of memory reconsolidation.

Change of dysfunctional relational schemas and memory reconsolidation

In healthy personality development, schemas are open to change in a constant process of assimilation and accommodation (Piaget & Inhelder, 1966/1990). Assimilation is the process of adapting new events and situations to existing schemas. An individual interprets events and reacts to them based on previous experience and in this way new information and experience is assimilated into the existing schemas. But sometimes new events and situations are so different from previous experience that the individual notices the difference. This triggers the process of accommodation and the person modifies schemas based on new information. Relational schemas are thus constantly in a state of flux and open to change. In adaptive functioning, relational schemas are open to change; any activation of a schema constitutes a potential entry point for new information.

This process of change can be explained by the mechanisms of *memory reconsolidation*. The process of memory reconsolidation is based on neuroscience research, which shows that old emotional learning, including implicit emotional schemas, can be revised at the level of the "physical, neural synapses that encode it in emotional memory" (Ecker et al., 2012, p. 13). Memory reconsolidation can be understood as the "brain's innate process for fundamentally revising an existing learning and acquired behavioral responses and/or state of mind maintained by that learning" (Ecker, 2015, p. 4). The neurological process of memory reconsolidation can be understood as a unifying mechanism of change in the various psychotherapies that promote transformational change (Ecker, 2018; Ecker et al., 2012; Lane et al., 2015).

Figure 6.1 illustrates the process of change of relational schemas. Certain internal or external stimuli trigger and activate certain schemas. Their activation is manifested in specific self-states, which are the basic units of subjective experience and behaviour (top arrow). Self-states can reinforce a certain schema (process of assimilation) or trigger its change (process of accommodation), illustrated in the figure by the bottom arrow. Individuals experience many different states, which change from moment to moment. These self-states are influenced by the state of the organism and its needs, relational schemas (influence of past experience), and specific influences of the present moment. Present moment events and

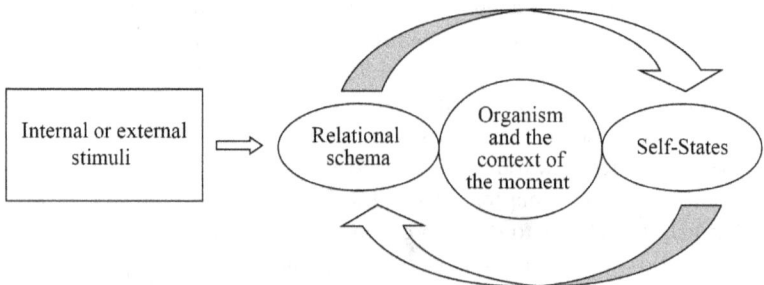

Figure 6.1 Activation of relational schemas and self-states

interpersonal relationships can induce self-states that we have not experienced before and that are not part of our accumulated relational schemas.

Even though the activation of schemas brings patterns of past experience into the present, each present situation is different. It is a mixture of various influences, not only those of relational schemas. Each time a schema is activated, it is activated under slightly different circumstances. This is precisely what makes the constant process of schema change possible.

If this were not the case, we would be completely trapped in the patterns of past reactions. Self-states paradoxically represent a reawakening of past experience and, at the same time, a new experience that a person has never had before in quite the same form. If the new experience and the related self-states are similar enough to past experiences, a process of assimilation occurs, and the structure of the schema is preserved. However, if the new experience is radically different from the experiences that have become a part of a relational schema, the schema itself is changed (accommodation). This process of schema change is congruent with the process of memory reconsolidation that describes how memories are not fixed and perfect accounts of our past but are constantly revised and reshaped (Lane et al., 2015).

For memory reconsolidation, it is important that relational schemas are activated and that the person has a new experience, which is juxtaposed with old learning (Ecker et al., 2012). This provides a "mismatch experience", where the individual notices the difference between old schema learning and the new experience. Relational schemas are through this process transformed and changed. Each activation of a schema is an opportunity for that schema to change based on new information entering the system. Schemas are changed and transformed in psychotherapy through the process of memory reconsolidation.

The client Emma, for example, had a relational schema related to "feeling unsafe in relationship with men", which had developed following experiences with an abusing father and two previous boyfriends who sexually and physically abused her. New relationships with the therapist and with her new boyfriend provided a new experience of "being safe" in relationship with another person, which helped her to change the dysfunctional schema.

Ecker and colleagues (2012) have translated the neurological process of memory reconsolidation into psychotherapy practice. They have described the necessary phases of psychotherapy in order to promote memory reconsolidation. The therapeutic reconsolidation process occurs in three main phases: (1) Accessing sequence, (2) Transformation sequence, and (3) Verification phase. In the first phase, the old emotional learning is activated and brought to conscious awareness. It has to be experienced as a felt experience that is verbalised. Just cognitive understanding is not enough; the relational schema has to be activated and experienced. In the second transformation phase, the old emotional learning is juxtaposed with the new contradictory experience. In this process, both old and new experiences have to be brought to awareness at the same time. Such mismatch creates a *prediction error* experience that unlocks the synapses. The repeated juxtaposition experience between old and new learning re-writes and changes the dysfunctional schema. The verification phase consists of observations to confirm if memory reconsolidation has occurred. This shows in emotional non-reactivation, symptom cessation, and effortless permanence (Ecker et al., 2012).

The process of memory reconsolidation helps us to understand the necessary steps to promote transformational change. It can guide therapists in using the processes of change and related interventions. In MCIP, memory reconsolidation occurs through various methods and interventions connected to different processes of change. New experiences that contradict old learning may be: insight, new emotional and body experience, new behaviour, and new relational experiences. Mindfulness and compassion processes are in our approach to integrative psychotherapy central to schema change as they provide fundamentally new experiences in contrast to dysfunctional schemas – the experience of present moment awareness, acceptance, decentred perspective, and compassion. Working with several processes of change potentiates the effects of schema change.

It is crucial that a relational schema is fully activated because this is the only way that change of the schema is possible. If a relational schema is not activated, the change is only cognitive and behavioural, an attempt to control activation of dysfunctional schemas that shows in different symptoms. Ecker et al. (2012) describe this as *counteractive change*, where psychotherapy promotes new learning that exists alongside old emotional learning. The old emotional learning is not changed but is regulated through different methods and techniques, such as relaxation techniques, affect regulation, cognitive reappraisal (Ecker & Vaz, 2019). New learning, in this case, competes with old learning. Counteractive change results in partial symptom reduction and takes effort to maintain and can result in relapses of symptoms. Therefore, change must reach all the elements of a schema – not just the verbal level but also the subsymbolic ones (sensory, visceral, and motor) – so that the individual actually sees and feels the world differently (Bucci, 1997). It is not enough to talk about emotional experiences and beliefs; they must be experienced and felt in the body. Activation and decentred awareness of schemas is a crucial precondition for transformational change, which is attributed to memory reconsolidation. In this case, the dysfunctional relational schemas are revised, which results in the elimination of symptoms and permanent change which is effortless to maintain (Ecker et al., 2012).

Dysfunctional schemas, although they are not adaptive in the present, serve an important intrapsychic function. They give a person a feeling of predictability, identity, continuity, and stability (Erskine et al., 1999). A change of schemas can shake our experience of stability and continuity, and when such change occurs, a client may experience temporary instability and a feeling of identity loss. Old beliefs and experiences of the self and others stabilise our psychic organisation. A change of dysfunctional schemas is sometimes experienced as a dying of the old and the birth of something new.

Corrective relational experience and change of dysfunctional schemas

Activation of a relational schema in an interpersonal setting means that a person will experience the other in a way that is similar to how they experienced a significant other in the past. In psychotherapy, this corresponds to the concept of transference. This makes it possible for the schema either to change or to be reinforced. For memory reconsolidation to occur, it is important that the individual has new experiences that are fundamentally different from old learning. New corrective relational experiences with the therapist may be one such experience that is different from old schema expectations.

Relational methods of inquiry, attunement, and involvement may provide the client with new relational experiences that are in stark contrast with previous experiences and expectations in a relationship. This creates a *juxtaposition* experience between the old relational memories and new attuned relationship with the therapist (Erskine, 2015). Erskine (1993) describes how such a juxtaposition between the therapist's attunement and memories of a lack of attunement in previous significant relationships can produce "intense, emotional memories of needs not being met" (p.184). Erskine (1993) further explains:

> Rather than experience those feelings, the client may react defensively to the contact offered by the therapist with fear, anger, or even further dissociation. The contrast between the contact available with the therapist and the lack of contact in the original trauma(s) is often more than clients can bear, so they defend against the current contact to avoid the emotional memories.[2]

Understanding and working with a juxtaposition experience is crucial in integrative psychotherapy so that clients can integrate the new relational experience and for memory reconsolidation to occur. Even though the juxtaposition experience may be difficult and painful for the client, it is also crucial for profound personality change and memory reconsolidation.

Mindfulness and memory reconsolidation

For memory reconsolidation, a mismatch is essential between old learning and new information that contradicts the old learning. This means that old emotional learning needs to be juxtaposed with new information. We propose that mindful awareness is the core new experience that provides a juxtaposition to old learning and promotes memory reconsolidation. In MCIP, through the use of different psychotherapeutic methods we activate the clients' dysfunctional relational schemas and bring mindful awareness and compassion to their experience. Dysfunctional relational schemas are by definition connected to avoidance of experience, negative beliefs about self, and unpleasant emotions. Mindful awareness and compassion provide radically new information and experience. Most of our clients have negative beliefs about themselves – that they are not OK as persons. With mindful awareness and compassion, clients can have an entirely new experience that could be described in words such as "you are accepted as you are". Such new information and experience can provide the necessary juxtaposition experience, which is essential for memory reconsolidation and schema change.

Mindfulness and compassion challenge the foundation of dysfunctional relational schemas – the process of avoidance of internal experience – by enabling a client to establish contact with the experiences that would otherwise be dissociated. Thus, therapy is a process of integration, of re-association of experiences that would usually be dissociated because of dysfunctional schemas. In this way, new connections between dysfunctional schemas and new adaptive experiences can be formed.

For example, a client can access the grief he was keeping in because his schema was related to being strong in relation to a depressed mother. Decentred awareness and compassion related to the schema "I have to be strong and take care of others" helped him to develop a new experience of "I have a right to be vulnerable and comforted". This opened the way for him to feel the grief, which provided new emotional/body experiences that promoted memory reconsolidation.

Decentred perspective may also contradict old learning. Decentred perspective and contact with the observing self enable the client to relate to their negative beliefs and ideas as "just thoughts" and not reality itself. This provides a fundamental deconstruction of negative beliefs about self. Contact with the observing self by itself provides a new experience that is fundamentally different from old emotional learning. Clients can observe their experience from different perspectives, which naturally brings new insights and experiences that provide an antidote to old experiences. For example, a client can relate to their experience from the perspective of their wise, future self or may relate to themselves from the perspective of a loving best friend. Such interventions usually promote new experiences and insights that contradict old emotional learning.

Developing new adaptive schemas

The process of psychotherapy involves not only decentred awareness and transformation of dysfunctional relational schemas; it also involves developing new adaptive schemas through the new relational experiences with the therapist or through developing a new mindful and compassionate relationship with the self. In this process, the new adaptive schemas can coexist with the old dysfunctional schemas. They provide new ways of relating to both self and others and extend the client's repertoire of relational experiences. As dysfunctional schemas are not necessarily changed, this process could be described as *"counteractive change"* (Ecker et al., 2012, p. 32), where new learning competes against old learning. New adaptive schemas can inhibit activation of dysfunctional schemas and provide more adaptive responses.

The relationship with the therapist enables the client to form new adaptive relational schemas. This is particularly important for those individuals who, in the past, experienced deprivation concerning inadequate interpersonal experiences, and as a result lack adaptive relational schemas. In this way, a client who is having difficulty regulating their emotions builds up this capacity in the relationship with the therapist. Through the repetitive experience of the relationship with the attuned and compassionate therapist, the client forms a relational schema of such interactions. The relational schemas of attuned contact with the therapist are recorded in the form of adaptive relational schemas. Such schemas enable the client to have new forms of relationship both with other people and with themselves. A new internal accepting relationship enables the client to regulate their own emotions.

In addition to the therapeutic relationship, new adaptive schemas can also be developed by other methods and techniques that are focused on the creation of the new intrapsychic relationship. With mindfulness and compassion processes, the client develops a new relationship with themselves, which is based on awareness, acceptance, and compassion. Such a relationship is gradually represented in the new adaptive relational schema.

Notes

1 Adapted from the article "Between self and others: Relational schemas as an integrating construct in psychotherapy" by G. Žvelc, 2009, *Transactional Analysis Journal, 39*(1), 22–38 (https://doi.org/10.1177/036215370903900104). Copyright 2009 by Taylor & Francis Ltd. Adapted with permission of the publisher (Taylor & Francis Ltd, www.tandfonline.com

2 From "Inquiry, attunement, and involvement in the psychotherapy of dissociation," by R. G. Erskine, 1993, *Transactional Analysis Journal, 23*(4), p. 187. (https://doi.org/10.1177/036215379302300402). Copyright 1993 by Taylor & Francis. Reprinted with permission of the publisher (Taylor & Francis Ltd, http://www.tandfonline.com).

7   Beyond ordinary unhappiness: From personal to observing self

In Chapter 3, we describe the two main senses of self: a *personal sense of self* and the *observing/transcendent self*. The personal sense of self refers to the experience of ourselves as a particular person with an autobiographical history. It is a sense of self that gives us an experience of continuity flowing through our past, present, and into the future. We know that we are a particular person and that we have certain personality characteristics and phenomenological experiences. These include beliefs about ourselves, memories about the self in the past, and fantasies about the future. It represents our identity – this is who I am. When I (Gregor) introduce myself to new students of psychotherapy training, I usually say:

> I am a psychologist, I have a PhD in clinical psychology, and I am a prac-tising psychotherapist and supervisor. I am married, I have two sons, one is 19 years old and the other is 16. I am also a keen reader and have a long-time interest in spirituality.

When I (Maša) speak to new colleagues at a conference, I may say:

> I am an integrative psychotherapist, very involved in supervising and teach-ing psychotherapy. I have two sons. I adore going to the mountains, I do dance classes, and I love to go for long walks with my husband, sons, friends, and our dog. I very much enjoy reading literature.

These descriptions include the words "I am", which is followed by some statement of personality characteristics. The personal self refers to our identifi-cation with our self-narrative and could be described with the formula: I am = self-narrative.

However, the personal self does not represent our whole experience of self. It represents only aspects related to our identity. In addition to the personal self, we also have another experience of self, that we call the observing/transcendent self. The observing self is our experience of being an aware and conscious human being. In the background behind all of our experiences, there is a sense of I – the sense that I exist and I am aware. Take a moment and reflect on this. While you are reading this book, just become aware that there is a certain sense of "I am aware, I exist", a sense of I who is aware of thoughts, emotions, current behaviour, and external environment, leading you to an awareness that you are alive and that you enjoy having time for reading and contemplating the nature of the human mind. Behind our every experience, there is a constant presence of awareness. It is simple, non-conceptual awareness that is phenomenologically experienced as "I am aware". The observing self, as an experience of ourselves as being aware and conscious, could be described with the formula: I am = awareness.

The personal sense of self

We propose the following definition of a personal sense of self:

The personal sense of self is the lived and embodied experience of the self-narrative that is continually self-reinforcing and maintaining itself. While self-narrative refers to a sense of self as mentally represented, we define the personal self as the lived and embodied experience of being a "person" in relationship with others. The personal sense of self is: (a) Lived and embodied, (b) An expression of self-narrative, and (c) A self-reinforcing system.

The personal sense of self as lived and embodied experience

In the previous chapter, we describe the formation of the self-narrative, which integrates numerous relational schemas into an overarching autobiographical narrative. The personal sense of self describes our lived and embodied experience of this narrative organisation. It refers to the phenomenological experience of our self-narrative. We live our life based on our self-narrative and networks of related schemas that provide lenses through which we process every experience. This process is mostly out of awareness. We experience ourselves and others based on schemas, without knowing that schemas determine our experience. Our experience of self, who we are, who we were in the past, and who we will be in the future, is largely the result of our self-narrative and related schema networks.

The personal sense of self as an expression of self-narrative

In the course of growing up, we develop a story about ourselves, which answers the questions: "Who was I, who am I and, who will I become in the world with other people?" Mitchell (2012, p. 145) writes, "we are stories, our accounts of what has happened to us … No stories, no self". Such stories refer to our self-narrative – our narrative identity (McAdams & McLean, 2013). Although this narrative is usually understood as a verbal story, following both Stern (2004) and Lichtenberg (2017) we conceptualise the narrative as both verbal and nonverbal. Lichtenberg (2017) describes how narratives "capture both the implicit and explicit aspects of lived experience" (p. 3). Part of our self-narrative is conscious and is expressed in different narratives that we tell to others and ourselves. However, our self-narrative is not only a conscious story about our life; it is also unconscious and nonverbal. The nonverbal aspects of our life-story are elements of our nonverbal schemas coded in implicit memory. Nonverbal relational schemas are a constant part of our experience and tell an important story about the experience of self and others. Erskine (2015) describes how an unconscious and nonverbal life-story is often enacted in behaviour, entrenched in the person's affect, and embodied in physiology. This is congruent with Stern (2004), who described how children create emotional narratives of their experience before the development of language. These emotional narratives are not verbalised in stories but are emotionally felt. Stern (2004) described such narratives as *lived stories*, which are "experiences that are narratively formatted in the mind but not verbalized or told" (p. 55). Some of these *lived stories* are translated later into language and become stories that we tell to others. However, some of our emotional narratives are never symbolised and stay unconscious. They may be expressed in physical sensations, emotions, body expressions, and movements.

In childhood, autobiographical narratives are co-created in relationship with parents, siblings, and significant others (Stern, 1998/2018). Parents constantly ask their children to tell stories about their experiences: "How was today in kindergarten?", "What did you do at the party?", "Did you get any marks in school?" The resulting narratives are co-created in relationship with parents (Stern, 1998/2018). Stern (1998/2018, p. xxiv) argues that child and parent collaboratively "gather the pieces of the story" and "order them sequentially" into a coherent narrative. This autobiographical narrative is developed in relationship with others, so it is by nature relational, embedded in contexts with other people and culture. The autobiographical narratives that we tell to self and others become the official history of our life (Stern, 1998/2018).

Throughout the course of our life, we develop our self-narrative, which refers to an overall life-story that integrates discrete events in a temporal sequence in a meaningful way (Angus & Greenberg, 2011) and provides us with identity. McAdams (2001) proposed that "identity itself takes the form of a story, complete with settings, scenes, character, plot and theme" (p. 101). He argues that people "reconstruct the personal past, perceive the present, and anticipate the future in terms of an internalized and evolving life-story, an integrative narrative of self" (p. 101). This story provides us with "unity, purpose and meaning" (McAdams & McLean, 2013, p. 233) and is co-constructed in relationships and cultural context (McAdams, 2001; McAdams & McLean, 2013). It is through telling our narratives that our life-story is continually updated and re-written. Bluck and Habermas (2000) proposed that although a life-story schema is a stable organisation it may also be updated and changed during our life. The personal sense of self as an expression of our self-narrative includes both verbal stories about self as well as nonverbal "lived stores" that are expressed in emotions and body experiences.

The personal sense of self as a self-reinforcing system

The personal sense of self can be described as a self-reinforcing system. It needs constant reinforcement to maintain itself. This view is influenced by Černigoj's

(2007) theory of self in which he proposed that self is "the continual process of maintaining the self-concept as a special cognitive structure" (p. 213). According to this view, the self is an "*autopoietic*" system, which does not exist physically as a living organism, but it could be described as a "virtual autopoietic system" (Černigoj, 2007, pp. 210–211). Such a system has its own autonomy and dynamics. It is continually changing, with all changes being subordinated to maintaining its own organisation. In this way, self as an autopoietic system maintains its own identity.

Černigoj (2007) describes how the autonomy of the self is seen in the human experience of being separated from nature and other people. However, autonomy does not mean total independence. As an organism needs food and nutrients from the environment, the self needs its "food" from the social environment in the form of symbolic confirmations of its existence and value (Černigoj, 2007).

Based on Černigoj's (2007) theory of self, we propose that the personal sense of self is a process of continual maintenance and reinforcement of our self-narrative. We become identified with our life-story and start to live it in the world. We are unconsciously continually reinforcing our life-story by selectively ignoring and avoiding certain aspects of subjective reality that do not fit our life-story. At the same time we are also actively seeking experiences that would confirm or enhance our self-narrative. We start to live our story of life and behave in a way that is consistent with our story and invite others to reinforce it. This is congruent with the self-confirmation theory (Andrews, 1993), which assumes that each person maintains "self-consistency by arranging his or her interactions with the environment so that they form a negative feedback loop" (p. 166) that returns a system to its previous equilibrium. In this way our personal sense of self is a system, which is continually reinforcing itself.

The personal sense of self has important functions that are crucial for our existence. Erskine et al. (1999) describe how we maintain our habitual patterns of experience and behaviour because they serve the psychological functions of predictability, identity, consistency, and stability. Although these functions were described in relation to defensive patterns related to life-scripts (Erskine, 2016) they are important also for understanding the nature of the personal sense of self. The personal sense of self provides us with a sense of identity, continuity of existence, stability, and gives a sense of predictability about ourselves and others:

> *Identity*. The personal sense of self provides a sense of personal identity; this is "me" and this is how I am.
>
> *Continuity*. We know that we were such a person in the past, are in the present, and will be in the future. Autobiographical memories provide us with a sense of continuity of existence.
>
> *Stability*. The personal sense of self gives us a sense of stability and a sense of control in our life.
>
> *Predictability*. The personal sense of self gives us a sense of predictability about ourselves, others, and the world. We know how we will probably react

in different situations and how other people will probably behave towards us in a particular situation.

Because of these functions, the personal sense of self is a relatively stable organisation and gives us the foundation of experience: "This is me. This is how I have been in the past and will be in the future. I also know what to expect from myself and other people."

Identification with the personal sense of self and "ordinary unhappiness"

Even though the personal sense of self is necessary for our existence as human beings, at the same time it is also restrictive and limiting. In Buddhism, attachment to one's separate self is the main source of individual suffering (Engler & Fulton, 2012; Hanh, 1998). Attachment to self manifests as the "fixation on either positive or negative aspects of self" and viewing the self as fixed (Whitehead et al., 2018, p. 2). In acceptance and commitment therapy (ACT), attachment to a conceptual self is seen as the main cause of psychological inflexibility (S. C. Hayes et al., 2012) that is related to many psychological problems.

In line with Buddhism and ACT, we propose that identification with the personal sense of self is a source of human suffering. Identification with the personal sense of self refers to merging with our self-narrative. Our sense of "I" becomes merged with our life-story. We become so involved with our story that we forget it is no more than a story that we have constructed in the course of our life and not substantial "truth". We propose that identification with a personal sense of self is at the root of *ordinary unhappiness*, from which we all suffer. Freud (1895/2013) was the first psychotherapy author to write about ordinary unhappiness. He proposed that psychoanalysis helps people to transform suffering from neurotic to common unhappiness: "…much will be gained if we succeed in transforming your hysterical misery into everyday unhappiness" (Freud, 1895/2013, p. 168).

Identification with a personal sense of self that is related to ordinary unhappiness manifests in: (1) Living unconsciously according to our life-story, (2) Egocentricity and preoccupation with self, (3) Fear that our life-story will be disconfirmed, (4) Existential loneliness and feelings of separation, (5) Loss of present moment and experiential avoidance.

Living unconsciously according to our life-story

From childhood onwards, we start to identify with our self-narrative. Our sense of "I" becomes attached to our life-story. We usually live our story without knowing that this story is organising our life (Berne, 1972). We may become captives of our story, which was written very early in life through different experiences with self and others. Because of identification with our story, we may behave according to old patterns, not daring to behave differently and pursue new avenues in life. This limits psychological flexibility (S. C. Hayes et al., 2012) and autonomy

(Berne, 1967). For example, someone may follow a story that they must "work hard to be worthy", which can then result in neglecting other areas of life and possible burnout because of overwork.

Egocentricity and preoccupation with self

Identification with the personal sense of self appears in egocentricity and pre-occupation with ourselves. It can prevent us from having empathy and compas-sion for others and may be seen in narcissistic self-preoccupation. Since the personal self is focused on self-preservation and maintenance, it is fundamentally egocentric. It needs reinforcement from the social environment in terms of recognition of its value and existence (Černigoj, 2007). In this regard, Berne (1967), the founder of transactional analysis, talked about the need for recognition as one of the basic human needs. Maintaining our personal sense of self may become a priority in life, which may be the cause of suffering both for ourselves and others. We may be continuously preoccupied and concerned with ourselves. We may try to perfect our self-esteem or have the tendency of comparing our-selves with others (Engler & Fulton, 2012). Engler and Fulton (2012) describe how even "the 'healthy' narcissism characteristics of a well-adjusted, mature individual is a cause of distress" (pp. 178–179) because when relating from the perspective of self, we tend to judge our "experience as 'good' for me and 'bad' for me" (p. 179). Attachment to our personal sense of self is seen in desire and aversion. We grasp at things that support or enhance our personal sense of self and avoid things that can undermine it. We may, for example, become preoccupied with being admired, which can then be seen in excessive attempts to be liked and loved, while we are likely to avoid any situations that would disavow us. Because we have to continually maintain our personal sense of self, we all suffer from a lack of basic security in life.

Fear that our life-story will be disconfirmed

Identification with the personal sense of self may also appear in fear that our self-narrative will be disconfirmed or challenged. The personal sense of self is very vulnerable, as it is a story with which we are identified. It has the potential to become unstable, and we may fear that we might lose it. The possibility of any change in our narrative may disrupt our sense of predictability, identity, con-sistency, and stability (Erskine et al., 1999). We may become very aware of even the slightest attempt at disconfirmation of our self-narrative and try to maintain it at any cost. Because of identification with our story, we feel that rejection or dis-approval of our story means rejection of ourselves. Someone may, for example, feel threatened by the negative comments of others or may fear some imagined criticism stemming from a life-story related to "I am worthy, only if I am perfect". Positive change may also be feared, for example, a person with the self-narrative "I am a bad person, not worthy of love" may end a relationship with a person who is loving and kind.

Existential loneliness and feelings of separation

The personal sense of self gives us an experience of substantial and independent self-existence, that we are essentially separate and different from other people. Because of this, we may feel that we are fundamentally alone in the world and that nobody really understands us. Existential writers have described these feelings as existential loneliness that is related to the awareness of one's separateness from other people and nature (Ettema et al., 2010). It may also appear in fears of dying.

Identification with the personal sense of self can also be seen in self-isolation and identification with our suffering. It may prevent us from seeing what is common to all humanity – that all people sometimes suffer and experience pain (Neff, 2003b) – leaving us with the feeling that we are the only one who is suffering. Being merged with our self-narrative prevents us from experiencing self-compassion and from realising that we are all fundamentally interconnected (Hanh, 1998).

Loss of present moment and experiential avoidance

Because of identification with the personal sense of self, we may also lose contact with the present moment. We may feel guilty or ashamed because of our past experiences. A frequent example of this is the person who has a story that they have to be "strong", and who is then self-critical for feeling weak or not confident. We may also become preoccupied with the future, desiring things which could enhance our self-narrative and fearing things which might challenge it. When we are identified with our self-narrative, we will also avoid both internal and external experiences contrary to our narrative. The person in our last example may, for instance, avoid feelings of insecurity and weakness in order to maintain their narrative requiring them to be strong.

Ordinary unhappiness and the pursuit of happiness

We consider that many problems of human society can be understood from the perspective of identification with a personal sense of self and our continual attempts to maintain it. Because of attachment to the personal sense of self, people are suffering and are experiencing ordinary unhappiness. This means that our normal human condition is not happiness, bliss, and peace, but rather the constant flux of both pleasant and unpleasant experiences. At the level of our personal sense of self, we can never really be at peace, as our story has to be maintained at any price. Because of this, we don't feel a basic sense of safety. Threats to our story can appear in fear, sadness, shame, and rage. Even though affirming our personal sense of self may be experienced in temporary happiness, pride and a sense of achievement, these states are only temporary.

Harris (2007) describes how we live in a culture of "happiness". Our culture exists on the assumption that mental health is a natural state of the human being.

We try to pursue happiness and ease and feel that something is wrong with us if we do not find it. Experiencing pain and suffering is often viewed as pathological with the belief it should be eliminated by pharmaceutical drugs or psychotherapy. However, the avoidance of pain may make the pain worse and is connected to many mental health problems (S. C. Hayes et al., 2012).

This view is congruent with the core philosophical assumption of our approach – it is part of being human to experience ordinary unhappiness. This ordinary unhappiness is part of our human condition and is related to identification with the personal sense of self. We are "not guilty" for being in this state, it is simply a natural state of being human. This proposition helps us to develop a different approach towards ordinary unhappiness. Instead of attempting to avoid suffering and to "do" something to become happy, we advocate the importance of self-compassion and mindful awareness of our ordinary unhappiness. The aim is to come into contact with the *observing self* and become a loving witness to our pain and suffering.

Life-script as a dysfunctional aspect of our self-narrative

While self-narrative as a story about our life is a relatively new concept in psychology, in the field of psychotherapy it is not new. Berne (1961) wrote about life script as an "an extensive unconscious life plan [that] determines the identity and destiny of the person" (p. 23). In integrative psychotherapy, the life-script is one of the central constructs describing the unconscious and limiting part of our life stories (Erskine, 2015).

Erskine (2010) defines life scripts as a

> set of unconscious relational patterns based on physiological survival reactions, implicit experiential conclusions, explicit decisions and/or self-regulating introjections, made under stress, at any developmental age, that inhibit spontaneity and limit flexibility in problem-solving, health maintenance, and in relationship with people.
>
> (p. 91)

This definition implies that life-scripts are developed because of ruptures in contact between the person and significant others. The person develops unconscious relational patterns as a way of coping with the stress caused by failures in significant relationships. These unconscious patterns inhibit spontaneity and flexibility in life.

In terms of relational schemas, the life script is related to networks of dysfunctional relational schemas (G. Žvelc, 2010c). Life script describes dysfunctional and defensive aspects of our self-narrative. While it is clinically useful to distinguish between healthy and non-healthy aspects of our life story, we think it is important to bear in mind that even a "healthy" self-narrative is limiting as we describe in the previous chapter. Even if our life story is not based on trauma and neglect, the very nature of the personal sense of self is constricting. Regardless of whether our self-narrative is harmful and damaging or whether it is more positive, attachment to it prevents us from being truly autonomous (Berne, 1967) and psychologically flexible (S. C. Hayes et al., 2012).

The self-narrative system as a diagnostic and treatment planning tool

In integrative psychotherapy and transactional analysis, the concept of the racket/ script system is used as a diagnostic and treatment planning tool (Erskine, 2015; Erskine & Moursund, 1988; Erskine & Zalcman, 1979). It is defined as a "self-reinforcing, distorted system of feelings, thoughts and actions maintained by script bound individuals" (Erskine & Zalcman, 1979, p. 53). It describes how we live our life script in daily life and how our life script is continually reinforced. The script system is very useful in psychotherapy when the aim is to analyse and change the content of the client's script.

We think that the concept of the script system describes not only the nature of our life script but also the reinforcing nature of the personal sense of self. As we have already proposed, the personal sense of self is a system which has to be continually reinforced in order to maintain itself. Based on these ideas, we have adapted the original script system (Erskine, 2015; Erskine & Moursund, 1988; Erskine & Zalcman, 1979) and developed the *self-narrative system*, which can be used for understanding not just the more pathological but also the healthy aspects of our self-narrative (see Figure 7.1). The model is consistent with the relational schema theory and can be used as a model for diagnosis and treatment planning. The self-narrative system describes various elements of our self-narrative and relational schemas, their activation and reinforcing experiences. The self-narrative system could be defined as a *self-reinforcing, lived and embodied life-story, which gives the experience of identity and continuity of existence.*

The self-narrative system describes how we continually maintain our story through:

- Living according to our life-story and reinforcing experiences that maintain the story.
- Remembering the past and imagining the future that is consistent with our story.
- Avoidance of experiences that are not congruent with our story.
- Enactments in relationships – we act in a way that draws others into reinforcing our story.

Figure 7.1 presents an example of the self-narrative system in the case of Anna. It shows three interconnected elements of the self-narrative system: (1) Internalised self-narrative, (2) Lived and embodied experience, and (3) Reinforcing experiences.

INTERNALISED SELF-NARRATIVE	LIVED AND EMBODIED EXPERIENCE	REINFORCING EXPERIENCE
Relational Schemas: **Self:** I'm not worthy of love. I am not important. **Others:** Other people are more important. **Quality of Life:** Life is empty of love.	**Behaviour:** Avoids intimate relationships. Pleases and adapts to others. Works hard. Speaks silently with little eye contact. Avoids conflict and confrontation.	**External Events:** Boss does not recognise my hard work and praises a co-worker. My boyfriend abandons me after three months of being together.
Autobiographical Memories:	**Verbal Narratives:** I am not made for relationships. I am a kind person.	**Internal Experiences:** Criticising myself for the loss of my boyfriend.
Mother and father ignored me – I felt invisible. Brother is more important for parents. Father was humiliating me and joking about me being fat. Father distant. Mother criticising me for being lazy. Grandmother telling me that I am kind and a "good" girl.	**Emotions:** Anxiety, shame, loneliness, emptiness. **Body Experience:** Frequent headaches. High blood pressure.	
Experiential Avoidance: **Emotions:** Anger, sadness, dignity and pride.	**Fantasies and Expectations About the Future:** Meeting a perfect man – a soulmate on my holidays and having a wonderful time with him. I will die alone.	
Body Sensations: Difficulties with feeling body sensations.	**Remembering Autobiographical Memories:** Being alone as a child.	
Needs: Being close, seeking support.	**Dreams:** Recurring dreams related to being alone, waiting and searching for someone.	

Figure 7.1 The self-narrative system of Anna[1]

Internalised self-narrative

The first column presents the core elements of the internalised self-narrative: relational schemas, autobiographical memories, and experiential avoidance.

Schemas about self, others and quality of life describe our central personal story of how it is to be in relationship with others and the world. Schemas about self describe our conceptual identity and are expressed in the words: "I am …". These schemas often unconsciously organise and influence our daily life. Schemas can be negative as with a person who believes that she is bad and unworthy, or can be positive ("I am good looking", "I am competent", "I am healthy"). Schemas about self are connected to schemas about others, which represent generalisations of experience of other people ("Other people are mean"). Internalised self-narrative also includes schemas that express our generalised experience of the quality of life ("Life is hard", "Life is meaningless").

Clinical psychology and psychotherapy have usually focused on a negative self-concept as a focus of treatment. Negative self-concept is indeed related to many psychological difficulties. However, we think that positive self-concept can also be limiting. Think, for example of a woman, who has the belief "I am competent and good looking" based on her experience of parents who were admiring her as a child. This concept of self can help the person to be successful in her work and to feel attractive in relationships with other people. However, because the personal sense of self has to be maintained, this belief can compel her to think that she must be successful in what she does and may be afraid of making a mistake at work. She may try to engage in activities that show her competence and may neglect other areas of life, which are also meaningful (like being with her family). She may try to look impeccable and good looking and be afraid of negative comments about how she looks or dresses. When getting older and finding her first grey hairs or seeing the first wrinkles on her face, she may be devastated, fearing that her belief that she is "good looking" is being undermined. This illustrates how attachment to our positive beliefs may manifest in fears that we may lose them. The personal sense of self is not something pathological; it is something we all have. We are all in the same boat regarding the limitations of our personal sense of self and the possible suffering that comes with it.

Autobiographical memories refer to specific explicit memories, which are the basis for our identity and life-story. Core relational schemas and autobiographical memories are interrelated. For example, Figure 7.1 describes the self-narrative system of Anna, who developed a relational schema that she was not worthy of love and that other people were more important than her. This was based on her autobiographical memories of her parents ignoring her and giving more importance to her brother.

Experiential avoidance describes the process of avoidance of emotions, body sensations, and needs in order to maintain the self-narrative and to protect the person against unpleasant experiences. By identifying with certain aspects of our life-story, we inevitably try to avoid other specific experiences which are incongruent with our self-narrative. In the case of Anna, she was avoiding feelings of sadness and anger and had difficulties in feeling her body sensations. She was also avoiding her needs for intimacy and support.

Lived and embodied experience of the self-narrative

The second column of the self-narrative system describes our lived and embodied experience of our self-narrative. The self-narrative is expressed through our behaviour, in the stories that we tell to others, emotions, body experiences, and dreams. We live our life story through the fantasies, expectations about the future, and our memories of the past, which are congruent with our self-narrative. We are our life-story, and this story is expressed in our subjective experience and behaviour. Anna, for example, was living her belief that she was not worthy of love and that other people were more important, by avoiding close relationships, pleasing others, and working hard. In therapy, she often expressed this, saying that she was not made for relationships. In her relationships with other people, she experienced anxiety related to fears of not being accepted and being unimportant. She often felt emptiness and loneliness. When she felt lonely, she often reflected on being alone all her life and having fantasies that she would die alone. She also had recurring dreams related to being alone.

Reinforcing experiences

Lived and embodied experience of our self-narrative can manifest in experiences that reinforce our self-narrative and related schemas. The personal sense of self needs constant reinforcement in order to maintain its stability, continuity, and predictability. Reinforcing experiences can be both external events that reinforce the self-narrative or internal experiences. Anna, for example, would talk very quietly and had little eye contact. Because of her appearance and behaviour, she was often overlooked. Even though she was an excellent worker, her boss did not recognise that and praised her co-workers instead. These experiences reinforced her self-narrative that she was not important and that other people are more important than her. Her boyfriend also abandoned her. She criticised herself, saying that she was guilty for her boyfriend leaving, as she was too cold and critical of him. Both internal criticism and abandonment reinforced her self-narrative related to "not being worthy of love".

Beyond ordinary unhappiness

We have described how the personal sense of self is an expression of our self-narrative. There is also another sense of self existing in the background behind all of our experiences – the observing/transcendent self. It is awareness itself that is the perceiver of all our experiences. This awareness is not identified with concepts, thoughts, emotions, and body sensations. It is simple awareness that we are, that we exist. It is a sense of being, a sense of presence. This awareness could be described as pure awareness, as it is not identified with the contents of awareness. It is the context of all our experiences. While we use the word "self" for this experience, it is not self in the usual conceptual sense. It is an experience of ourselves as awareness itself, which is non-conceptual. It is experienced as our own awareness, something we have always been and which is present in all of our experiences (Josipovic, 2019). In Chapter 3, we describe how the observing/transcendent self is a crucial aspect of ourselves that is the basis of psychological health and healing. This experience of self is described by different names in philosophy, different spiritual traditions, and modern psychology. In spiritual traditions, this aspect of ourselves is often described as the essential self, spiritual self, no-thing self, or simply as Self. We understand the observing self as the essential self (Salvador, 2019), which has spiritual qualities. Our clients and students often describe the experience of the observing self with words such as: "like it is always there", "peace", "sense of meaning", "being fully present", "sense of safety – everything is OK", "like a universe".

From personal sense of self to the observing self

Although we have described both main senses of self as if they are separate, they are in reality interconnected and intertwined. The observing/transcendent self is the ground of all of our experience. When we are identified with the personal sense of self, we are not aware of the observing self. We are "looking" through the lenses of the personal sense of self. The observing self is always present in the here and now, even though we may not be aware of it. Many different spiritual traditions aim at recognising awareness as a ground of all experience.

In our ordinary human state, the observing self is attached to and identified with a personal sense of self. This view is congruent with different spiritual traditions, which have described how suffering is the result of attachment to our "name and form", to our "ego". Different spiritual and mystical traditions describe the personal sense of self as illusory. Buddhist psychology for example "identifies the persistent illusion of a separate, enduring self as a primary source of psychological distress" (Engler & Fulton, 2012, p. 177). People suffer because they mistakenly take their self as "real". Albahari (2006) has proposed a "two-tiered" illusion of self, based on Buddhism and Advaita Vedanta. The first tier of the illusion is that the person's awareness identifies with the bounded self. Because awareness itself is inherently unbounded, it cannot be the bounded self that it takes itself to be. From this perspective, the self as distinctly separate and unique is a mental construct and illusory (Albahari, 2014). The second tier of the illusion is that the bounded self, which is a construct, takes itself to be unbounded awareness. However, a personal sense of self is constructed in relationships and cannot be an unconstructed self.

In terms of our theory, "I" as awareness is identified with the personal sense of self. We could say that awareness "dresses" in the clothes of personality. The original meaning of the word *persona* is connected to the masks worn by actors. We may say that we identify with the mask we wear. The phrase "I am" signifies awareness itself. It describes a simple sense of "being" without being tied to forms. However, as the personal sense of self develops, we identify with the contents of awareness such as emotions and beliefs and our self-narrative. We say: "I am Peter, I am a depressed person, I have no luck …". "I am" becomes identified with different contents which appear in awareness. Contact with the observing self helps us to decentre from our personal sense of self and recognise the observing self as awareness itself. This helps us to develop a new relationship with the personal sense of self, based on mindful awareness and self-compassion. By being a loving witness in relation to our personal sense of self, we may overcome ordinary unhappiness and radiate qualities of peace, compassion, and wisdom.

Whilst most approaches to psychotherapy are focused on changing different aspects of our self-narrative, acceptance and commitment therapy (ACT) has proposed an alternative to this idea (S. C. Hayes et al., 1999, 2012). The goal of psychotherapy in ACT is not changing the story itself, but developing a new relationship with our story – to become less attached to the story itself. We think this is one of the significant contributions of this approach to psychotherapy. In MCIP, we also embrace this new paradigm (See Table 7.1).

Table 7.1 Acceptance oriented versus change oriented paradigm

Old change oriented paradigm	Negative self-narrative is the source of the problem. The goal: change of self-narrative.
New acceptance oriented paradigm	Both positive and negative aspects of the self-narrative are limiting, causing ordinary unhappiness. The goal: mindful awareness and compassion of self-narrative. Change of self-narrative paradoxically happens through acceptance of what is.

In MCIP, we invite our clients to activate their observing self and then to form a new relationship with the personal sense of self, based on mindful awareness and compassion. We think that even if mindfulness and compassion are not aiming to change the self-narrative, changes in our self-narrative often happen as a by-product of accepting awareness and compassion. When clients start to see themselves from a different perspective, and they bring love and compassion to their experiences, this may act as a new experience, which has the power to change their self-narrative and related relational schemas.

Note

1 Adapted from *Relational patterns, therapeutic presence: Concepts and practice of integrative psychotherapy* (p. 124), by R. G. Erskine, 2015, Karnac Books. Copyright 2015 by R. G. Erskine. Adapted with permission.

8 The multiplicity of mind, states of consciousness, and treatment planning

The idea that the self is unified and whole has been challenged by a number of psychotherapy authors, neuroscience research, and spiritual traditions such as Buddhism. Although we usually experience ourselves in our everyday life as unified and whole, this experience can be described as an illusion (Bromberg, 1996; Safran & Muran, 2000; D. J. Siegel, 1999). Bromberg (1996), for instance, suggests that the experience of a unitary self is "an acquired, developmentally adaptive illusion" (p. 515).

The personal sense of self consists of various self-states that are, in healthy functioning, integrated and give us an experience of continuity and a coherent sense of self. Our experience of self is the flow of different states that are more or less integrated into the whole. From this perspective, the personal sense of self can be viewed as a system of different states. During our day, we are likely to experience many different self-states, according to different situations and contexts. We may be, for example, in an anxious state of self, when we are talking to our boss. When we come home and talk with our children, we may be in a nurturing self-state, and in the evening we may be in a "playful sexy state" with our wife. All these different self-states serve different functions in everyday life. Berne (1961), for example, described controlling, nurturing, problem-solving, adapted, and natural ego states. Schwartz (1995), in his internal family system therapy, described parts of self, such as exiles, managers, and firefighters. The idea of the multiplicity of mind has been part of psychotherapy practice for many years and has been described through different concepts, and given different names such as subpersonalities (Assagioli, 1965/1993), ego states (Berne, 1961), self-states (Bromberg, 1996), parts (Schwartz, 1995; van der Hart et al., 2006), or states of mind (D. J. Siegel, 1999).

In Chapter 6, we describe how activation of relational schemas is seen in different self-states. Self-states are patterns of phenomenological experience and behaviour that are related to moment-to-moment activation of relational schemas. In healthy personality development, we are usually only momentarily aware of individual self-states and their realities because each of them functions as part of our cohesive identity (Bromberg, 1996). In a healthy personality "each self-state is a piece of a functional whole, informed by a process of internal negotiation with the realities, values, affects, and perspectives of the other" (Bromberg, 1996, p. 514).

D. J. Siegel (1999) from a neurobiological point of view, similarly argues that the idea of a "unitary, continuous 'self' is an illusion our minds attempt to create" (p. 229). He proposed that we experience many different states of mind that are clusters of activity of the brain at any given moment in time. With repeated activation, states of mind develop "into a specialized, goal-directed set of cohesive functional units" (p. 230) that he defines as self-states.

Ego states, integrating Adult, and mindfulness

Eric Berne developed a unique and influential theory of ego states (Berne, 1961, 1966, 1967, 1972) that is based on psychoanalytic ego-psychology and object relations theory. Berne (1972) defined "ego-states as coherent systems of thought and feeling manifested by corresponding patterns of behaviour" (p. 11). He described three main ego states: Parent, Adult, and Child ego states. There are different models of ego states in transactional analysis, such as functional and structural models (Stewart & Joines, 2012; Trautmann & Erskine, 1981). In integrative psychotherapy, the concept of ego states is based on Berne's (1961) original structural model, which provides a comprehensive model for treatment planning and interventions (O'Reilly-Knapp & Erskine, 2003). In this model, Child ego states are the manifestation of the *archaeopsyche* and refer to patterns of thoughts, feelings, and behaviour from previous developmental phases. An Adult ego state is the manifestation of the *neopsyche* and refers to current patterns of thoughts, emotions, and behaviour adapted to current reality. Parent ego states refer to manifestations of the *exteropsyche* and describe thoughts, emotions, and behaviour introjected from significant others. In this model, only the Adult ego state presents a healthy state of mind adapted to the current situation and congruent with the person's developmental age. Parent and Child ego states represent non-integrated states, which are split off from the neopsychic ego. This model of ego states is referred to as the "integrating Adult" model (Summers & Tudor, 2014b; Tudor, 2003), where the goal is the integration of exteropsychic and archaeopsychic states into the neopsychic ego. Erskine (1991) described the Adult ego state as consisting "of current age-related motor behavior; emotional, cognitive and moral development; the ability to be creative; and the capacity for full contactful engagement in meaningful relationships" (p. 66). The Adult ego state functions "without the intrapsychic control of introjected parent or archaic Child ego states" (Erskine, 2015, p. 237).

Tudor (2003) further expanded this concept and described the integrating Adult as present-centred and as a continual process of integration. The Adult ego state is characterised by a "pulsating personality, processing and integrating feelings, attitudes, thoughts and behaviors appropriate to the here-and-now—at all ages from conception to death" (p. 201). Tudor (2003) described the following characteristics of the integrating Adult: autonomy, relational needs, consciousness, reflective functioning, critical consciousness, maturity, motivation, and spirituality.

G. Žvelc (2010c) further developed this theory of the integrating Adult with his concept of the mindful Adult. He proposed that mindfulness is a feature of the

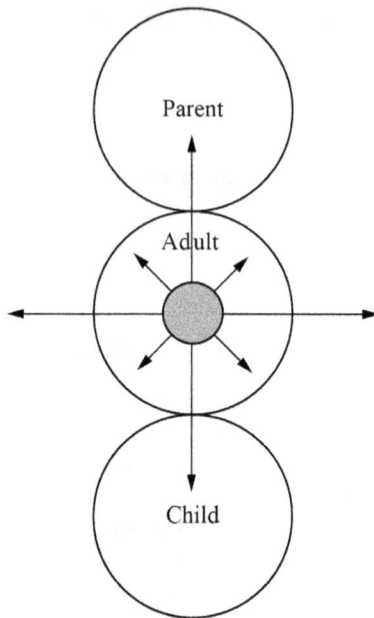

Figure 8.1 Mindful Adult
Source: "Relational Schemas Theory and Transactional Analysis" by G. Žvelc, 2010, *Transactional Analysis Journal*, *40*(1), p. 19 (https://doi.org/10.1177/036215371004000103). Copyright 2017 by Taylor & Francis Ltd. Reprinted with permission of the publisher (Taylor & Francis Ltd, http://www.tandfonline.com).

integrating Adult that is crucial for the integration process. Figure 8.1 illustrates the mindful Adult model of ego states, with the central inner circle representing the mindful Adult, which refers to mindful awareness. The arrows from the mindful Adult illustrate the mindful awareness of Parent, Adult, Child ego states and the external environment.

In MCIP, we have further developed and integrated the model of the integrating Adult with the theory of the personal sense of self and observing self. It became clear to us that mindfulness is not a property of the Adult ego state, but refers to the observing self. Parent, Adult and Child as "states of ego" are related to the personal sense of self. In the next subchapter, we describe how the model of Four States of Consciousness (FSC) provides integration of the integrating Adult model of ego states with the theory of the personal sense of self and the observing self.

The model of the Four States of Consciousness (FSC)

In the previous chapters, we present in detail the concepts of the observing self and the personal sense of self. However, the question remains, how the observing self and personal sense of self are related, and how can the observing self promote transformational change and well-being? We want to address this through the development of a new model that we call the model of the Four States of Consciousness (FSC) which is based on the integration of concepts of ego states with our theory of the personal sense of self and observing self. In the FSC model, we talk about self-states, which is a term more congruent with our description of relational schemas and the concept of the personal sense of self. We use the term ego state when referring to the theory of transactional analysis and the term self-state when referring to our specific model.

The FSC is a model of the human psyche that explains:

1   The structure and functioning of the personal sense of self in terms of self-states.
2   The relationship between the observing self and self-states.
3   Different states of consciousness: restrictive state of consciousness, Adult state of consciousness, mindful state of consciousness, and nondual awareness.

The FSC model is based on the integrating Adult model of ego states, developed by M. James and Jongeward (1971/1996), Erskine (1988), Tudor (2003), G. Žvelc (2010c), and Summers and Tudor (2014a, 2014b). In this model, Adult refers to present-centred states, whereas Child and Parent refer to non-integrated aspects of ourselves. In his elaboration of the integrating Adult model of ego states, Keith Tudor proposed the "two ego states model" (Summers & Tudor, 2014b). In this model, he distinguishes between present-centred relating which manifests in health and past-centred relating that is connected to pathology. He distinguishes between two main ego states: present-centred ego states (*Neopsyche*) and past-centred ego states (*Archaeopsyche*). The archaeopsyche consists of introjected Parent ego states and archaic Child ego states since both ego states are historical in origin. We find Tudor's classification of ego states very thoughtful and congruent with our own relational schemas theory in which there are two main categories of self-states: self-states that are the manifestation of adaptive relational schemas, and self-states that are the manifestation of dysfunctional relational schemas. Based on Tudor's ideas (Summers & Tudor, 2014b), we propose that the personal sense of self can function in two main modes: integrating Adult self-mode and past self-mode.

Integrating Adult self-mode describes our current present-oriented self, which is adapted to the current situation and congruent with a person's developmental age. This mode is connected to adaptive relational schemas and manifests in self-states that are adaptive to the present moment – Adult self-states. These states are continually integrated and enable healthy functioning.

Past self mode is related to our past self-states, which are not adapted to the current situation and are related to earlier developmental periods. Past self-mode is the manifestation of dysfunctional relational schemas and consists of non-integrated, dissociated, or introjected self-states. These self-states developed because of unbearable traumatic experiences, which could not be tolerated and integrated into the Adult self. These self-states were defensively dissociated or introjected. The past self-mode consists of archaic Child self-states and intro-jected self-states.

Figure 8.2 illustrates the Four States of Consciousness model (FSC). It presents the interrelationship between the observing self and personal sense of self with its two modes: integrating Adult and past self-mode. The observing self is represented by the central sphere and the personal sense of self with the two rings around it.

The outer ring represents the past self-mode with its archaic Child and intro-jected self-states. The inner ring represents the integrating Adult self-mode, which includes a number of overlapping circles showing the constant process of integration, which is based on Tudor's (2003) illustration of the integrating Adult. The integrating Adult consists of self-states that are related to the present situation and are continually updated based on current experiences. The observing self is shown in the centre of the model with rays (illustrated by straight arrows) pointing outwards in different directions. These rays symbolise the observing self being mindfully aware of Adult self-states and past self-states. The horizontal rays pointing out beyond the outer ring represent mindful awareness of the environment. The model also includes an arrow of the observing self pointing back at itself, which is awareness of awareness itself.

This illustration of the observing self is similar to our diamond model of the observing self, where the observing self is illustrated in the centre, with rays pointing out in different directions (see Figure 3.1, Chapter 3). As we describe in Chapter 3, an important influence on the development of the illustrative figure of the diamond model of the observing self was D. J. Siegel's (2007, 2018) visual metaphor of the *wheel of awareness*, where the central hub of the wheel describes

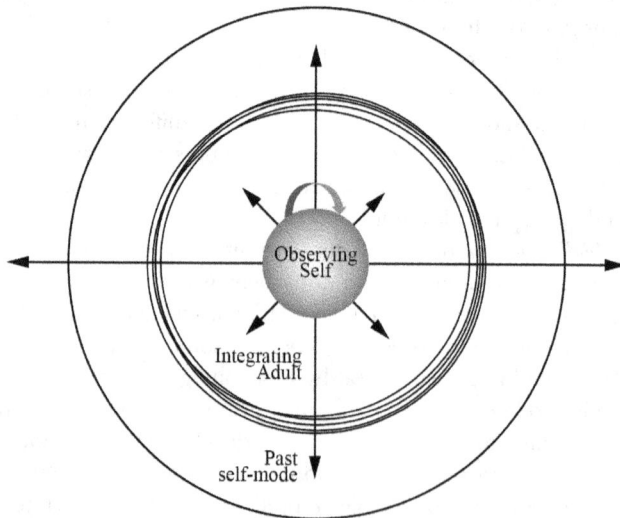

Figure 8.2 The model of the Four States of Consciousness (FSC)

the experience of being aware, while the rim represents the elements of awareness.

In the following sections, we describe different elements of the model. First, we describe the structure and functioning of the personal sense of self: past self mode and integrating Adult self-mode. Then we focus on the observing self and the four different states of consciousness.

Past self-mode: Archaic Child self-states and introjected self-states

The outer ring in Figure 8.2 represents past self-mode which is connected to the activation of dysfunctional relational schemas. There are two main poles of relational schemas: the schema of the self and the schema of the other (G. Žvelc, 2010c). "The schema of the self refers to aspects of how we experience ourselves, and the schema of the other refers to how we experience the other person" (G. Žvelc, 2010c, p. 10). Past self-states can appear either as self-states stemming from identification with the "self pole" of the dysfunctional relational schema or the "other pole" of the schema. In line with transactional analysis and integrative psychotherapy (Berne, 1961; Erskine, 1988; O'Reilly-Knapp & Erskine, 2003; Tudor, 2003), we propose two main categories of such self-states: *archaic Child self-states* and *introjected self-states*. Activation of schemas of the self is seen in archaic Child self-states and activation of the schemas of the other in introjected self-states. In transactional analysis and integrative psychotherapy, they are colloquially referred to as Child and Parent ego states.

Archaic and introjected self-states are actually not separated states, but are interconnected (Little, 2006). They are both manifestations of dysfunctional relational schemas that are structures of relationship and not of the separate experience of self and other. G. Žvelc (2010c) describes how Child and Parent states are manifestations of different poles of the same dysfunctional relational schema: the schema of the self and the schema of the other. Congruent with Little (2006) we could describe archaic Child and introjected self-states as "self-states relational units". When one self-state is observed, we should also look for the other part of the unit (Little, 2006). Both states can be either experienced intrapsychically or attributed to other people or situations.

Archaic Child self-states and introjected self-states are historical in origin, psychologically inflexible and limit our adaptive functioning. We do not feel safe in these states and activation of these states is seen in either hyperarousal or hypoarousal of our ANS. When we are identified with these states, our consciousness is in the "restricted" state.

Archaic Child self-states

Activation of the schema of self in dysfunctional schema units appears in an experience of archaic Child self-states. In transactional analysis and Erskine's integrative psychotherapy these states of self are defined as Child ego states, that is, fixated emotions, thoughts, and behaviour from previous developmental phases

(Berne, 1961; Erskine, 1988, 1991). When these self-states are activated, we behave, think, and feel in the same way as we did in the past. Even though it may appear that we are reacting to the current situation, we are actually experiencing the world with the capacities of a child on the developmental level of unresolved traumatic experience (Erskine & Moursund, 1988). Erskine (1988) describes Child states as "the entire personality of a person as he was in a previous developmental period of time" (pp. 16–17). This may include needs, physical sensations, defence mechanisms, emotions, thoughts, and behaviour.

For example, our client Cathy was sexually abused by her uncle when she was 11. During therapy, her Child self-state would sometimes reappear related to that abuse. In such moments she felt frozen, young and speechless. She had difficulties in communicating and was withdrawn from contact with the therapist. She was in a state of immobilisation, related to re-experiencing the trauma of the abuse.

Child self-states are the result of traumatic experiences that were not processed and integrated. Because of the person's inability to tolerate such experiences, they were dissociated as separate states of self. Child self-states are therefore dysregulated and related either to hyperarousal or hypoarousal of ANS. Although these self-states are often from our early childhood, they can also be from other times in our lives, as traumatic experiences can occur during any developmental period (Erskine, 1988). We may, for example, display the experiences and behaviour of a nonverbal infant, three-year-old child, or confused adolescent. Although in psychoanalytic terms, re-experiencing the past is related to the concept of regression, we think that regression is not the most appropriate term, since the person is not returning to the past. It is, in fact, just the opposite. Self-states, which are the result of unresolved traumatic experiences, reawaken in the present through activation of dysfunctional relational schemas. They represent reawakening of the past in the present.

Introjected self-states

Introjected self-states result from identification with the schema of the "other person" in the dysfunctional relational schema unit (G. Žvelc, 2010c). When we identify with the schema of the other person, our sense of self becomes the other as represented in the relational schema. We may feel, think, and act as we experienced one of our significant other people in the past.

In both transactional analysis and Erskine's integrative psychotherapy, these states correspond to Parent ego states that were developed as a result of introjections of significant other people. Parent ego states are "an actual historical internalization of the personality of one's own parents or other significant parental figures as perceived by the child at the time of introjection" (Erskine, 1988, p. 17). Introjected contents are often irrational and coloured by the child's experience of authority. They may remain in our personality as a foreign body and are unaffected by later learning (Erskine & Moursund, 1988). They are non-integrated introjects and not adaptive to the current situation. Although useful, the metaphor "Parent ego-state" can be limiting as a person can have various introjects related to different significant people. So, for instance, people can have introjected self-states such as "angry priest self-state", "abusing neighbour", "depressed sister", "critical teacher", or "humiliating peer".

In our model, introjected self-states are related to activation of the dysfunctional schema of the other person. As dysfunctional schemas are not updated and represent rigid structures, the schema of the other person could be described as an introject. Although we find the word "introject" clinically useful, it is important to keep in mind that there is nothing that is taken from outside to inside. These schemas are developed from the inside – they are a child's experience of significant others (Stern, 1995). Introjects are our experiences of significant others that become part of our personality structure. When we identify with these schemas, we experience these self-states as "I".

Introjected self-states can function as active self-states or as an intrapsychic influence (Berne, 1961; Erskine & Moursund, 1988). An active manifestation of introjected self-states means that people behave and experience the world as they experienced their parents or other significant figures in the past. In couple therapy, for example, one husband criticised his wife in the same way his father used to humiliate him and his mother. He used similar words and gestures. He told her that she was lazy and incompetent in taking care of the house. In this example, an introjected self-state manifested as an active state directed at the wife. In the case of the intrapsychic influence of an introjected self-state, the person may react towards themselves in the same way as their parents or other authority figures had once behaved towards them. The husband from the previous example also humiliated himself as he was humiliated by his father and was saying to himself, "You are useless!". In such a case, both Child and Parent self-states are activated at the same time, the Child who experiences the humiliation and feels shame, and the Parent, who is inflicting humiliation.

Trauma and development of dissociated and introjected self-states

Archaic Child and introjected self-states may exist on different levels of integration. We understand dissociation on a continuum stemming from nearly "normal" phenomena to pathological dissociation that is seen in dissociative disorders (Bromberg, 1996). We can say that we all have some unresolved experiences that appear in past self-mode and corresponding archaic and introjected self-states. However, in a healthy personality these states are part of our verbal self-narrative. They are part of our adaptive illusion of continuity, as Bromberg (1996) describes it. Even though these states are not necessarily adaptive to the present moment, they are accepted as part of our identity – the personal sense of self. We can, for example, describe ourselves as a person who sometimes becomes very angry and is capable of humiliating other people. Although this may not be an aspect of ourselves that we particularly like, it is, nevertheless, still part of our sense of self – of "who we are". But there can also be some experiences that we experience as "not me" that are dissociated to such an extent they are excluded from our verbal self-narrative. Someone may, for example, not remember the time when they were acting abusively to their partner or may have an experience that at that moment they were not themselves. These experiences are part of dissociative disorders.

Integrating Adult self-mode

The personal sense of self can also function in integrating Adult self-mode, which refers to present-oriented self, congruent with a person's developmental age and situation in the here-and-now. In Figure 8.2, this is represented as the inner ring, which symbolises the integrating Adult self-mode. Adult self-mode refers to current thoughts, emotions, and physical sensations adapted to the current reality. In Figure 8.2, the outer edges of the integrating Adult ring are illustrated with a number of overlapping circles, which symbolically describe the "integrating" nature of this self-mode.

While past self-mode relates to our historical experiences, related to dysfunctional relational schemas, integrating Adult mode is connected to adaptive relational schemas. In integrative psychotherapy, integrating Adult self-mode presents a healthy adaptation to life's present circumstances. Introjected and archaic self-states represent re-awakening of experiences from the past that are not adapted to the current situation. They were adaptive in the past as a creative way of coping with unbearable situations; however, in the present, they are dysfunctional. They are the source of many symptoms and problems with which clients come to psychotherapy. Introjected and archaic self-states are self-states that are not integrated with our Adult personality, presenting non-processed and undigested experiences, which were developed and are maintained because of defence mechanisms. Dissociation and introjection were "normal" responses to non-normal circumstances, but in the present they limit our flexibility and choice.

One of the goals of integrative psychotherapy is wholeness and integration of personality, meaning here the integration of introjected and archaic self-states into Adult self-mode. This does not mean that self-states will cease to exist. Integration means that parts of self are in this process transformed, and take on new functions that are congruent with the integrating Adult. Integration means harmony and coherence of the *personal sense of self*. Ideally, the *personal sense of self* would function only in integrating Adult self-mode, where all dissociated and introjected self-states would be integrated (Erskine & Moursund, 1988; Erskine, 1988). Tudor (2003), in this sense, proposes an expansion of Adult functioning to include previously dissociated and introjected self-experience.

When something happens to us that is outside of our normal experience, we may feel the pain and unpleasant emotions connected to that event.

Peter, for example, worked as a nurse in a hospital. One day he found one of his patients had hanged themselves. He was deeply shaken by the experience and experienced lots of fear and sadness. He talked about the experience with his co-workers and with his therapist. He managed to stay with the experience and tolerate its intensity. He cried deeply during psychotherapy sessions and accepted the emotions of helplessness that "he could not save him". He even dreamt about the event. After a few weeks, he was able to process the experience and integrate it into his personal sense of self. The experience was assimilated as a "sad story that happened in the past".

Mindful awareness is crucial in this integrating process. It enables the person to be present with a painful experience without avoidance or merging. Mindful awareness also brings the person into the window of tolerance and related ventral vagal system that is crucial for processing and integration.

If a person cannot tolerate their painful experience, dissociation will follow, and the experience will not be assimilated in the Adult self-mode. It becomes a separate part, which is not integrated with the Adult personality. Cathy, who experienced abuse at 11, never talked about it. Her uncle had threatened her that he would kill her mother if she did, so she remained silent and alone with enormous pain she could not process and integrate.

Our personal sense of self may be better or less well integrated. The integrated self is seen in an experience of coherence and continuity of self-states. The process of integration can be described as the continual process of assimilation and accommodation of our relational schemas, and with it the separate self-state becomes part of our sense of self, which is welcomed and accepted by other self-states. In this process, the previously dissociated self-states re-organise and transform.

Observing self and the Four States of Consciousness

The observing self is in Figure 8.2 represented by the central sphere. Illustrating the observing self in the centre symbolically shows that the observing self is our *essential self.* In spiritual traditions, it is often described as *inner essence, heart, spiritual sun,* or *centre of ourselves.* Even though we have illustrated the observing self in the centre, the observing self cannot be localised as it is the perspective through which we are aware and conscious (Deikman, 1982; S. C. Hayes et al., 2012). The observing self is ever present, behind every experience, as a sense of "being" and "existing". It is within every self-state, both Adult or past self-states. However, when we are identified with a particular self-state, then we "become" that self-state and look from its perspective, unaware of the observing self, and our consciousness is limited.

The FSC model describes four primary states of consciousness: (1) Restricted consciousness, (2) Adult state of consciousness, (3) Mindful state of consciousness, and (4) Nondual awareness. The first two states are related to our ordinary consciousness of the personal sense of self, where the observing self is identified with the personal sense of self. The remaining two are more or less free of identification with the personal sense of self.

In Figure 8.2, the outer ring is related to restricted consciousness, the inner ring to the Adult state of consciousness, and the central sphere to the consciousness of the observing self, which can manifest in either mindful state of consciousness (straight arrows pointing in different directions) or nondual awareness (arrow pointing back at the observing self). The inner and outer rings act like filters through which we view ourselves, others, and the world. The distance from the centre symbolically illustrates states of consciousness in terms of restrictiveness. The further we are from the centre, the more restricted our consciousness becomes and our perceiving is less clear. The distance from the centre also represents the degree of the multiplicity of the mind. The restricted consciousness of the outer ring is related to the highest degree of the multiplicity of the mind that appears in non-integrated self-states. In contrast, the nondual awareness of the central sphere is related to a sense of oneness where there is no multiplicity.

Restricted consciousness

The outer ring in Figure 8.2, represents the most limited state of consciousness, which is related to the identification of the observing self with the past self-mode and its archaic or introjected self-states. In this state, we look at ourselves and others through the prism of dysfunctional schemas and react to current stimuli based on archaic or introjected self-states. This restricted state of consciousness is related to the highest degree of the multiplicity of the mind which manifests in separate and non-integrated self-states.

"Living" in the past self-mode is the source of suffering and is related to the clinical problems with which many clients come to therapy. In terms of the autonomic nervous system, the restrictive state of consciousness is related to defensive autonomic states that manifest in hyperarousal or hypoarousal of the autonomic nervous system. At the most severe end of the continuum, there are clients who have suffered complex trauma, and experience altered states of consciousness related to dissociation, such as depersonalization, derealisation, identity alterations, and interruptions in awareness (Lanius, 2015). Restricted consciousness is here related to severe discontinuity and lack of integration in terms of the four dimensions of consciousness: time, thoughts, body, and emotions (Lanius, 2015).

Adult state of consciousness

This state of consciousness is related to the identification of the observing self with Adult self-states and their related adaptive relational schemas (inner ring in Figure 8.2). In this state of consciousness, we perceive ourselves, other people and the world from the perspective of adaptive relational schemas. The consciousness of the Adult self-mode, in comparison to restrictive consciousness, is flexible and adaptive, as our adaptive relational schemas are open for change and are continually updated. Compared to restrictive consciousness, the Adult state of consciousness is related to a lesser degree of multiplicity and appears in greater integration and continuity of consciousness.

Living in the Adult self mode is an essential goal in psychotherapy. Compared to past self-mode, which is related to hyperarousal or hypoarousal of ANS, the Adult self-mode is also related to the social engagement system and functioning within the window of tolerance. This enables social connection and compassion.

The Adult state of consciousness is also related to accurate neuroception (Porges, 2017).

The Adult state of consciousness has its virtues and shortcomings. Even though this state of consciousness is one of the main goals of psychotherapy, it is nevertheless still related to ordinary unhappiness, as we remain identified with our self-narrative and related schemas. It is predominantly related to the "doing" mode (Segal et al., 2002) and what Fromm (1976) describes as the "having mode". Šumiga (2019) in his analysis of Fromm's work, describes how modern society is dominated by this having mode, which is seen in egocentric possessiveness of objects, people, or ideas.

Mindful state of consciousness

The mindful state of consciousness is an essential state of consciousness related to the observing self. It is related to pure awareness and is the most direct, as we do not perceive through the filters of our self-states and we are not identified with them, being able to observe both past and current self-states from a decentred perspective. In comparison to the Adult state of consciousness, mindful awareness is related to the "being" mode (Segal et al., 2002) – awareness and acceptance of "what is". In this state of consciousness, we relate to our experience in a fundamentally different way – in the present moment, with acceptance and decentred perspective (see Chapter 3).

In terms of the multiplicity of mind, the mindful state of consciousness is experienced as a continuous and integrated stream of awareness. When we are in this state of consciousness, we experience ourselves as a whole, even though there is a slight separation between "us" who are aware and the contents of our awareness.

In Figure 8.2, the mindful state of consciousness is represented as rays pointing from observing self to the external environment, Adult self-mode, and past self-mode – the rays symbolically representing processes of the present moment, acceptance, and decentred perspective. When we are in contact with the observing self, we are a "loving witness" to our experience. Rays of mindful awareness pervade our experience and nourish it with awareness, acceptance, and love. The left and right rays portray mindful awareness of the external environment. This manifests in an experience of mindful presence and present moment awareness of what is happening in our environment. For example, someone walking in the forest may experience nature more fully, seeing colours more vividly, feeling the air on their skin and the scent of flowers nearby – almost as if for them nature is more "alive". They don't have to change anything; in touch with nature, they can just "be".

The arrows pointing from observing self to the past self-mode describe mindful awareness of the archaic Child self-states and introjected self-states. For example, a person can mindfully observe, even when their introjected self-state related to "mistrust" is activated. They can decentre and observe with curiosity thoughts such as "don't trust men, they will disappoint you". Or they can observe their

Child self-state related to fear of abandonment. The arrows pointing towards the integrating Adult self-mode portray mindful awareness of different Adult self-states. Such states are manifested by present-centred thoughts, feelings, and physiological reactions that arise from moment to moment. The person in the gym may, for example, be mindfully aware of sensations in their body such as pain in their thigh muscles, pleasure in doing exercise, and satisfaction at being part of the gym group.

In MCIP, one of the main process goals is to invite the client into a mindful state of consciousness. During the therapy session, the therapist continually invites the client to activate this state of consciousness and bring mindful awareness to their experience.

Nondual awareness

Figure 8.2 also shows the arrow pointing from the observing self back onto itself. This illustrates mindful awareness of awareness itself. It refers to the recognition of the nondual nature of awareness. As we describe in Chapter 3, awareness itself cannot be localized; it is without boundaries and all-encompassing. Recognition of the nondual nature of awareness manifests in this fourth state of consciousness: nondual awareness. It is found in spiritual experiences such as a sense of inter-connectedness and oneness with others and the world. Josipovic (2019) describes nondual awareness as the "foundational aspect of consciousness, consciousness itself alone without any other phenomenal content, an empty awareness that is non-conceptual and without subject-object structuring, hence nondual" (p. 275). Nondual awareness appears to the conceptual mind as empty of any reification, as awareness without thoughts, emotions, body, space, time, and the usual sense of self (Josipovic, 2019). Josipovic (2019) proposes that nondual awareness is conscious of itself without the mediation of concepts and representations. This suggests one property of nondual awareness is non-conceptual reflexivity in contrast to the "ordinary" Adult state of consciousness, which depends on concepts. Josipovic (2016) proposes that love and compassion are intrinsic properties of nondual awareness. When nondual awareness is realised, love and compassion arise spontaneously as part of authentic being.

The concept of nondual awareness has become in recent years the subject of scientific discourse and research (Fucci et al., 2018; Hanley et al., 2018; Josipovic, 2010, 2014, 2016, 2019; Krägeloh, 2018; Mills et al., 2018; Vieten et al., 2018). While there is considerable research on mindful awareness, there is only a small amount of research investigating nondual awareness. Josipovic (2014) researched Tibetan Buddhist practitioners, who were experienced in the nondual form of meditation. He describes how nondual meditation increases functional connectivity between intrinsic and extrinsic networks in the brain, which may be related to subjective accounts of "decreased fragmentation of experience into subjective versus objective or self versus other" (Josipovic, 2014, p. 16). The mindful state of consciousness is in comparison to nondual awareness manifested in the subtle dualism of experience where there is this "I" being aware of the internal and external environment. In nondual awareness, we recognise that at the level of the observing/transcendent self, we are not separated from each other and the world – we are the universe itself.

Phases in mindfulness- and compassion-oriented integrative psychotherapy

The model of the Four States of Consciousness can serve as a guide for treatment planning in MCIP, which proceeds in phases that orient our psychotherapy work. Figure 8.3 presents the phases of MCIP and specific therapeutic tasks that are fundamental to each phase. Therapeutic tasks include different interventions that encourage and facilitate the particular psychotherapy process. Even though therapeutic tasks are related to specific phases, most of the tasks are important throughout the whole therapeutic process. For example, developing an attuned relationship, the therapeutic alliance, developing mindful capacity, and promoting self-regulation are essential in all phases of therapy. The phases often do not proceed in linear order and can also be interlinked. During the psychotherapy process, we often have to attend to previous phases, or we may work with several phases simultaneously. Phases are meant to be guidelines for the psychotherapist and should not be used rigidly.

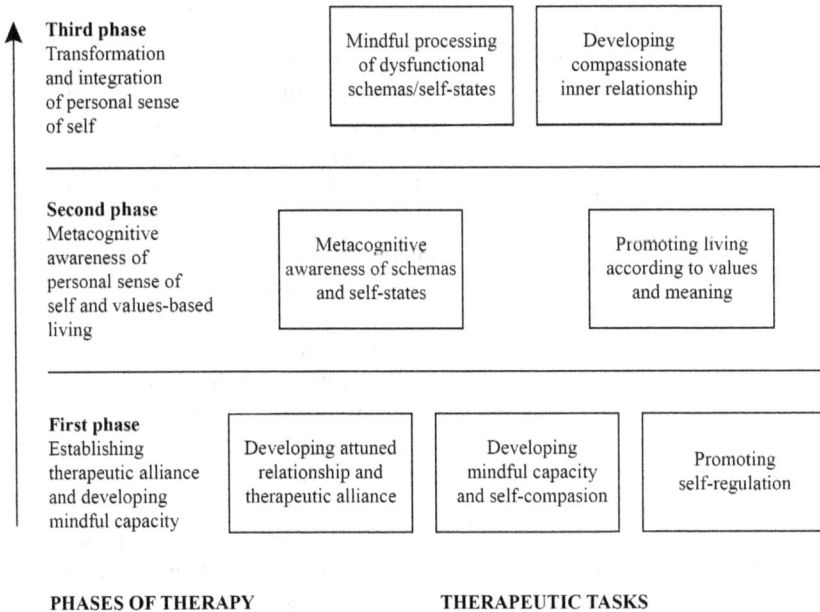

Third phase
Transformation and integration of personal sense of self

| Mindful processing of dysfunctional schemas/self-states | Developing compassionate inner relationship |

Second phase
Metacognitive awareness of personal sense of self and values-based living

| Metacognitive awareness of schemas and self-states | Promoting living according to values and meaning |

First phase
Establishing therapeutic alliance and developing mindful capacity

| Developing attuned relationship and therapeutic alliance | Developing mindful capacity and self-compasion | Promoting self-regulation |

PHASES OF THERAPY   **THERAPEUTIC TASKS**

Figure 8.3 Phases of MCIP and related therapeutic tasks

The first phase: Establishing therapeutic alliance and developing mindful capacity

In Chapter 7, we describe how most people live in a state of *ordinary unhappiness* which is the result of identification with the personal sense of self. We live our life more or less unconsciously according to our life-story. Our life is driven by our beliefs about ourselves, memories of the past and hopes and fears for the future. The suffering related to ordinary unhappiness increases when people identify with various archaic and introjected self-states. Specific internal and external triggers may activate past self-states, and the person "becomes" that self-state. In this case, we are not reacting to the present reality, but according to old experiences and preconceptions that colour our perceiving. This is a state of restrictive consciousness, related to the outer ring in Figure 8.2. Many of our clients constantly live in the "outer ring", identified with various past self-states that are activated by different internal or external triggers. In this state, we are not living our life – our life is "lived". For example, our client Nina started to feel helpless and speechless whenever somebody raised their voice. This was a trigger that activated her Child self-state when she experienced physical abuse by her father. Identification with archaic and introjected self-states is seen in psychological inflexibility and lack of autonomy.

The state of restrictive consciousness is related to the lack of mindful awareness. People have difficulties staying in the present moment and in establishing a witnessing stance towards their experience. They are either distanced or merged with their experience. They usually want to get rid of certain aspects of themselves, such as negative beliefs and painful memories. They lack self-compassion and are often extremely critical of themselves. In terms of the autonomic nervous system, they are dysregulated and suffer from emotional and physiological dysregulation, displaying either hyperarousal or hypoarousal.

In this phase of therapy, there are three main tasks: (1) Developing an attuned relationship and therapeutic alliance, (2) Developing mindful capacity and self-compassion, and (3) Promoting self-regulation. These tasks are fully elaborated in Chapters 9, 10, and 11.

Developing a secure and trusting relationship and therapeutic alliance are the prerequisites for all other therapeutic tasks and are essential throughout the whole therapeutic process. Inquiry, attunement, and involvement provide the compassionate therapeutic relationship, which invites clients into the exploration of their inner world (Erskine, 2019c; Erskine et al., 1999). Mindfulness processes and compassion are gradually introduced through contact in a therapeutic relationship. Clients with the help of an attuned therapeutic relationship develop mindful awareness of their experiences and aspects of the personal sense of self. An attuned relationship and mindful awareness are also essential for the regulation of the client's emotions and physiology. The aim is the regulation of the client's dysregulated states, which helps clients to activate their social engagement system (Porges, 2011, 2017). The task of self-regulation is essential throughout the whole therapeutic process, as clients often present dysregulated autonomic and emotional states.

The second phase: Metacognitive awareness of the personal sense of self and values-based living

In the second phase of therapy, the goal is to develop metacognitive awareness of the personal sense of self and to start living according to one's deepest values and aspirations. In terms of the model of the Four States of Consciousness, this corresponds to increasing the client's ability to stay in Adult self-mode and enhancing their capacity for mindful awareness. The second phase of therapy is related to two main tasks: (1) Metacognitive awareness of schemas and self-states and (2) Promoting living according to values and meaning. These two tasks are fully elaborated in Chapter 10.

Dimaggio et al. (2015) describe how metacognition involves "human ability to understand one's own and other's mental states, as well as the ability for reflection and mastery" (p. 33). In our model, metacognitive awareness refers to the ability to decentre from our self-states and schemas and to reflect on how these structures shape our lives and relationships with other people and the world. This results in greater inner freedom and psychological flexibility. Metacognitive awareness is in our model connected to the observing self and the related processes of mindful awareness and mentalisation (see Chapter 2).

Metacognitive awareness helps clients to develop insight into and understanding of their personal sense of self. This is related to the growing *ability of mentalisation*. Clients start to understand and become aware of different self-states and activation of these states in response to internal and external stimuli. They start to differentiate between their past self-states and Adult self-mode, which is our present related self.

For example, Nina understood that her response to the angry feelings of other people triggered her experience from the past when she was physically abused. She also started to understand that when she identified with her abused Child self-state, she perceived other people as dangerous, even if they were just acting assertively. She came to realise that she often looked at other people from the perspective of her frightened and helpless Child self-state.

Metacognitive awareness and related mentalisation help clients to reflect upon the impact of their self-states on both their experience and interpretation of other people. Metacognitive awareness is also related to the growing capacity for being in the mindful state of consciousness. Clients gradually become a *loving witness* in relation to their experience, instead of being merged or distanced in relation to self-states and schemas. They start to differentiate the observing self from self-states and schemas. From the position of observing self they can mindfully observe various self-states and dysfunctional schemas. This helps them to become less identified with their archaic and introjected self-states. When those states are activated, clients can relate to them with a decentred perspective, openness, and acceptance. This helps clients to stay in Adult self-mode, even if archaic and introjected self-states are activated.

For example, at the end of this phase of her therapy, Nina could stay in her Adult self-mode, even if people were talking loudly and appeared angry. She could observe how she was sweating, her heart beating and the heat in her body. At the same time, she had clear awareness that she was re-experiencing a memory from the past. She could stay in Adult self-mode and react accordingly, even though her archaic Child self-state was activated. In Figure 8.2, this is illustrated by the inner ring symbolising the Adult state of consciousness.

Metacognitive awareness is also crucial for the second task in this phase – *living according to one's values and meaning.* In MCIP, we do not focus only on the problem and our clients' difficulties in life, we are also curious about the client's values that give meaning and purpose to their life. Metacognitive awareness promotes living according to one's values, as clients become less identified with their past self-states and dysfunctional schemas. We invite the client to go beyond the symptoms and imagine a life lived in contact with meaning and purpose. With the help of a therapist, clients can focus on what is important to them and start to live a more meaningful life.

At the end of this phase, clients show greater stability, have better self-regulation skills and can stay more easily in the present moment. In terms of the FSC model, clients start to live in integrating Adult self-mode (see Figure 8.2). Contact with the observing self and mindful state of consciousness also help clients to undermine attachment to the personal sense of self. However, in this phase, archaic and introjected self-states are not yet integrated. In times of higher stress, a person can still identify and react from these states. The difference is that the person can quickly recognise these shifts and come back more quickly to the Adult self-mode, as these states no longer exert so much power over an individual. This is related to increased psychological flexibility and a lessening of symptoms, which is a highly desirable goal in psychotherapy and is, for example, the main goal in acceptance and commitment therapy.

The third phase: Transformation and integration of the personal sense of self

In this phase of therapy, the goal is transformation and integration of the personal sense of self. In terms of the FSC model, the clients are in this third phase more grounded in a mindful state of consciousness, which helps to transform the personal sense of self. This phase is related to memory reconsolidation and results in an in-depth psychological change. There are two main tasks related to this phase: (1) Mindful processing of self-states and dysfunctional schemas and (2) Developing a compassionate inner relationship. Mindful processing is fully elaborated in Chapter 12 and developing a compassionate inner relationship in Chapter 13.

Although integrative psychotherapy uses various methods and techniques for processing, in MCIP we give primacy to the processes of mindful awareness and compassion. Mindful awareness and compassion can transform our personal sense of self. They not only help us become less attached to our life-story, but they are also at the heart of the processes of change. Mindfulness and compassion processes are essential for the processing of traumatic memories and transformation and integration of dissociated and introjected self-states. They help us also to transform our restricted life-story. In this way, they promote the integration of the personal sense of self.

The *task of mindful processing* refers to the processing and integrating of disturbing experiences and self-states with the help of mindful awareness. G. Žvelc (2012) proposed that "mindfulness promotes natural healing of the organism, where the change comes spontaneously by acceptance and awareness of internal experience" (p. 46). Mindful awareness promotes acceptance of experience, which was previously avoided. In Chapter 6, we describe how mindful awareness may be essential for the process of memory reconsolidation. When, for example, Child self-states are activated and we embrace them with acceptance and kindness, this may promote a new experience that is juxtaposed with old emotional learning that these states are dangerous and need to be avoided. This experience promotes their integration.

The second task of this phase refers to *developing a compassionate inner relationship*. In this phase of therapy, the client is more in contact with the observing self, which is seen in greater compassion for themselves and others. From the position of the observing self, clients can actively engage with different Child and introjected self-states. With the help of the therapist, they can acknowledge their existence, validate their function, and normalise their experience. They start to understand and acknowledge the pain and suffering of different self-states. In this way, clients are able to develop compassion for their self-states that were split-off, which can promote their integration. Our client Nina gradually started to develop compassion for her helpless Child self-state, who experienced abuse. Step-by-step her Child self-state started to feel more secure and integrated with the rest of her personality. One of the tasks of this phase of therapy is therefore the development of a new internal relationship between the observing self and various self-states. Such internal relationship is based on compassion and love for different self-states. Through this process, the personal sense of self is transformed and becomes more integrated.

Figure 8.4 represents the goal of MCIP – the integrated personal sense of self, where archaic and introjected self-states have been integrated into the Adult self-mode. We are aware that this is an idealised goal and that most of us will have

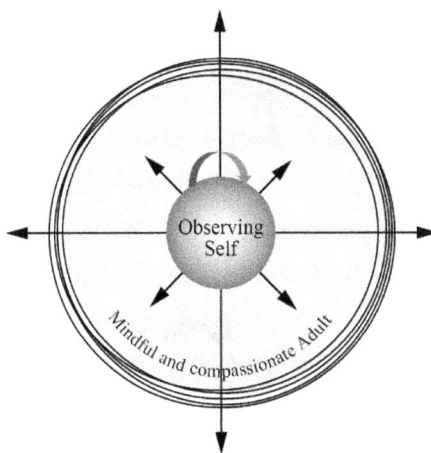

Figure 8.4 The integrated personal sense of self and observing self

certain self-states that are not integrated; however, these states can be tolerated and self-regulated by the observing self. The aim in this phase is to develop a harmonious inner world, in which the observing self is differentiated from our personal sense of self, although in a dynamic relationship with it.

Figure 8.4 also represents the transformed Adult self-mode. The observing self not only promotes the integration of past self-states but transforms the Adult self-mode as well. Xiao et al. (2017) write that mindfulness practice can change the self. They describe such a changed self as the *mindful self*. With greater mindfulness and compassion, personality can be changed at the level of beliefs, emotions, behaviour, physiology, and brain functioning. Through mindfulness and compassion, people become calmer, more peaceful, compassionate, and show qualities of equanimity. We describe such a transformed personal sense of self as the *mindful and compassionate Adult*. The processes of mindfulness and compassion become personality traits. Such a person shows greater ability to be in the present moment, is more compassionate, accepting, and displays signs of inner wisdom. This person also realises that the personal sense of self can never become perfect or in a state of permanent happiness, developing insight into the *ordinary unhappiness* of a personal sense of self, which means living with human limitations. From this perspective, they can be more compassionate towards their limitations and failures. They can also experience a greater connection with other people and understand that they cannot be perfect, and in this way they may eventually stop trying to change other people in order to perfect them.

Beyond three phases: Spiritual development and nondual awareness

Even if we are living in an integrating Adult self-mode and our life is not troubled by past self-states, we are still living in what we call *ordinary unhappiness*, identifying with our life-story. In some people, a deep-seated desire for spiritual growth is awakened, and they may start to search for a deeper meaning of life. In psychotherapy, this is usually seen in a greater focus on themes related to spiritual development. This potential fourth phase is usually not the domain of psychotherapy but is an intrinsic part of different spiritual traditions.

Historically, mindfulness and compassion have been part of different spiritual traditions, and their primary goal was not an enhancement of the personal sense of self, but non-attachment to self or ego (Hanh, 1998; Malachi, 2005). Nondual spiritual traditions also propose that behind our everyday experience, there is nondual awareness, which we describe as the observing/transcendent self. The goal of spirituality in these traditions is to recognise nondual awareness as a ground of being (Albahari, 2006; Ganesan, 2017; Josipovic, 2019; Malachi, 2004, 2005). In Figure 8.4, this is shown by the arrow pointing back at the observing self. Grounding in nondual awareness may present this potential fourth phase of MCIP.

Even though we propose this potential fourth phase of therapy related to spiritual development, we must emphasise that spiritual experiences are often present in all phases of therapy. As MCIP is focused on enhancing mindful awareness and compassion, spiritual experiences often spontaneously emerge. Contact with the observing self is often related to experiences of deep connection with the essence, a sense of oneness, with feelings of trust, meaning, and inner peace. Spiritual experiences often occur when the client makes a profound and compassionate connection with their own vulnerability and is open to contact with the compassionate therapist.

What is the role of the therapist during this phase? We think that the role of the psychotherapist is to be open for any spiritual issues that may emerge during psychotherapy. Whilst the psychotherapist is not a spiritual teacher, it is important that the client is heard and understood regarding the spiritual dimension. This opens the way for an authentic I–Thou relationship, which may have a spiritual quality. We also see the role of the therapist in helping the client to integrate spiritual experiences with everyday life. Some clients have the idea that the goal of spiritual development is detachment from personal identity in a way that may be harmful. Some clients start to neglect their physiological needs or try to retreat from the world. We think that this "spiritual bypassing" can create an imbalance in our daily living. People have numerous roles in the world and have to function in different contexts. Detachment from a personal sense of self can create an illusion of being above all this. We think that the observing self has to be embodied and lived through our personal sense of self. In our opinion, healthy spirituality involves a transformation of the personal sense of self, and an ongoing relationship between the observing/transcendent self and personal sense of self. The spiritually minded therapist may help the client to integrate the spiritual path with everyday living.

Having described the main concepts, theories, and phases of MCIP, we now turn to the third, practice-oriented part of the book. The concepts and theories of the MCIP provide us with a solid foundation for our understanding of the therapy process and the use of mindfulness and compassion-oriented methods and interventions.

Part III

Methods and interventions

9 Methods of relational mindfulness and compassion

In this chapter, we describe the fundamental methods of relational mindfulness and compassion that are crucial in all phases of MCIP and are important for all of the therapeutic tasks described in Chapter 8. Methods of relational mindfulness and compassion integrate the processes of mindfulness and compassion with the *keyhole model* developed by Erskine and colleagues (Erskine & Trautmann, 1996; Erskine et al., 1999; Erskine, 2015) (see Figure 9.1). The keyhole model is a comprehensive model of the relational methods of integrative psychotherapy that describes three fundamental methods: *inquiry, attunement,* and *involvement.* These methods provide an in-depth relational model that invites the client into contact with self and others and promotes the integration of split-off parts of self.

The fundamental assumption underpinning the methods of relational mindfulness and compassion is that mindfulness and compassion can be developed and facilitated within an attuned relationship. In this way, our model differs from other approaches that use mindfulness and compassion primarily as techniques to be learned and used by the client. In our approach, the therapist, through the power of a mindful and compassionate therapeutic relationship, acts as a guide for the client to embody present moment awareness, a decentred perspective, acceptance, and self-compassion. The therapist embodies these qualities themselves and relates to the client from the position of the observing self. Through the power of such a mindful and compassionate relationship, the client brings qualities of mindfulness and compassion into their life and to their self-states.

Our model combines the power of the attuned therapeutic relationship with the processes of mindfulness and compassion. The synergy of both creates a powerful healing relationship in which both processes are mutually enhanced. An attuned therapeutic relationship is essential for clients to feel safe to attend to their inner world with mindful awareness and compassion. The mindful and loving presence of the therapist provides the context of safety, which enables the clients to relax their defences and dive deep into their experience. The processes of mindfulness and compassion enhance the relational processes. If both the client and the therapist are mindfully present, this will have an impact on the relationship itself. Such a relationship is characterised by aliveness, vitality, presence, and a sense of interconnection. It may be evidenced in moments of meeting, of deep I–Thou contact (Buber, 1999).

Mindfulness and compassion processes

INQUIRY

INVOLVEMENT

Phenomenology	Awareness	Acknowledgement
History/expectations	Acceptance	Validation
Coping/choices/decisions	Self-compassion	Normalisation
Vulnerability	Observing self	Mindful presence

Relational   Developmental   Cognitive   Rhythmic   Affective   Physiological

ATTUNEMENT

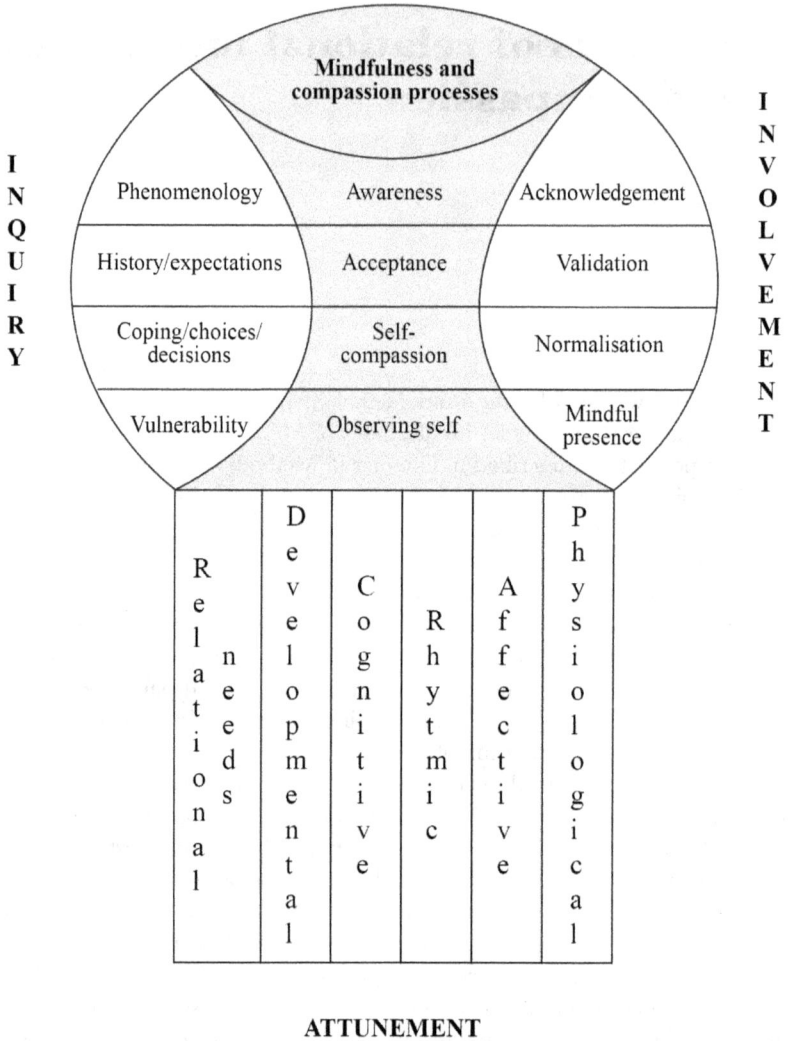

Figure 9.1 Keyhole model of relational mindfulness and compassion
Source: Adapted from *Beyond empathy: A therapy of contact-in-relationship* (p. 159), by R. G. Erskine, J. P. Moursund, and R. L. Trautmann, 1999, Brunner/Mazel. Copyright 1999 by Taylor & Francis. Adapted with permission of the publisher (Taylor & Francis Ltd, www.tandfonline.com).

Meditation practices are often used to develop mindfulness and compassion. As research shows, such practices are beneficial for mental health and can be very useful for clients and for progress generally in psychotherapy (Goldberg et al., 2018, 2019; Khoury et al., 2013). For some clients, however, meditation practices are challenging and may not be appropriate, especially if they are suffering from a severe traumatic experience or are experiencing high distress. Many people have difficulties in bringing mindful awareness to painful experiences during their meditation practice. It may not be so challenging to be mindfully aware of positive, neutral, or even mildly negative stimuli, but when we are in contact with a painful and traumatic experience, we may quickly lose our witnessing stance and move out of the window of tolerance. We may start to dissociate or become flooded by unpleasant emotions and thoughts. Metaphorically, we can say that it is difficult to be alone in hell. Methods of relational mindfulness and compassion provide a new context in which "two aware minds are more powerful than only one" (G. Žvelc, 2012, p. 47). By adopting these methods, the client is not left alone with their painful experiences. The mindful and loving presence of the therapist helps the client to attend to them with curiosity, openness, acceptance, and love (D. J. Siegel, 2007). When two people are together and one is becoming lost, the first one can help the other to be found again. The therapist helps the client to be in the present moment, to adopt a decentred perspective, to accept their experience, and to bring compassion to their self-states. Inquiry, attunement, and involvement (Erskine et al., 1999) are the main methods that invite the client into mindful awareness and compassion.

Keyhole model of relational mindfulness and compassion

Figure 9.1 shows the keyhole model of relational mindfulness and compassion, which is an adaptation of Erskine's original keyhole model (Erskine et al., 1999). It illustrates the processes of mindfulness and compassion connected to the relational methods of integrative psychotherapy: *inquiry*, *attunement* and *involvement* (Erskine et al., 1999).

Over the years of using Erskine's model of the keyhole with our clients and teaching it to our students, it became clear to us that these methods enhance processes of mindfulness and compassion. As this was not explicit in the original keyhole model, we decided to connect interventions related to inquiry and involvement to the processes of mindfulness and compassion. In the centre of the diagram (see Figure 9.1), we have added the main processes of mindfulness and compassion: awareness (present moment and decentred perspective), acceptance, self-compassion, and the observing self. Each process is related to the corresponding interventions of inquiry and involvement that promote the described process. Awareness is related to phenomenological inquiry and acknowledgement. Acceptance is related to the inquiry into history/expectations and validation. Self-compassion is related to the inquiry regarding coping strategies and the intervention of normalisation. And finally, we have added the observing self that is related to the inquiry into the client's vulnerability and the therapist's mindful presence. We have also redefined Erskine's concept of *presence* as *mindful presence*, to make explicit the connection between the therapeutic presence and mindfulness.

In the original keyhole model, interruptions to contact were listed in the centre of the diagram: existence, importance, resolution, and the self (Erskine et al., 1999). In our adapted model, we have exchanged interruptions to contact for the processes of mindfulness and compassion, to show how the processes of mindfulness and compassion are connected with the corresponding methods of inquiry and involvement. In this way, the whole model of relationally focused therapy becomes centred on the facilitating processes of mindfulness and compassion. By making these processes central, this also opens the way for further integration of mindfulness- and compassion-oriented interventions with the relational methods of integrative psychotherapy.

We would like to emphasise that changes to the original model do not invalidate the original model, quite the contrary. We think that adding processes of mindfulness and compassion to the model complements the original model. Mindfulness and compassion processes enhance contact with self and others and are an antidote to the interruptions to contact listed in the original model.

In the original model, there were only five aspects of attunement listed. We have also added *physiological attunement* as an important facet of the attunement process that is crucial in MCIP. It enables the therapist to synchronise with the client's physiology, expand the awareness of physiological processes (both in the client and themself) and accordingly respond in terms of physiological regulation.

Inquiry and involvement: Methods for enhancing mindful awareness and compassion

On the left side of the diagram is the *inquiry* method, and on the right side is the *involvement* of the therapist. Inquiry and involvement are the two main relational methods for inviting the client into the present moment, decentred awareness, acceptance, and self-compassion. With inquiry, we invite the client to explore their experience (Erskine et al., 1999). Through this process of phenomenological inquiry, the client becomes increasingly aware of their current experience and its connection with related past experiences and expectations about the future. It also involves an exploration of the client's protective mechanisms and the vulnerability that lays behind the defences.

The therapist not only inquires about the client's current experience, but also provides an involved response that acknowledges, validates, and normalises the client's experience (Erskine et al., 1999). Involvement is an expression of the therapist's full internal and external contact (Erskine et al., 1999). It is "the result of the therapist being fully present, with and for the person, in a way that is appropriate to the client's developmental level of functioning" (Erskine, 2015, p. 18). This underlines the importance of the mindful presence of the therapist and their responsiveness based on genuine interest and attunement to the client.

Involvement is conveyed by *acknowledgement, validation, normalisation* and *presence.* With involvement, the therapist invites the client to be fully present with their experience. With *acknowledgement*, the therapist invites the client to become aware of their experience, with *validation* to accept the experience and with *normalisation* to develop compassion for themselves. The therapists' *mindful presence* invites the client to come into contact with the observing self; to become a loving witness to all of their experiences. The interventions related to involvement invite the client into present moment awareness, acceptance of their experience, self-compassion, and contact with the observing self.

Attunement as a foundation for mindfulness and compassion

At the base of the diagram (see Figure 9.1), is the therapist's *attunement*, which provides the foundation and texture for all methods and interventions.

Erskine and Trautmann (1996) give the following definition of attunement:

> It begins with empathy – that is, being sensitive to and identifying with the other person's sensations, needs, or feelings – and the communication of that sensitivity to the other person. More than just understanding or vicarious introspection, attunement is a kinesthetic and emotional sensing of the other – knowing his or her rhythm, affect, and experience by metaphorically being in his or her skin, thus going beyond empathy to provide a reciprocal affect and/or resonating response.[1]

In this definition, attunement goes beyond empathy (Erskine et al., 1999). It starts with empathy, with deep sensing of the client, and then proceeds further through a resonating response. For instance, if the client is feeling scared, the therapist will provide the reciprocal response of security that will be mirrored in the therapists' gaze, facial expression, tone of voice, and gestures that all communicate safety. In this process, the therapist is not merging with the client. For effective attunement, the therapist has to be aware of the boundary between themselves and the client (Erskine et al., 1999). They also have to decentre from their own experience, so that they can be present with the client. While words may be important in conveying attunement, nonverbal communication is the primary channel through which attunement is expressed.

Erskine et al. (1999) have described different aspects of attunement: cognitive, affective, rhythmic, and developmental. We have added to this list physiological attunement that is crucial for physiological regulation (see Figure 9.1).

Cognitive attunement

Cognitive attunement goes beyond a simple understanding of the contents of the client's narrative and the client's meaning-making processes. It involves a deep immersion into the client's frame of reference to understand the client's unique way of thinking and logic. It is profound listening to the client's use of words and implicit messages the client is unconsciously communicating.

Affective attunement

Affective attunement involves empathic sensing of the client's affect and responding with reciprocal affect (Erskine & Trautmann, 1996). For example, the therapist responds to the client's sadness with compassion or the client's expression of joy with vitality and expressions of pleasure.

Rhythmic attunement

Rhythmic attunement refers to sensitivity to the client's rhythm and tempo and responding accordingly. It involves pacing the rhythm of the therapy to facilitate the optimal processing of both internal and external stimuli (Erskine & Trautmann, 1996). For facilitating the processes of mindfulness and compassion, the therapist and client must slow down and give time and space for "being" with experience. Rhythmic attunement also promotes regulation of the client's autonomic nervous system.

Developmental attunement

Developmental attunement refers to understanding the developmental level of the client and responding to the client in a way that is sensitive to the client's developmental age at a particular point in therapy. Clients may manifest different archaic Child self-states from different developmental periods, usually from early childhood. With developmental attunement, the therapist looks through the eyes of the "child" of the client and tailors therapeutic interventions based on that understanding.

Attunement to relational needs

Attunement to relational needs involves responding to relational needs that emerge in the course of the therapeutic relationship (Erskine & Trautmann, 1996). This means that the therapist adapts and responds flexibly to the client's relational needs. For example, when there is a *need for authenticity*, the main task would be to establish a sense of safety, validation, and respect for the client's uniqueness. When there is a need for *shared experience*, the therapist may selectively disclose their personal experience (see Chapter 4).

Physiological attunement

We propose that physiological attunement is another crucial aspect of attunement that is essential in our approach to integrative psychotherapy. It refers to attunement to the client's autonomic nervous system. Physiological attunement is sensing the physiological arousal of the client and providing the corresponding response. If the client's physiological state is regulated, then the therapist's adaptive response is physiological synchronisation. If the client is in a hyperarousal or hypoarousal of ANS, then the therapist should stop the physiological synchronisation and lead the client towards physiological regulation. In Chapters 5 and 11, we present the detailed theoretical and practical implications that highlight the importance of physiological attunement and physiological regulation in MCIP.

Inquiry, attunement, and involvement all go hand in hand in promoting the client's mindful awareness and self-compassion. The keyhole model of relational mindfulness and compassion provides a useful map for applying the methods of MCIP in clinical practice. In the following pages, we will describe how relational methods facilitate the main processes of mindfulness and compassion: present moment awareness, decentred perspective, acceptance, and self-compassion.

Inviting the client into present moment awareness

The process of present moment awareness is facilitated by *phenomenological inquiry* and *acknowledgement* of the client's experience (see Figure 9.1).

Phenomenological inquiry

Phenomenological inquiry is a process of "respectful exploration of the client's phenomenological experience" (Erskine, 1993, p. 186) that invites the client into present moment awareness. Inquiry invites the client to explore their experiences through questions and by the therapist's nonverbal communication, expressed with gestures, facial expression, and tone of voice that communicate to the client interest in knowing their experience (Erskine et al., 1999). Inquiry starts with the premise that the therapist knows nothing about the client's experience and that the client can teach the therapist so that they can explore it together (Erskine et al., 1999). In the process of inquiry, the therapist is open to the client's particular experience and decentres from their own assumptions and expectations. The fundamental principle is that the therapist is free of any expectations, preconceived ideas, and goals for the client (Erskine, 2015). The therapist is there for the client bringing curiosity, genuine interest, and respect in relationship with the client. The therapist is like an empty vessel to be filled with the client's phenomenology while simultaneously remaining in full contact with themselves (Erskine, 2001).

Phenomenological inquiry is focused on the client's moment-to-moment experience. The therapist in this process, while following the client and their phenomenological experience, also leads them based on their curiosity and internal felt experience. The purpose of such inquiry is primarily for the client and not the therapist (Erskine et al., 1999). The aim is for the client, through respectful inquiry, to discover aspects of themselves that they were previously not aware of (Erskine et al., 1999). In this way, inquiry increases present moment awareness and contact with self and others.

We think that for effective inquiry, it is essential for the therapist to be in contact with the observing self and to bring qualities of mindful awareness and compassion into the therapeutic relationship with the client. They have to be fully present and attuned to their own and to their client's ongoing experience. In terms of the *triangle of relationship to experience* (see Chapter 3), the therapist adopts the witnessing stance towards both their own and their client's experience, which involves present moment awareness, decentred perspective, and acceptance.

Erskine et al. (1999) describe how inquiry involves for each client many different experiential areas including physical sensations, physical reactions, emotions, memories, thoughts, conclusions and decisions, meanings, expectations, hopes, and fantasies. We would also add to this list inquiry connected to the spiritual dimension. This involves inquiry about clients' values, the meaning of life and inquiry about the nature of awareness itself – the observing/transcendent self. Inquiry is in this way related to all the dimensions of human experience as represented in the *diamond model of the observing self* (see Chapter 3).

A fundamental inquiry question, which relates to all dimensions of human experience is:

> "*What are you experiencing now?*" or
> "*How is that for you when you speak about ...?*"

Such open questions invite the client into present moment awareness. In order to access the present moment, it is important that the therapist slows down the process and makes space for mindful observation. The therapist is also careful to ask questions in the present tense about the client's experience.

Inquiry can focus on any specific dimension of human experience: cognitive, affective, physiological, relational, or spiritual.

Cognitive inquiry

The therapist may inquire about thoughts, beliefs, memories, and images that the client is experiencing at the moment.

CLIENT: *I feel so embarrassed* (looks down).
THERAPIST: *What thought just comes to your mind?*
CLIENT: *That something is wrong with me, and you will see that.*

Affective inquiry

Inquiry may be focused on awareness of emotions with questions such as:

> "*What are you feeling now?*"
> "*Which emotion do you feel now?*"

Physiological inquiry

Inquiry can focus on physiological sensations or body movements.

> "*What do you feel in your body now?*"
> "*Where in your body do you experience anxiety?*"
> "*What would your legs like to do?*"

Relational inquiry

> "*How do you feel in our relationship?*"
> "*How is it for you telling me about the loss of your mother?*"

Inquiry about values and meaning in life

This involves inquiring about the client's values, which give purpose and meaning to the client's life.

> *"When you think about that important moment in your life, what meaning has it for you and your life?"*

Inquiry into the nature of the observing self/transcendent self

We have described inquiry directed towards the contents of awareness such as cognitions, emotions, body sensations, relational field, and values. There is, however, another vital area of inquiry – inquiry about the nature of awareness. Such inquiry invites the client to become aware of awareness itself, and also promotes a decentred perspective. While the contents of our experience are always changing, our observing/transcendent self is always in the here-and-now.

> *"You are aware now of the thought 'I am a bad person'. Just become aware of who or what is aware of this thought?"*
> *"In this exercise, you were aware of your thoughts, emotions, and body sensations. Now ask yourself: 'who or what is aware of all these?'"*

For some people, such an inquiry may at first be experienced as strange and confusing. We are not used to such questions in everyday life. Even in meditation practice, most mindfulness practices focus on the contents of awareness, such as perceptions, thoughts, emotions, or body sensations. Inquiring about awareness itself may be experienced as unusual. It is important to be attuned to the client's experience when using such inquiry. D. J. Siegel (2018) includes awareness of awareness as part of his Wheel of Awareness mindfulness practice. He has found that while for some people such experience may be unusual, lots of people report a sense of expansiveness, love, joy, peace, and timelessness. In our experience, there is often a sense of spacious awareness, inner peace, love, and compassion. Being centred in the observing self helps clients to decentre from the contents of their mind and bring acceptance and compassion to all experience. The observing self enhances mindfulness processes and compassion.

Such inquiry is part of various nondual traditions of spirituality, for instance Advaita Vedanta. Ramana Maharshi calls it self-inquiry (Ganesan, 2017). In most psychotherapy traditions, this type of inquiry is not part of psychotherapy practice. The exception is acceptance and commitment therapy, where the transcendent/perspective-taking self is one of the main therapeutic processes (S. C. Hayes et al., 2012; S. C. Hayes et al., 2019).

The diamond model of the observing self and the *triangle of relationship to experience* guide our mindful interventions. The diamond model of the observing self (see Figure 3.1, Chapter 3) helps the therapist to determine on which dimension the client is open or closed to contact at any particular moment during therapy. In this way, the therapist is able to flexibly choose which areas of client experience may be important for inquiry. The triangle of relationship to experience (see Figure 3.2, Chapter 3) also orients us in this process. Whenever the client is in the distant mode or merged mode, the client is losing contact with the present moment. Inquiry and acknowledgement help the client to become aware of the present moment and invite them into a witnessing stance towards their experience.

Acknowledgement

Another important method for promoting present moment awareness is *acknowledgement*, which is part of therapeutic involvement (see Figure 9.1). The therapist does not merely inquire about the client's experience, but is fully present and provides an involved and unique response. With acknowledgement, the therapist is communicating to the client that they are aware of the client's experience or behaviour (Erskine et al., 1999), and in this way the client can become increasingly aware of their own experience. The therapist is in this process multidimensional. The therapist is not only following the client's narrative but is at the same time attentive to the client's emotions and nonverbal communication, such as body gestures, tone of voice, breathing patterns, facial expression, and eye movements. We can never be fully aware of the totality of our experience and behaviour, since a lot of these happen spontaneously and unconsciously. The therapist with acknowledgement helps the client to become aware of the experience and their nonverbal behaviour, which the client is usually unaware of. Acknowledgement has to be attuned to the client and has to be an expression of the mindful and loving presence of the therapist. Only in this way can an acknowledgement be taken by the client as beneficial.

Acknowledgement can take many forms. It is often expressed in the form of *empathic reflection*:

> "*You are feeling really sad.*"
> "*I imagine that this has to be very painful for you.*"

It can also be a simple statement of *observation of the client's behaviour*:

> "*I just noticed that when I asked you how you experience our relationship, you started to talk very quietly.*"

It can be directed towards awareness of nonverbal body behaviour:

> "*I am aware that when you talk about your father, you are clenching your fist.*"
> "*I just noticed that when you mentioned your girlfriend, you looked down and away from me.*"
> "*Your eyes started to water just now.*"

In providing acknowledgement, attunement to the client's continuing experience is crucial. Acknowledgement has to be attuned to the client's unique way of experiencing the world. Some clients may be struggling with shame and may find such acknowledgements at the beginning of therapy too intrusive. Some may feel as if they are too transparent – and that their therapist can see right through them. It is crucial to follow the client and check continually with them the impact of our interventions.

Promoting a decentred perspective

When clients are merged with their experience, this is a marker for promoting a decentred perspective. Without a decentred perspective, there can be no real contact, as contact requires someone who is in contact with something else. When we are merged with our experience, we become one with our experience. We look at ourselves, other people, and the world through that experience. Phenomenological inquiry and acknowledgement described in the previous section not only promote contact with the present moment but are important also for a decentred perspective. For some clients this alone is not sufficient and we have to use additional interventions that are focused on creating an observing stance towards their experience.

A decentred perspective can be promoted with a simple acknowledgement of the client's experience, followed by an invitation to observe that experience mindfully.

> "*You are feeling anxiety in your chest. Just become aware of this anxiety and pay attention to it with curiosity ...*"
> "*So you are having these dark thoughts that you're a bad person, and you do not deserve to live. Just observe those thoughts ...*"

Decentred awareness can also be promoted by *using the language of the self-states*. Relating to inner experience like a self-state promotes decentring. We can invite the client to observe their self-states with mindful awareness.

In the following example, our client Cathy was merged with a Child self-state and experienced deep loneliness. Relating to her loneliness as being part of her helped her to establish a decentred perspective towards her loneliness.

CLIENT: *I feel very alone. Like there is no one there for me. I know rationally that my husband and kids love me, but loneliness is still there.*
THERAPIST: *It looks like there is one part of you who feels very alone. Just become aware of that part of you ... (pause) What are you experiencing now?*

By using the language of parts, the therapist promotes decentred awareness.

CLIENT: *It is a small girl. Sitting in a hospital bed and crying. I was hospitalised when I was a child.*

By having an image of a small girl, the client is no longer merged with the Child self-state, as there is now the perspective of the loving witness.

THERAPIST: *How old is that part of you?*
CLIENT: *Small, about four.*

Our client Simona, who was suffering from depression was often feeling very judgemental towards herself, especially in situations with her children. She was merged with a self-critical introjected self-state and corresponding Child self-state that felt that she was a bad person.

CLIENT: *I just feel like I am a bad person. You should never yell at other people!*
THERAPIST: *It looks like there is a part of you that tells you that you are a bad person and you should never yell at other people.*
CLIENT: *Yes, I am torturing myself – you are bad … Like I don't deserve to live … It is so strong. I would never do anything to myself, but it is difficult to live with that.*
THERAPIST: *Are you willing to do a little experiment regarding that part of you, so that we can know it better?*
CLIENT: *Yes, I want to work with this.*
THERAPIST: *Just be in touch with that part of you that tells you that you are bad. And now just stand up and examine the basket where I have soft toys. Just look at each toy and find a toy that represents this part of you.*
CLIENT: *It is a crocodile.* (smiles)
THERAPIST: *Just put it in front of you and observe this part of you.*
CLIENT: *It is a very nasty, torturing crocodile.*
THERAPIST: *And now find a toy that represents part of you that feels a bad person.*
CLIENT: *It is a small mouse.*

In this example, the therapist in addition to using the language of parts, has also invited the client to *externalise* her internal experience by finding a toy that symbolised part of her.

Externalisation can also be promoted by inviting the client to imagine that their experience is in the space outside of them:

CLIENT: *I don't know what I feel. It is just very uncomfortable like it is all over my body. I cannot stand it.*
THERAPIST: *Imagine that this feeling is in the space outside of you. Where would it be? How does it look?*
CLIENT: *It is behind me … It is just darkness behind me … it is chasing me.*
THERAPIST: *Just observe the darkness, which is now behind you. And ask what it would like to tell you.*

Inquiring about physical properties of emotion or physical sensations also provides the experience of decentring:

THERAPIST: *You are feeling this uncomfortable sensation in your body. Just focus on it. And let me know what colour could it be?*

CLIENT: *It is red.*

THERAPIST: *What shape is it?*

CLIENT: *It is a large circle …*

THERAPIST: *If you could hear it … How would it sound …*

CLIENT: *Like the sound of sirens.*

Distance from the contents of awareness can also be enhanced by *exercises in mindful observation* of the contents of awareness, such as observing the thoughts as they would appear on a screen, or imagining that thoughts are like clouds in the sky.

> "*Imagine that this thought 'Something's wrong with me' is on the screen in a cinema. And you are sitting in the cinema observing the thought.*"

Decentred perspective can also be promoted by an *invitation to contact the observing self – loving witness.*

> "*So you have this uncomfortable sensation in your stomach as if you would like to throw up. Just become aware that there is You who is aware of this sensation. There is someone observing it. Just become aware of the observer. That you are an observer who is looking at this sensation with curiosity and loving eyes.*"

Contact with the observing self promotes a safe space from which clients can observe their experience. As we have already described in Chapter 3, the observing self is not touched by experiences, as it is a fulcrum of our perspective. This promotes decentred awareness and the ability to contain and accept our experience.

Promoting acceptance

Although clients may be well aware of their experience, they may try to avoid it and try to escape from it. For mindfulness, awareness alone is not enough; it must be coupled with acceptance of the experience (Černetič, 2005, 2017). The relational methods of integrative psychotherapy invite the client to pay attention to and accept their experience. With these methods, we are reversing the cycle of experiential avoidance (S. C. Hayes et al., 1999).

The model of the *triangle of relationship to internal experience* (see Figure 3.2, Chapter 3) can help the therapist to track the client's experience. When the client is becoming distant from their experience, the therapist can invite the client to attend to their experience and accept it.

There are two main interventions that promote acceptance: *validation* and an *invitation to the clients to willingly attend to their experience.*

Validation

The primary intervention related to acceptance is *validation* (see Figure 9.1). Validation is an acknowledgement of the significance of the client's experience (Erskine et al., 1999). It communicates to the client that their experience is significant and valuable. Even experiences that seem strange and we would rather not have them, have a story to tell. We should never ignore or throw away any aspect of our experience. This is also true for the parts of us that we experience as unfavourable, like for example, the harsh critic or a part of us which is very withdrawn from the world. These self-states may be serving an important function within the whole personality system. They may be communicating an important message or story, which is usually out of conscious awareness. The symptoms that brought the client into therapy have their own internal logic and are communicating something important.

Validation is a form of acknowledgement; the difference is that acknowledgement communicates to the client the existence of their experience, whereas validation also communicates significance (Erskine et al., 1999). Acknowledgement and validation go hand in hand in promoting accepting awareness. The first promotes awareness of experiences and the latter acceptance. Validation can be simple: "*These are important tears,*" or "*Let's appreciate that sensation in your body, it is not random that it is here.*"

The therapist's validation also communicates that the client's experience is not happening in isolation but is related to something significant (Erskine & Trautmann, 1996). In this way, validation promotes connections between separate experiences and links cause and effect. Validation communicates: "What you are experiencing has meaning and is significant!"

CLIENT: *I am starting to feel sad, I don't want to cry again.* (tears start to run down her cheeks)

The client Eva is aware of the experience, but she is trying to avoid it. She is moving towards the distant pole of the triangle of relationship to experience.

THERAPIST: *Sadness and tears are telling an important story, how alone you have been in your childhood. And how you missed your parents.*

The therapist validates the client's experience and, in this way, promotes acceptance of her experience. With validation, the therapist also makes a connection between experiences and gives meaning to them.

CLIENT: (starts to cry)
THERAPIST: *Let the tears come, they are important tears. Let's appreciate them.*

Another validation.

CLIENT: *Yes, I have been alone all these years, and there was nobody there for me. I am feeling sad for what I have missed ...* (cries again)

THERAPIST: *Just make room for this sadness ...* (handing her a tissue) *It is important and this time you are not crying alone.*

The therapist is promoting processes of acceptance and new relational experiences.

To be effective, the validation has to be congruent with the therapists' subjective experience of acceptance and compassion. The therapist, in this way, communicates with all their being that they accept the client's experience. Sometimes the validation is not even expressed in words or sentences, just the therapist's look and facial expression can communicate to the client acceptance and valuing of their experience. This is in line with Rogers (1957), who wrote that unconditional self-regard is crucial for the client's acceptance of themselves and their experience.

Invitation to willingly attend to the experience

In addition to validation, the therapist also invites the client to willingly attend to their experience and not to run away from it. In the previous example, the therapist communicated: "*Just make room for this sadness*". This form of intervention invites the client to willingly and with acceptance experience emotions or other internal experience. This intervention originally comes from gestalt therapy (Perls et al., 1951).

Some other examples of this would be:

"*If you are willing, just allow yourself to feel this emotion.*"
"*Let's stay a few moments with sadness. Allow yourself to feel it fully. It is an important part of you.*"
"*Focus on that sensation and embrace it with acceptance.*"

Validation and invitation to attend to experience have to be attuned to the client's experience. There are situations when acceptance of some specific experience is too much to bear for the client. This is especially the case with unresolved traumatic experiences. If the clients are dysregulated, we first help them to regulate their autonomic nervous system (see Chapter 11). Physiological attunement to the client's nervous system is essential in the process of awareness and acceptance of the client's experience.

Developing the capacity for acceptance often takes time and has to be done in small steps. The client has to be ready to experience painful material. Some clients need to develop their capacity for regulating and containing their emotions first before they are invited to attend to painful material. They have to develop what has been termed *integrative capacity* in order that they can safely experience the dissociated experience (van der Hart et al., 2010). The practice of mindfulness and compassion meditations are important in developing integrative capacity, which will enable them to approach and accept painful experiences. With mindful awareness, clients are widening their window of tolerance so that they can gradually contain and tolerate their painful and traumatic experiences.

In the process of therapy, the therapist continuously tracks the client's experience and regulates it so that the client can function within the window of tolerance connected to the ventral vagal system (Porges, 2011, 2017). *The model of the triangle of relationship to experience* enables the therapist to "fine tune" their interventions (see Chapter 3). If the client is moving towards the distancing or merging part of the triangle, the therapist helps the client to come back to the position of *loving witness*. In the case of moving to a position of distance, the therapist invites the client back to present moment awareness and acceptance of their experience. In the case of merging, the therapist helps the client to decentre from their experience, and to attend to a broader field of present moment awareness.

Enhancing self-compassion

Self-compassion is in the relational mindfulness and compassion model related to the intervention of *normalisation* (see Figure 9.1). Clients often blame themselves or feel ashamed because of their experiences or coping mechanisms. They often experience themselves as pathological and not-normal. Normalisation is an intervention that de-pathologises the clients' definition of their internal experiences or coping mechanisms (Erskine, 2015). With normalisation, the therapist conveys to the client that "his experience is a normal and not pathological reaction" (G. Žvelc, 2012, p. 45).

As Neff (2003a) noted, self-compassion consists of three main components: Self-kindness, Common humanity, and Mindfulness. In order to experience self-compassion, mindful awareness is essential. Self-compassion is connected to the previously described interventions that enhance the processes of present moment awareness, decentred perspective, and acceptance, which facilitate mindful awareness. The therapist with *inquiry* invites the client to present moment awareness, with *acknowledgement*, the therapist communicates that they are aware of the client's experience, and with *validation* helps the client to accept their experience. *Normalisation* takes the process a step further. Normalisation helps the client to embrace themselves or their self-states with compassion. This goes against the client's negative self-definition and view of themselves. It conveys to the client a sense of common humanity – that all our experiences are part of being human. It is also related to the fundamental principle of MCIP that people experience ordinary unhappiness and are not perfect. We all experience pain and other unpleasant emotions, make unwise decisions, and (often unintentionally) hurt others.

Clients frequently criticise or blame themselves because of their ways of coping and surviving in the past. They often define themselves as crazy:

> "*My main problem is that I don't let anyone be close. Something is really wrong with me!*"
> "*I am a real borderline … Every slight criticism makes me yell …*"

"Since I was seven years old, I talk with an angel! I am crazy ..."

The intervention of normalisation helps the clients to develop compassion for their way of coping. It conveys to the clients that their coping with the situation and the world was their best attempt to survive in that particular situation. With normalisation, the therapist communicates

> fully and genuinely, that the client has done the absolute best that he or she could, given the circumstances, and that anyone at this developmental level, with access to these resources, would probably have made the same sorts of decisions. (Erskine et al., 1999)[2]

In integrative psychotherapy, we are not confronting defences and wanting the client to change – quite the opposite. In MCIP we bring acceptance and compassion towards the totality of all of our clients' experiences, including protective mechanisms. By showing compassion for the client's way of coping and surviving, the client often paradoxically relinquishes old patterns of defence. When clients' protective mechanisms are accepted and looked at from the position of compassion, clients spontaneously drop their defences and are willing to risk contact with vulnerability, which is like a flower hiding behind the wall of protection. Only when clients feel safe, accepted, and respected, they are willing to let go of protection. Clients in this way come into contact with the experience, which they previously avoided. Normalisation helps them to accept and embrace their defences.

CLIENT: *My father was like a Nazi; we were all terrified of him. I remember that I was strange already back then. I started to avoid social contacts and had my own world. Like I lived on the "other side"... In my world everything was fine.*
THERAPIST: *You were strange?*
CLIENT: *Yes, I felt different from others. I didn't tell you about my inner world, for a long time I felt that you would think I am crazy and will put me in a psychiatric hospital.*
THERAPIST: *So you were very afraid of your father, who was often drunk and violent. And at that time you started to live on the other side where everything was ok. So this "other world" in which everything was fine helped you to survive and keep you sane in the "insane world".*

The therapist acknowledges and validates the client's coping mechanisms, which promotes the client's awareness and acceptance.

CLIENT: *Yes, it helped me to survive, definitely.*
THERAPIST: (with a kind and compassionate voice) *Let's appreciate this strategy of a five-year-old that helped you to survive.*

Another validation, which helps the client to experience self-compassion.

CLIENT: *I feel touched, I never thought about this in this way ...*

THERAPIST: *Maybe this strategy was the most clever strategy to survive in a family where there was no one to hold on to* ... (short pause) *What do you feel now?*

The therapist conveys the normalisation of the client's past coping strategy.

CLIENT: *I feel like I would embrace this younger part of me* ... *telling him I love him and care for him.*

THERAPIST: *Just do this, take your time.*

CLIENT: (crying) *I feel sad for what I have gone through* ... (pause) *Now I understand that having my own world actually saved my life* ... *I feel appreciation for this. However, I also understand that I am not there anymore, I am safe now.*

In this process, clients come to realise that they were for many years sticking to decisions, choices, and coping strategies which were developed in childhood as a means of coping with stress. When they are able to feel compassion towards themselves for doing this, they develop a new internal relationship which is built on safety and compassion. They realise that this mechanism of protection belongs to the past when it was necessary; however, in the present, it is often not needed any more in most situations. In this way, they can flexibly choose whether old strategies of protection are still useful in current situations.

In conveying this intervention of normalisation, it is crucial that the therapist is feeling compassion towards the client. If not, the interventions will be purely technical and will not have the intended effect. If the therapist feels compassion towards the client, this will be mirrored in their facial expression, tone of voice, and gestures. Normalisation will be conveyed compassionately with the whole of the therapist's being. The compassion of the therapist helps the client to feel kindness towards themself.

It is also important for the therapist not to introduce normalisation too soon, which could leave the client feeling that the therapist does not understand their point of view. The client's experience must first be acknowledged and validated so that the client feels deeply understood.

Phases of relational mindfulness- and compassion-oriented interventions

We have described the main relational methods and interventions that enhance mindfulness and compassion processes in the psychotherapeutic relationship. But, how are these methods related? In Figure 9.1, the main processes of mindfulness and compassion are presented in the following order from top to bottom: awareness, acceptance, and self-compassion. At the foot of the diagram is the observing self. In the diagram, these main processes are related to the corresponding methods of inquiry and involvement. The order of the processes describes the four main phases of relational mindfulness- and compassion-oriented interventions:

Phase 1: Promoting present moment and decentred awareness.

Phase 2: Promoting acceptance.
Phase 3: Promoting self-compassion.
Phase 4: Being a loving witness to a client's vulnerability.

These phases correspond to Erskine's four phases of integrative psychotherapy connected to the keyhole model: starting point, making connections, choices and decisions, and full contact (Erskine et al., 1999). As Erskine and his colleagues (1999) describe, these phases are not linear. Progression from one phase to the next can sometimes happen in only a few minutes; another time, one phase may be more dominant and take the whole therapeutic hour.

The first phase: Promoting present moment and decentred awareness. This phase is related to the enhancement of the client's mindful awareness of the present moment and decentred perspective. It invites the client into a mindful state of consciousness and corresponds to Erskine's phase of "starting point", where the focus is on the client's awareness of phenomenological experience (Erskine et al., 1999). At the beginning of therapy, clients are usually not aware of their phenomenological experience. They may be unaware of their thoughts that are behind the symptoms, emotions, or sensations in their body. In this phase, the therapist facilitates the processes of present moment awareness and decentred perspective. Phenomenological inquiry, acknowledgement, and interventions related to a decentred perspective all promote awareness of experience that the client was previously unaware of. They help the clients to become aware of their thoughts, emotions, memories, body sensations, or body movements. The client Anna, for example, became aware of her deep sadness that she had been avoiding by taking care of others and appearing "strong and happy".

The second phase: Promoting acceptance. This phase is related to promoting the clients' acceptance of their experiences. The aim of this phase is that clients start to accept experience that was previously avoided. The therapist with *validation* promotes acceptance of the client's experience. The therapist also uses interventions that help clients to "willingly attend to their experiences". The client Anna, for example, allowed herself first to feel sadness and then to cry after a long time in her life.

In addition to acceptance, this phase is also related to making connections between experiences (Erskine et al., 1999). The therapist with validation communicates that present experiences are not random but are connected to other similar experiences. With the help of *inquiry*, the therapist helps the client to make connections between present experiences, memories, and expectations about the future. In this way, clients can become aware of the influence of their past experiences on their present life and future expectations. Anna, for example, became aware that her sadness was connected to the divorce of her parents in childhood and that this experience was continuing to influence her present life.

The third phase: Promoting self-compassion. This phase is related to promoting the client's self-compassion. It corresponds to Erskine's phase of "choices and decisions" (Erskine et al., 1999). The therapists' inquiry is focused on the client's way of coping and surviving with painful and disturbing experiences. The therapist explores survival reactions, as well as the conclusions, choices, and decisions that the clients made under stress and are now protecting them from pain. For example, Anna became aware of how, after the divorce of her parents, she felt alone and missed her father. As her mother was depressed, she started to take care of her psychologically and outwardly appeared as a "happy child". Awareness of coping strategies and ways of surviving "not-normal" circumstances often spontaneously awakes self-compassion.

Just being aware of protective mechanisms is often not enough. Anna, for example, often criticised herself for being naive and having difficulty in saying "no" to other people. The therapist's normalisation helped her to start to feel compassion for her Child self-state, which had coped with the pain by being "happy and strong" and taking care of others. Compassion also helped her to feel more secure and to realise that her *façade* of happiness that was useful in the past is not always needed in the present. This allowed her to come into contact with vulnerability, sadness, and anger.

The fourth phase: Being a loving witness to a client's vulnerability. This phase corresponds to Erskine's phase of "full contact" (Erskine et al., 1999). Through compassion towards their ways of coping and surviving, clients come into contact with a vulnerability that lays behind their protective mechanisms. In this process, the clients reintegrate parts of themselves that were hidden and rejected a long time ago. Dissociated, denied, and disavowed experiences are gradually welcomed back into awareness (Erskine et al., 1999). Schwartz (1995) describes how certain parts of us live in exile. Mindful awareness and compassion towards our "exiled" self-states help our clients to become whole again. Erskine et al. (1999) write that in this phase defences are:

> melting in the face of growing appreciation of and compassion for all the parts of self that have been hidden away for so long … There is tenderness about these moments, a feeling of awakening, almost of rebirth …. And each of those long-repressed, long-hidden parts of self has a kind of fragility, like a flower bud freshly opened or a butterfly newly escaped from its hard cocoon.[3]

Anna progressing step-by-step in her therapy came into contact with her wounded Child self-state, something that she had been running away from since the divorce of her parents. Compassion helped her to embrace the sadness and anger of that self-state and opened the way for the transformative affects (Fosha, 2000a; Fosha & Conceição, 2019) of worthiness, dignity, and pride.

When a client's vulnerable self-state emerges, the therapist needs to be a *loving witness* to it. The therapist's mindful presence is like a midwife at the rebirth of a part of the client, which was hidden long ago. The therapist embodies a witnessing stance towards the client's experience and is fully there, without any expectation, relating to the client from the position of the observing self. The therapist is witness to an emerging part of the client, which has finally returned home from exile (Schwartz, 1995). We can say that this is like a meeting of two souls, of *shared conscious presence* (see Chapter 4). Both the client and the therapist are fully present and aware. These moments can be described as *moments of meeting* (Stern, 2004), moments of the vulnerability of the I–Thou relationship (Buber, 1999).

Notes

1 From "Methods of an integrative psychotherapy", by R. G. Erskine and R. L. Trautmann, 1996, *Transactional Analysis Journal, 26*(4), p. 320 (https://doi.org/10.1177/036215379302300402). Copyright 1996 by Taylor & Francis. Reprinted with permission of the publisher (Taylor & Francis Ltd, www.tandfonline.com).

2 From *Beyond empathy: A therapy of contact-in-relationship* (p. 171), by R. G. Erskine, J. P. Moursund, and R. L. Trautmann, 1999, Brunner/Mazel. Copyright 1999 by Taylor and Francis. Reprinted with permission of the publisher (Taylor & Francis Ltd, http://www.tandfonline.com).

3 From *Beyond empathy: A therapy of contact-in-relationship* (p. 172), by R. G. Erskine, J. P. Moursund, and R. L. Trautmann, 1999, Brunner/Mazel. Copyright 1999 by Taylor and Francis. Reprinted with permission of the publisher (Taylor & Francis Ltd, www.tandfonline.com).

10 From mindful awareness and self-compassion to values-based living

In this chapter, we describe three interrelated tasks of MCIP: (a) Developing mindful capacity and self-compassion, (b) Developing metacognitive awareness of schemas and self-states, and (c) Promoting living according to values and meaning. These tasks are fundamental in the first two phases of MCIP (See Chapter 8). In the first phase, clients develop their capacity for mindfulness and become more self-compassionate. In the second phase, mindfulness capacity and self-compassion are crucial for metacognitive awareness of schemas and self-states. Metacognitive awareness is related to the ability to recognise schemas and self-states, decentre from them and to reflect on how schemas and self-states influence one's life. Clients and therapists working together come to recognise the client's core schemas and reflect on how they influence their perception of themselves and others. Mindfulness skills and self-compassion help clients in their daily life to decentre from their schemas and self-states when they become activated. This helps our clients to develop greater inner freedom so that they can actively engage in living according to their values and meaning.

In Chapter 9, we have described methods of relational mindfulness and compassion that develop mindful capacity and enhance self-compassion through an attuned therapeutic relationship. Mindfulness and self-compassion can also be explicitly introduced to the client in the form of mindfulness and compassion practices and mindful metaphors. In the following sections, we describe different ways in which mindfulness and compassion can be explicitly enhanced in psychotherapy.

Developing mindful capacity

Mindfulness practices

The client's mindful capacity can be significantly enhanced by mindfulness meditation. We may introduce clients to traditional mindfulness practices, such as sitting meditation, body-scan and three-minute breathing space (Kabat-Zinn, 1990; Segal et al., 2002). We inform the clients about the benefits, and may point them to further resources regarding mindfulness practices. For clients taking part in regular psychotherapy, an eight-week mindfulness-based programme is helpful.

Mindfulness practice is not a prerequisite for our approach, as mindfulness capacity is primarily developed through methods of relational mindfulness and compassion.

We may start the session with a short mindfulness exercise, like awareness of the breath, short body-scan, or awareness of the external environment. Such practices often colour the rest of the session, which may then proceed at a slower tempo that facilitates contact with inner experience.

"For a few seconds become aware of your breathing, each in-breath and out-breath."
"Become aware of your body as you are sitting here. With attention travel from your toes to the top of your head."

We regularly use brief *mindful pauses* during the session, which helps to provide awareness, self-regulation as well as deeper contact with both body and emotions.

"Take a few seconds and become aware of what you are experiencing inside your body now."

We have developed a mindfulness practice based on the *diamond model of the observing self* (see Chapter 3). This practice invites the client towards mindful awareness of the different dimensions of human experience and awareness of the observing self. The practice starts with mindful awareness of the body, followed by awareness of emotions and thoughts. In the next step, we then invite the client to focus their awareness on other people in their life (interpersonal dimension) and on their interconnectedness with the rest of humanity and natural environment (ecological and spiritual dimension). The final step promotes awareness of the external environment through different sensory modalities. Through this exercise, we invite the client to become aware of the observing/transcendent self (spiritual dimension).

Exercise: The diamond of mindful awareness

"Becoming aware of your breathing – each in-breath and out-breath. You are breathing. Becoming aware of where do you feel the breathing in your body. Maybe you feel it more in your nostrils, chest or stomach. (pause)
Now bringing attention to the whole of your body. Simply becoming aware of the sensations that might be present. There is no need for changing them or doing anything about them. If you can, allowing them to be as they are. (pause)
Now moving the focus of attention to your emotions. Noticing if there are any emotions present for you right now. If there are, just making space for them and welcoming them all. It is OK as it is. (pause)
Now turning attention to your thoughts. Being aware of each thought coming and going. Becoming aware of the tendency to either cling to or avoid specific thoughts. Just allowing them to be as they are, a passing event in our minds, continually arising and disappearing. Observing them with loving eyes. (pause)

> *You are aware of body sensations, emotions and thoughts. Notice that there is someone or something aware of all these... Become aware of awareness itself. (pause)*
> *Now becoming aware of other people in your life, people you have a close relationship with (e.g. your family, close friends) (pause)... and now people you don't perceive as close (e.g. acquaintances). (pause)*
> *Noticing that in you and each human being, there is a presence of awareness. There is a conscious presence that we all share. (pause)*
> *Now becoming aware that we all exist on the earth together with other life forms, such as animals, plants. Becoming aware of the earth and the interconnectedness of all people with earth and space. We can all only exist because of air, food, water, sun ... We are part of a greater whole. (pause)*
> *Now bringing attention to the external environment.*
> *Turning attention to smells in the room ... (pause)*
> *Noticing sounds arising and disappearing .... If you perhaps notice your attention wandering, just gently bringing it back to awareness of sounds. It is normal that the mind wanders, that is the nature of the mind. If you notice that you are lost in your thoughts, be aware of that and gently bring them back to awareness of sound. (pause)*
> *Who or what is aware of all these? Don't try to answer the question intellectually, just let the question lead you towards an experience of awareness itself ... The awareness is not body sensations, emotions, thoughts, or perceptions. These are passing events in the field of awareness. It is I who is aware of it all. (pause)*
> *Now bringing attention to your breath and expanding it to your body as a whole. Becoming aware of your posture as you sit in the chair and the points of contact with the chair. Now putting one hand on your body and one hand on the chair, holding them at the same time. (pause)*
> *As we are coming to the end of this practice, opening your eyes (if they were closed) and having a look at the room... Trying to see the room with fresh eyes as if seeing it for the first time just now ...."*

When this exercise is done in groups, we invite participants to look at each other; if not, the client is invited to look at the therapist.

> *"Look at your colleagues as if seeing them for the first time in your life. Becoming aware that there is a presence of awareness in each one of you. And when you catch another person's gaze, becoming aware that you are both seeing each other from the place of awareness itself."*

Use of metaphors

Metaphors, enlightening stories, and poetry can all be powerful ways of introducing clients to mindful awareness, self-compassion, and the observing self. They point the client towards the experience, rather than just conceptual understanding. The therapist can use different metaphors and stories that were developed within different mindfulness-based therapy approaches and different spiritual traditions. One example is "the limitless sky" – a metaphor and mindfulness exercise that points to the observing/transcendent self.

Limitless sky

> "*Imagine that you are the limitless blue sky, while thoughts, emotions, and physical sensations are like clouds in the sky. Become aware of thoughts, emotions, and sensations as clouds that appear in the sky. Become aware of each cloud with acceptance and kindness. Thoughts, emotions, and sensations are coming and going, continually changing. You, as a witness of them, are always there as the unchanging sky. You are not touched by clouds; clouds appear and disappear in you ...*"

In MCIP, we may creatively use different metaphors and stories that point to mindful awareness and compassion. We have found particularly useful metaphors that were developed within acceptance and commitment therapy such as the Chessboard metaphor, Passengers on the bus, the Polygraph metaphor, and the Tug of war with the monster (S. C. Hayes et al., 2012). Therapists may also wish to creatively develop their own metaphors, related to their client's experience. Sometimes we may also use stories or poetry, such as Rumi's Guesthouse (Segal et al., 2002).

Enhancing self-compassion

To be able to bring compassion to themselves, clients first need to recognise and be aware that they are suffering and that they have the ability to stay mindfully present while attending to a painful state (Neff, 2011). Compassion and mindfulness go hand in hand. There is no compassion without mindful awareness and presence. Furthermore, the essential part of mindfulness is acceptance and in the depth of that acceptance there is always love and compassion. To help our clients bring the light of mindful awareness and self-compassion to their painful states and their rejected or exiled parts is, in our opinion, the essential healing process in psychotherapy. Clients' motivation for self-compassion develops when they recognise the value of being accepting, kind, and compassionate towards themselves (P. Gilbert, 2010). Some clients can access self-compassion easily, while some have difficulties.

There are different ways to enhance self-compassion (Desmond, 2016; P. Gilbert, 2010; Tirch et al., 2014). In Chapter 9, we have described how self-compassion can be developed within a therapeutic relationship with the help of normalisation of clients' experience and their protective mechanisms. In addition to such relational interventions, we may promote self-compassion by (a) *compassionate interaction with the body* and (b) *internal compassionate dialogues*. In all these interventions, we invite our clients to bring self-compassion to themselves. We believe that self-compassion is a state within all of us; it only has to be awakened, and a compassionate therapist can help the client with this.

Compassionate interaction with the body

When promoting self-compassion, mindful awareness of inner states, particularly body awareness, is needed. When introducing compassion to our clients, we often use *supporting breath* and *loving hand* exercises that promote a *compassionate interaction with the body*. Such exercises encourage the bottom-up process of self-compassion. We may also use exercises that involve imagination, such as the sun behind the heart.

Supporting breath

> *"Direct your attention to your breathing. The in-breath … the out-breath … Be aware, that every single breath is supporting you, is here with you … cares for you … supplying the oxygen to your body, to the cells … giving you the energy, the strength you need… and taking away waste substances … Be aware of your breath; the supporting and caring nature of your breath … being with you throughout your life."*

(adapted from part of Kabat-Zinn body scan meditation)

Loving hand exercise

The loving touch of the body, especially of the chest, is part of our human experience and our innate wisdom. Other authors also describe a similar exercise (Germer, 2012; van der Brink & Koster, 2015).

The therapist invites the client into the *loving hand exercise* by speaking slowly and gently the following words:

> *"Put your hand on your chest in a kind and loving way. Feel the touch of your hand; feel the warmth of your hand on your chest. Be aware of the gentle, loving, accepting touch. Feel the touch of your hand on your heart, the touch of love, compassion, and forgiveness."*

The therapist's state of being and the way they are talking is crucial for this exercise. The therapist also puts the hand on their chest and is mindful of each word they are speaking. During the practice, they are bringing self-compassion also to themselves. Their heart is opening; their voice is touching. The therapist state of compassion is conveyed to the client through the process of physiological synchrony. The therapist, while saying these words, is also observing the client and noticing if their words and voice are helping to promote self-compassion. As self-compassion begins to emerge, the client's face gets softer; usually the eyes get a little wet, or tears start to fall, the breath is smooth and sometimes deeper. If the exercise is not activating self-compassion, the face is tense and breathing shallow. The therapist afterwards asks the client: *"What are you experiencing right now?"* or *"How was that exercise for you?"*

The sun behind the heart

Another exercise that promotes self-compassion is *the sun behind the heart* that is often used in different spiritual traditions (Malachi, 2004).

"Imagine that within and behind your heart there is a sun. A warm, loving sun that embraces and accepts everything. Imagine that this sun shines and touches with love your body, emotions, and thoughts … The sun also shines all around you and with its rays is bringing love and compassion to every living being."

Internal compassionate dialogues

Self-compassion can be enhanced with self-compassionate internal dialogues. The interventions that promote perspective-taking are often used to promote such dialogue because self-compassion is often spontaneously awakened when we can see ourselves from a different perspective. These interventions are related to the observing self that has the ability to shift perspective across time, place, and the person (S. C. Hayes et al., 2012). Such interventions may invite the client to move their perspective between an older and younger self. The client can be invited, for example, to observe themselves through the eyes of an older self in the future or to talk to a younger Child self-state. We may also invite the client to look now with loving eyes back at themselves to a time when they were suffering. These interventions can be creatively used to facilitate decentred perspective and self-compassion.

Looking at yourself with loving eyes of compassion

> "*Look at yourself with loving eyes like a mother would be looking at her beloved son or daughter when they are in pain. What would you be saying to yourself that would be kind, loving, and supporting? And how are you feeling when you are saying these words of compassion?*"

Clients can also be invited to imagine a visit from their wise and compassionate self from the future. They are invited to look at themselves through the perspective of this wise self.

> "*Imagine yourself in the future. You are old, wise and compassionate. Look at yourself through the eyes of your wise and compassionate self. What do you feel? Is there something you would like to tell yourself?*"

Receiving compassion from other people or resources

When clients cannot find compassion towards themselves on their own, we can help them with "bridging"; clients are invited to imagine that they are receiving compassion from someone or something else (Desmond, 2016). For instance, we can ask our clients to recall something or someone that invokes in them uncomplicated feelings of warmth or love (Desmond, 2016). We may say to our client:

> "*Imagine a compassionate figure who cares for you. Imagine this figure is there with your pain. (pause) What would this figure be saying to you? (pause) Imagine that you are looking at yourself with the eyes of that compassionate figure.*"

Different compassionate figures may be used that embody wisdom and love: a universal child, universal mother, a fairy, a particular tree, mother earth, or an animal. Figures from different spiritual traditions may also be used (like Jesus, an angel, Mary, Buddha, a spiritual teacher …). The client may also look at themselves with the eyes of a real beloved person, like a mother, grandfather, partner, a friend. In this case, we have to bear in mind that a real person can also trigger unpleasant feelings.

We can also invite our clients to remember their experiences of receiving compassion from others (P. Gilbert, 2010). This can be a valuable resource for developing self-compassion. Awareness of others being compassionate to us may awaken our sense of connection to other people, which increases our sense of safety. And last but not least, our client's self-compassion is encouraged by the compassion of the therapist.

Self-compassionate phrases

If a client is having difficulty with finding self-compassion, it is useful to try different approaches, knowing that some may be more acceptable than others. Phrases which carry a positive wish towards the self can also promote self-compassion. The client may be invited to say to themselves, for example, the following *metta* phrases "*May you be happy. May you be healthy. May you be safe. May you be loved*" (Desmond, 2016, p. 192). The client can also choose kind and wishing words by themselves (Neff, 2011).

Awareness of the source of self-compassion

When clients become compassionate towards themselves, we can direct their awareness to a stream of self-compassion or onto that aspect of themselves which they feel is the source of their self-compassion. We may say:

> "*Be aware of the flow of self-compassion you are experiencing right now …. How is that for you? (pause) Where is the compassion coming from? Be aware of that aspect of you that is pouring out self-compassion.*"

Awareness of the source of compassion leads to a recognition of the compassionate aspect of ourselves that we call the observing/transcendent self. The awareness of our compassionate observing self may invoke feelings of being cared for, not being alone, connectedness, trust, safety, and gratitude. These feelings may lead to spiritual experiences.

Barriers to self-compassion

For some of our clients, self-compassion may be a threatening process. Following the philosophy of MCIP, when this happens we help clients to acknowledge, accept, and understand the anxiety connected to self-compassion. There is a significant reason for fear of self-compassion, and behind the fear, there is an important story. So we do not fight with the anxiety; we do not force the client to be self-compassionate; we are compassionate with the client's fear and avoidance of being compassionate. In that way paradoxically the client's protective mechanism softens (Erskine et al., 1999). Sometimes the main focus is on working with anxiety and blocks related to compassion (P. Gilbert, 2010).

Guidelines for the therapist

Accept the client's current inability to find self-compassion; it has an important intrapsychic function. Remember that barriers to self-compassion are protecting the client from something.

Acknowledge and validate that the client currently cannot bring compassion to themselves. By acknowledging, the client will become aware of their protective mechanism, and by validating, they will understand that the protective mechanism has a meaning.

Together with the client in a kind and accepting attitude, explore the intrapsychic function of the barriers to self-compassion. Seeing the obstacles to self-compassion as a part of the client, which has a protective role, leads to understanding and acceptance. With this process, the barriers may vanish or transform.

Metacognitive awareness of schemas and self-states

The central goal in the second phase of MCIP is the mindful recognition and understanding of the core relational schemas and self-states that are behind the client's experience (see Chapter 8). Clients' experience of the present moment and future expectations are based on implicit relational schemas, which are the generalisations of past relationship experiences. Schemas, if unreflected, unconsciously influence our experience and behaviour. Because of this, we help clients to become aware of their schemas, understand how they were constructed, and recognise the effects of schemas on their lives. The aim is for clients to develop a decentred perspective and decentred relationship towards their schemas. When schemas and related self-states are activated, clients can then relate to them from their new decentred perspective, with acceptance and in the present moment. In this way, the schemas lose their grip on the client's life, and the client may come to see themselves, others, and the world differently from how they used to. This manifests in greater autonomy and psychological flexibility. From a neurobiological perspective, we can say that the probability of activation of different neural network patterns heightens (D. J. Siegel, 1999). Without mindful decentred awareness, the activation of dysfunctional schemas rigidly fires limited network patterns, which is seen in rigidity and psychological inflexibility.

In addition to decentred awareness and understanding, the task of metacognitive awareness also includes promoting connections between separated or dissociated experiences. The client is invited to make connections between emotions, sensations, thoughts, and behaviour through the time frame of past, present, and future. This process enhances the capacity for mentalisation. The therapist also helps the client to identify specific autobiographical memories that shaped the client's understanding and construal of the world. Connections between separate experiences enhance personality and brain integration (D. J. Siegel, 2012, 2018).

The psychotherapeutic work of promoting metacognitive awareness of schemas and self-states consists of the following psychotherapeutic subtasks: (1) Psycho-education about schemas, (2) Mindful recognition of core relational schemas, (3) Recognising the influence of schemas on client's life, and (4) Promoting decentred awareness of relational schemas and self-states.

Psycho-education about schemas

Educating clients regarding the existence, nature, and function of their schemas is an important step in developing a decentred awareness of them. Psycho-education has to be tailored according to each client's educational and cultural background. It can be provided by explanation or metaphors. One metaphor that we use is the Matrix metaphor, which is related to the cult film by Lana and Lilly Wachowski. The metaphor can be easily adjusted to people who do not know the original film.

Matrix metaphor

"*Maybe you know the film 'The Matrix'. In the film, people live in a simulated virtual reality called the Matrix. Their life is preprogrammed and determined according to the Matrix. You can imagine that our schemas are like the Matrix through which we experience reality. We are usually not aware of this Matrix; however, it determines our everyday life and experience. For example, a person may have a schema – 'I am incapable of relationships' and may live life according to this schema – avoiding relationships and being alone all their life. This schema colours a person's everyday reality and the person is usually not aware that their experience is determined by their schema.*

However, we can become aware of schemas and can decentre from them, so that our life is not driven by them. In the film, Neo represents a person who is liberated from the Matrix. Morpheus offers him two pills, a blue pill and a red pill. The blue pill represents our life lived unconsciously in the grip of our schemas. The red pill represents awareness and liberation from our schemas – our Matrix. It is related to insight into the nature of the Matrix and living life freely without the grip of our schemas. Mindful awareness is a red pill. It helps us to disidentify and decentre from our schemas so that we can more freely live according to our values and purpose.

So, would you like a red pill or blue pill? If you choose the red pill, what would your life look like? And if you choose the blue one?

In the film, there are also agents (like agent Smith) that do not want people to become liberated from the Matrix. They represent obstacles to our way of living life more freely. What are your obstacles?"

Mindful recognition of core relational schemas

The next significant psychotherapeutic task is mindful recognition of the clients' core dysfunctional schemas. The aim is for clients to become fully and mindfully aware of their core schemas. The therapist encourages clients to observe with a decentred perceptive, curiosity, acceptance, and in the present moment, how the lenses of their mind are shaping their perception and experience and influencing their behaviour.

Core dysfunctional schemas are often formed as a result of the relational experiences between the child and significant others. They make their appearance later in life in the form of internal dialogue and relationships with other people. To help the client identify relational schemas and to understand their origins and function, we inquire about four main areas that are connected with the same relational theme:

1   The experience of past relationships.
2   Intrapsychic relationship.
3   Experience of present relationships with others, including the therapist.
4   Fantasies and anticipations about relationships in the future.

These areas of exploration are direct windows into the client's relational world.

Exploring the experience of past relationships

With historical inquiry, the therapist helps the client make connections to past autobiographic memories that are related to present experiences. This helps the client to recognise that the connection between past and present experiences is the relational schema that is activated in the course of the client's life.

THERAPIST: *In your relationship with your boss, you are feeling scared. You are afraid that he will act in a sexually inappropriate way, even if you rationally don't find him threatening … Does this fear of being sexually assaulted remind you of something?*
CLIENT: (silence) *My uncle. They look the same – small, with glasses and have the same tone of voice … My uncle often touched my bum when he was around and told inappropriate sexual jokes.*

After the connection has been made, and the client feels validated and heard in relation to a past episode, the therapist can proceed with helping the client to recognise the schema which is a link between the past and the present.

THERAPIST: *So we can see, how based on your experience with your uncle you constructed the schema that men cannot be trusted, they may sexually assault you and you are not safe.*
CLIENT: *Yes, we could say so.*

Sometimes clients have difficulties in finding connections, so the therapist may use the *affect bridge technique* (F. Shapiro, 2018; Watkins, 1971), where the connection is made through contact with affect and body experience.

THERAPIST: *Become aware of the fear and the thought "something bad will happen". Where do you feel it in your body now?*

CLIENT: *In my stomach ... It feels like a knot or a lump in my stomach; like something is heavy and is squeezing me.*

THERAPIST: *Mm-hm, mm-hm. Be aware of this lump in your stomach, the heaviness and squeezing ... and let this sensation take you back to the earliest time in your life when you experienced it ...*

Exploring the intrapsychic relationship

The client's intrapsychic relationship that manifests in the form of intrapsychic dialogue is also an important area of inquiry for the recognition of schemas. When relational schemas are activated they can appear in the form of an inner dialogue between different self-states.

CLIENT: *I am very strict with myself. I don't allow myself any pleasure.*

THERAPIST: *What do you say to yourself when you are strict and don't allow yourself any pleasure?*

With this inquiry, the therapist is exploring the client's internal dialogue.

CLIENT: *You don't deserve it because you are a bad person! You should suffer!*

THERAPIST: *That sounds like a really harsh criticism ... It sounds like somewhere in your life you developed the schema that you are bad, and you have to suffer ...*

The therapist makes a short pause to see the client's response.

CLIENT: (nods)

THERAPIST: *Take a moment and be aware of what is happening in you now.*

The therapist is inviting the client into mindful awareness.

CLIENT: *A memory has just come back to me ...* (starting to cry ...) *Something happened to my brother ... I should have taken care of him. He fell down, hit his head and was in a coma for a few days. I thought he would die. I was seven, and my brother was about three. My father was furious with me. I felt so guilty. Maybe I am punishing myself for not taking good care of my brother and hurting him.*

With mindful awareness of the schema and criticising self-state, connections with past experiences come spontaneously.

THERAPIST: *As a small child, how did you understand that? What did you conclude?*

CLIENT: *I am bad and guilty ... and I have to be on guard all the time. There is no rest for me.*

THERAPIST: *So as a young girl, you developed a schema that still influences your life: "I am a bad person, I am guilty, and others will punish me." And you concluded: "I don't deserve to enjoy, there is no rest, I have to be on my guard all the time to not make a mistake." How does that sound to you?*

The therapist in a collaborative manner is elaborating the dysfunctional relational schema with the client.

THERAPIST: (later in the session) *Would you like to write down the schema? And then read it again during the week, without trying to do anything with it?*

Through the practice of writing down and reading the schema, the client further develops a decentred perspective and awareness of the schema. The relationship to schema changes as the client is not merged with it anymore. The activation of the schema can be more easily recognised in daily life. Through accepting awareness, the schema loses its influence.

Exploring the psychotherapeutic relationship

An important area of inquiry is into the client's experience of the psychotherapeutic relationship. It is important to bear in mind that the client is viewing the therapist through the glasses of relational schemas that were developed in early relationships. Understanding their thoughts, emotions, and expectations regarding the therapist can help clients identify their main relational patterns that were constructed usually in early child–parent relationships. In this way, the client's transference can be explored. Erskine et al. (1999) wrote: "What one expects, hopes for, or fears from one's therapist is an echo of what has happened before with important people" (p. 167).

CLIENT: *I rationally know that you are on my side ... but here* (indicating the stomach and chest) *I do not .... I feel so unworthy and unlovable.*
THERAPIST: *Tell me more about that part.*
CLIENT: *I am the person no one wants to be with ...*
THERAPIST: *Do you feel that I do not want to be your therapist?*
CLIENT: *Yes, sometimes ... I fear that.*
THERAPIST: *Is there something which I did or did not do that makes you feel that way?*
CLIENT: (silence) *I don't think so. Actually no.*

According to the relational view, there is a mutual influence between the client and the therapist. Even though the client here said no, the therapist still holds in their mind the possibility of co-creation of this relational theme. However, at the moment the therapist focuses on the identification of the relational schema.

THERAPIST: *As you often feel this way in relationships, can we presume that through your life you developed the schema: I am unworthy, I am unlovable, others will reject me. How does that resonate with you?*
CLIENT: (silence, holding the breath)

THERAPIST: *What do you feel now in your body?*

CLIENT: *Pain and emptiness in my chest. Like an intolerable longing.*

THERAPIST: *Be aware of the thought I am unworthy, I am unlovable, and feel the pain in your chest; the emptiness, the longing. Does this remind you of something?*

CLIENT: (with eyes beginning to water) *I see my mother ... her still and cold face, passing by me ... taking care of my twin brother. He was very ill when we were small.*

Exploring fantasies and anticipations about relationships in the future

An important area of inquiry for identifying and understanding schemas is also expectations about the future. Through anticipation "the mind attempts to 'remember the future', based on what has occurred in the past" (D. J. Siegel, 1999, p. 30). Inquiring about expectations can help us to discover underlying schemas.

CLIENT: *As I told you, I have a new boyfriend. He is very attentive, loving, and kind. We enjoy very much our time together and have similar interests. The only thing that bothers me is this recurring thought: "He will leave me, and I will be alone again."*

THERAPIST: *"He will leave me and I will be alone again." What do you feel when you say that?*

The therapist, identifying anticipation about the future of the relationship that may be part of a dysfunctional schema, inquires about emotions connected to the client's expressed expectation.

CLIENT: (silence) *It hurts ... to be left.* (eyes starting to water)

THERAPIST: *Is this familiar?*

The therapist invites the client to search for similar experiences. Relational schemas are generalisations of numerous experiences, so this thought is probably not an isolated thought, but an expression of a recurring relational theme.

CLIENT: *I am always left in relationships ...* (silence) *My father left my mother and married another woman. Also, two previous boyfriends left me ...*

THERAPIST: *How do you interpret this?*

The therapist inquires about the conclusion that the client made out of these experiences.

CLIENT: *I am a person to be left ... like I am not worthy ...*

THERAPIST: *Just be aware of this conclusion: "Because my father left me, and two boyfriends left me, I am unworthy and expect to be left again."* (pause) *So this schema was created long ago and is now triggered in relationship with your boyfriend.*

The therapist identifies and educates the client about the dysfunctional core relational schema. According to the relational view, we want to emphasise that there is probably also something in the boyfriend's behaviour that triggers the client's relational schema even if the client has not mentioned it.

Recognising the influence of schemas on the client's life

After schemas are mindfully recognised, the therapist encourages an understanding of how schemas were constructed and how they influence the client's perception of themselves, others, and the world. They also explore the influence of schemas on their behaviour and anticipation of the future.

Collaboratively completing the Self-Narrative System

After schemas are collaboratively recognised, we may introduce the client to the diagram of the Self-Narrative System (Figure 7.1, Chapter 7). This intervention helps the client to develop an awareness of the impact of schemas on their lives. The Self-Narrative System shows how schemas are lived in everyday life and how we are continually reinforcing them. Filling in the Self-Narrative System is done together with the client starting first with filling in the first column related to the client's *relational schemas, autobiographical memories, and experiential avoidance.*

THERAPIST: *We have identified the core schema: "I am not worthy of love and others cannot be trusted", which was developed based on your childhood experiences of being with your depressed mother and your father who left the family. Which specific memories are connected to that?* (client and therapist write down specific memories). *Because of this schema, which emotions and needs do you avoid?* (client and therapist write down avoided needs and emotions).

Then we move on to the next column, which describes how schemas appear in everyday life.

THERAPIST: *Schemas can influence our lives, without our awareness that schemas are behind our everyday experiences. They are like glasses through which we look at ourselves, other people and the world. How does this schema influence your life? How does it appear in your behaviour, emotions, thoughts, expectations?* (The therapist and client together fill in the second column of the Self-Narrative System)

After that, we explore, together with the client how the schemas are reinforced in the client's life.

THERAPIST: *Schemas can become self-fulfilling prophecies. We live our life according to schemas and unconsciously behave in a way that reinforces them. In this way, we maintain the stability and predictability of our lives. In your life, which experiences are reinforcing your schemas?*

Promoting decentred awareness of relational schemas and self-states

After clients develop insight into the influence of schemas on their life, we can proceed with promoting decentred awareness of schemas and self-states.

Mindful awareness of Self-Narrative System

After the client completes their Self-Narrative System, we invite the client into mindful awareness of the whole diagram to promote decentred awareness.

THERAPIST: *Take a deep breath and observe what you have written. Remember that you are not your schemas and life-story. Schemas are constructions based on previous experiences. Take a few moments and become aware of what you are experiencing right now.*

We can promote decentred awareness with additional interventions, such as "Our life story in the cinema".

Exercise: Our life story in the cinema

This exercise invites clients to decentre from the Self-Narrative System by observing the elements of their life-story as if on a cinema screen.

"Take a few breaths … become aware of the diagram we just wrote. It shows how schemas are influencing your life and how they are reinforced. In this exercise, I will invite you to observe elements of your life-story as if they are appearing on a cinema screen.

Imagine that you are in the cinema and there is that big screen. And now imagine the first scene. The first scene has a subtitle: (name the schema). Now imagine briefly memories that influenced the development of the schema. First memory … second … third … Become aware that you are in the cinema watching memories. They are memories from the past …

The second scene is about living life according to the script of the schema. Imagine that it has the title: 'My life according to (name schema).' What do you see? What do you hear? And when you watch this film, become aware that you are in the cinema watching this. There is someone/ something observing this.

The third scene has the title: 'The curse of the schema.' It describes how the schemas are leading us into experiences that reinforce the schema. Become aware of these experiences … And remember that you are there, watching this film. And that this is just a film, a story that was written long ago …

Imagine that you can step out of this story, and you now have a free hand as a director. How would you envisage a story that would represent your deepest desires, wishes and values? This scene has a subtitle: 'My life lived in accordance with my values.' Just observe that on the screen … what do you see, hear? And how do you feel when you observe this new story? Become aware that you can be flexible about how you are living your life. You can choose which story you would like to live …"

Decentred awareness of self-states

Activation of relational schemas manifests in the self-states. As we described in Chapter 8, we are often merged with our self-states and look through their perspective. The first goal in working with self-states is developing a decentred perspective in relation to them, which is followed by acceptance and compassion.

In relationally focused integrative psychotherapy and transactional analysis, various methods of working with self-states have evolved, such as psychotherapy with the Parent ego state and methods for working with Child ego states (Erskine & Moursund, 1988; Erskine et al., 1999; McNeel, 1976; Moursund & Erskine, 2004; Zaletel et al., 2012). These methods can be useful for promoting metacognitive awareness of self-states and also for their processing. For example, psychotherapy of Parent ego states helps the client to decentre from introjects (Erskine & Trautmann, 2003). The client is invited to "become" one of the parents or other significant persons who influenced the client's development. The therapist then interviews the client as if they were one of their parents. This promotes metacognitive awareness of introjected self-states and promotes their integration.

In working with self-states, the therapist may talk directly to various clients' self-states, or they may invite the clients to relate to their self-states from their observing self. These methods promote mindful awareness of self-states.

In the following example, the therapist promoted decentred awareness and compassion towards a Child self-state that carried anxiety.

CLIENT: *I feel very anxious. I don't know what is going on.*
THERAPIST: *It seems like one part of you feels very anxious. How old is this part?*

By relating to anxiety as a part of the client, the therapist promotes decentred perspective.

CLIENT: *Very young … I am not sure.*
THERAPIST: *What are you seeing?*
CLIENT: *I see a small girl hiding behind the door and being terrified.*
THERAPIST: *When you look at that small girl, what do you feel towards her?*
CHILD: *Tenderness …*

Decentred awareness of vulnerable Child self-states by itself awakens self-compassion.

THERAPIST: *Let her know that you are here with her.*

Working with self-states proceeds according to the phases of relational mindfulness and compassion (see Chapter 9). The client first develops decentred awareness of their self-state and with validation conveys acceptance. In the next phase, the aim is understanding and normalisation of self-states that have a protective function, which is followed by being witness to emerging vulnerable self-states that were previously avoided and in exile. In Chapter 13, we provide examples of working with self-states related to the development of the compassionate internal relationship.

Promoting decentred awareness between sessions

Decentring from schemas can be further encouraged by different experiential exercises that the client can do between sessions. Clients may be invited to observe the activation of their schemas in daily life. They may pay attention to their internal dialogue, their experiences in interpersonal relationships, their fantasies ... They may also experiment with behaviour that is contrary to schema expectations and observe their experience when doing so. They may also write down their schema on a piece of paper and mindfully reflect on it during the week (Ecker et al., 2012), as we have seen in one of our earlier case examples.

Promoting living according to values and meaning

This therapeutic task aims to encourage clients to take action and start to follow their values. It may include different interventions that come from the practice of transactional analysis, acceptance, and commitment therapy (ACT) and different behavioural approaches. These interventions invite the client to commit to the specific behaviour that is congruent with their values. Promoting living according to values and meaning is related to the ACT process of committed action. S. C. Hayes et al. (2012) describe committed action as "a value-based action that occurs at a particular moment in time and that is deliberately linked to creating a pattern of action that serves the value" (p. 328). Promoting living according to values is related to the task of metacognitive awareness of schemas and self-states. Mindful awareness of painful emotions and thoughts enables clients to be more willing to try new ways of behaving.

Coming into contact with meaning and purpose

From the outset, we focus in the therapy not only on clients' problems and their difficulties in life, but we are also curious about the clients' values that give meaning and purpose to their life. We invite clients to go beyond the symptoms and imagine a life lived in full contact with meaning and purpose.

> "*If your problems could magically disappear, what would you do? What is important to you in life?*"

It is essential that values are rooted in the body-felt sense (Gendlin, 1981) and that clients experience values as inherently their own and not introjected from other people. For this reason, we invite clients to experience their values fully.

> *"When you think about the importance of connecting with your son, what are you experiencing right now? Just take a moment and feel this. (pause) What do you feel in your body?"*

The therapist also explores significant moments in their client's life that gave them purpose and meaning.

> *"Think of a moment in your life that gave you purpose and meaning. What comes to your mind?* (client shares it with the therapist) *Let your mind travel to that moment … What do you experience?"*

We may use techniques and exercises from ACT therapy, which invite the client into contact with their values (S. C. Hayes et al., 1999; S. C. Hayes et al., 2012; Luoma et al., 2007). A classic example is an exercise that invites clients to reflect on their life from the position of an older or deceased person (S. C. Hayes et al., 2012).

> *"Imagine that it is your 80th birthday and you are looking back over your life now. What would you say to yourself regarding what is important in life?"*

Contracts for mindful action

In comparison to behavioural therapy, in integrative psychotherapy we do not use the term "homework assignment" as it carries an implication of the therapist being a teacher and the client a student, who has to obey what the teacher says. In contrast, we use the term *contract*, which comes from transactional analysis (Berne, 1966). The contract is "an explicit bilateral commitment to a well-defined course of action" (Berne, 1966, p. 362). It implies the collaborative nature of the agreement. It is crucial that the client makes a contract with themselves rather than just pleasing the therapist. Contracts for mindful action are contracts that encourage clients to engage in a particular action while being fully present with their experience.

We first invite the client to discover different activities that are congruent with their deepest values:

THERAPIST: *When you imagine yourself living according to your value of taking care of yourself, how would your life look? What would you do?*
CLIENT: *Let's see: going to dance lessons, having at least half an hour a day for things I enjoy, meditation, going for a walk …*

When clients discover their values and the activities that are congruent with their values, we invite them to pick a few that they could bring into their life in the following weeks. Then we invite the client to commit to one of them.

THERAPIST: *You said that it would be important to you to take time at least half an hour a day for yourself, such as going for a walk, reading, or meditating. Are you willing to do this? To take half an hour just for yourself?*

CLIENT: *I would like to do it, but I feel anxious just thinking about it. When I try to do it, thoughts come: "I should do something more useful."*

THERAPIST: *Are you willing to take this time for yourself, even if anxiety and negative thoughts come? If a thought "I should do something more useful" comes, just notice it without trying to push it away. And then return your attention to doing the things you enjoy. It is similar to the mindfulness meditation that you practise; you focus on your breath, and when you get caught by some thoughts or emotions, you notice that and bring your attention back to your breath.*

Through such a response, the therapist is encouraging psychological flexibility (S. C. Hayes et al., 2012). Clients are invited to bring mindful awareness to their difficult experiences and at the same time to engage in an activity that is congruent with their values. The therapist emphasises the willingness to accept difficult experiences for the purpose of moving towards valued action. S. C. Hayes et al. (2012) defines willingness as "the choice to act in a value-based way while knowing full well that doing so triggers feared content" (p. 337).

Mindful contracts may be connected to different behavioural techniques such as exposure and behavioural activation. Congruent with ACT, we do not encourage behavioural change in order to get rid of unpleasant emotions. Quite the contrary, mindful contracts involve full acceptance of experience while engaging in the desired behaviour.

Mindful imagination of the desired action

Contracts for mindful action have to be specific. The client and therapist together specify when, where, and how the client will perform a specific action. We also invite the client to imagine doing this to make it more grounded in reality.

THERAPIST: *Let's imagine that you are going for a walk today. When and where would you go?* (wait for client's answer) *And now imagine that your walk has started. What do you see, smell, hear …* (wait for client's answer). *And what do you feel when you are walking? Accept whatever comes. If unpleasant thoughts or emotions come, accept them and return to walking.*

CLIENT: *It's beautiful, autumn colours in the forest … And now slight anxiety comes … "I have to do something at work, as we are approaching a deadline".*

THERAPIST: *Notice this anxiety and thoughts with acceptance and continue walking …*

When clients imagine that they are performing a particular action, which is contrary to their schemas, they may experience unpleasant thoughts, emotions, and sensations. We invite clients to be mindfully aware of such experiences while continuing with their particular action in their imagination. We track our clients through *the triangle of relationship to their experience* and accordingly encourage the client to stay as a loving witness in relation to their experience.

Mindful behavioural experiments

We can also devise *mindful experiments* that clients can try out either in the therapy session or between sessions. The client is invited to carry out some value related action while maintaining mindful awareness of any related painful experiences.

In the following example, the therapist invites the client to behave in a way which is contrary to her obsessive thoughts. The client Yasmin was an adolescent suffering from obsessive-compulsive disorder. In obsessive-compulsive disorder, we find an extreme lack of decentred perspective and avoidance of intrusive thoughts and images. Yasmin had intrusive images of seeing members of her family dead. She had numerous compulsions in seeking to avoid these intrusive images like counting in a particular order or turning on and off the lights. Although she enjoyed painting, she rarely used black as it triggered her intrusions. So the therapist invited her to experiment with drawing while maintaining mindful observation of what was happening within her while she was drawing.

CLIENT: (drawing nature, sea, house …)
THERAPIST: *When you draw, what are you experiencing in your body?*
CLIENT: *I feel anxiety and tension in my chest. Like I should not use black, so I instead choose green.*
THERAPIST: *Are you willing to do an experiment and try drawing with black? And when you do, you just let me know if intrusions come.*
CLIENT: *Ok. Will try.* (drawing black cat) … *Now came an image that my brothers will die in a car accident.*
THERAPIST: *Just observe this image. And be aware that it is just an image that comes and goes … Just let it be there without trying to keep it or push it away …. And draw further …*
CLIENT: *Now I am using red …* (draws a red roof) *Now comes the thought that something bad will happen to you … An image comes – that you will have a car accident.*
THERAPIST: *Just observe this image … It is just an image, you are observing it and coming back to drawing …*
CLIENT: *That calms me … They come and go. They do not stay. I'll try more with red and black* …

Such mindful experiments help clients to experiment with new behaviour that is congruent with their values and enhances psychological flexibility.

11 The therapist's mindful presence and physiological regulation in the therapeutic relationship

Therapy is an intersubjective process of mutual reciprocity and interdependence between the therapist and the client. In Chapter 5, we have described the "invisible" and subliminal interaction between the client and the therapist that exists alongside verbal and visible behavioural interaction. The therapist does not influence the therapeutic process through interventions alone (*what the therapist says and does in therapy*), but also through their way of being (*how the therapist is in the therapy*) (Geller, 2018; Geller & Greenberg, 2012; Ogden, 2018; D. J. Siegel, 2007). The therapist's "way of being" refers to mindful presence: awareness and acceptance of what is. The therapist's mindful presence influences the use and quality of interventions. We argue that for effective therapy, the therapist needs to be continually mindfully aware of their own internal states, the client's mental states, and the space between them, the therapeutic relationship. To be able to do this successfully, therapists need to "practise" mindful awareness and self-compassion. Self-compassion protects us from the process of self-criticism, which dysregulates us and leads us away from mindful presence. We propose that in psychotherapy training and supervision there should be a strong emphasis on recognising the importance of the therapist's mindful and compassionate state of mind and on helping the therapist to use these qualities in therapeutic practice.

"The therapist first": Therapists' mindful awareness as the foundation for effective psychotherapy

The psychotherapist's state of mind has a crucial impact on the psychotherapy process. In a therapeutic relationship in which the therapist is mindfully present and compassionate, the client can receive optimal interactions which address the client's needs, regulate the client's autonomic nervous system and bring the client into a state of safety.

We propose that the first thing psychotherapists need to do in each therapy session is to focus their mindful attention onto themselves. The theory of psychotherapy methods usually emphasises the client as the main focus of the therapist's attention, attunement, and regulation. We are suggesting that this mindful attention, awareness, and regulation during the session should be primarily turned to the psychotherapist themselves. In other words, mindful awareness of the therapist's own states and their physiological regulation comes before attention to and regulation of the client. The rationale is the same as with the situation on an aeroplane when the level of oxygen falls dangerously low. First we have to put the oxygen mask on ourselves and only then do we put the mask on the child. Because of this emphasis on the primacy of the therapist's mindful attention to themselves, we have entitled this section "The therapist first". By being mindfully aware of their inner states, therapists can come into contact with themselves. We suggest that the therapists' mindful awareness of their own states and internal contact with themselves is a foundation for effective psychotherapy.

To do this, therapists have to activate their mindful state of consciousness, which is a quality of the *observing self*. If therapists look at themselves only from the personal sense of self, they may quickly become self-absorbed: "Oh, I am anxious, I don't know what to do now, I am incompetent." This will result in the therapy not being productive. For the therapy to be effective, therapists need to activate the observing self; then they can mindfully, with the attitude of acceptance, observe and regulate both their own autonomic states and their clients'.

Once in this state of mindfulness, the therapist's mind is "flexible, adaptive, coherent, energized and stable" (D. J. Siegel, 2007, p. 78). These qualities allow the therapist to *think and act effectively*. Mindful awareness helps the therapist to recognise implicit, unconscious therapeutic processes, transference, the counter-transference, as well as enactments and ruptures in the therapeutic alliance (Safran & Muran, 2000). The therapist's observing self and related mindful awareness are therefore essential for building, maintaining, and repairing the *therapeutic alliance*. The therapist can mindfully track the quality of the therapeutic bond and can detect the first signs of any rupture in the alliance (Safran & Muran, 2000). Recognising a rupture is the first and most essential step within the process of rupture repair. Rupture repair strengthens the alliance and deepens its quality (M. Žvelc, 2008).

Mindful awareness enables *interoception*, awareness, and understanding of the body and its physiological states. Interoception is the foundation of all other levels of the therapist's awareness and is a vehicle for effective psychotherapy. Mindful awareness of the body and its physiological states helps the therapist to self-regulate and enables the therapist to be *aware of emotions* that may be present during the therapy session. Awareness of the emotions that arise before, during, or after therapy informs the therapist about their own emotional part in the countertransference. It enables the therapist to understand the counter-transference and if necessary, regulate it and wisely use it in a psychotherapy session. Mindful awareness of their emotional state prevents a therapist from acting out or withdrawal.

Mindful awareness is also a foundation for *wisdom and compassion* (Brach, 2012; R. D. Siegel & Germer, 2012). Within the compassionate state, the therapist recognises and understands the suffering of their clients. It is also essential for therapists to show compassion to themselves in the situation of self-criticism or other difficult moments, connected to psychotherapy work.

How can we, the therapists, during the therapy session, achieve and maintain a presence, pervaded with mindful awareness? We suggest that we need to learn about the concept of mindfulness in our training. We recommend practising mindfulness meditation regularly. This will strengthen the ability to be mindfully aware in our lives in general, as well as in the therapy session. Being mindful in action (Safran & Muran, 2000), during the therapy session, begins much earlier than the start of the session itself and refers to the way in which we live our daily lives (Geller & Greenberg, 2012).

The therapist's interoception and self-regulation

The therapist's interoceptive awareness of their own body signals including physiological states is of great importance for effective clinical practice. By awareness of their own physiological sensations, the therapist can, because of the process of physiological synchrony, infer and understand the client's states, which is the basis for empathy and efficient attunement (Erskine et al., 1999; Fosha, 2000b; Iacoboni, 2009; Prochazkova & Kret, 2017; D. J. Siegel, 2007). The therapist also needs to develop mindful interoceptive moment-to-moment awareness to be able to self-regulate. With self-regulation, the therapist modulates their physiological state of arousal and keeps their autonomic nervous system (ANS) out of states of defence, within the window of tolerance (Geller & Porges, 2014; Ogden et al., 2006; Porges, 2017; D. J. Siegel, 2012). Within this state, cognitive processing is organised, the therapist can reflect and mentalise, and flexibly decide which intervention to use. Emotional acting out or withdrawal of the therapist is prevented. Self-regulation of the therapist also enables regulation of the client.

By interoception within the therapy session, the therapist detects their own physiological states which inform them about the level of ANS arousal. The therapist by noticing that their heart is beating fast, their body restless, and that they are feeling impatient, becomes aware that they are in a dysregulated defensive autonomic state, in hyperarousal. Alternatively, the therapist may notice that their breathing is shallow, posture bent and still, and that they are feeling blocked and have no idea what to say next. These can be the signs of hypoactivation of their ANS. The therapist, by being mindful of their dysregulated states, *already starts to self-regulate*. Mindful awareness and the compassionate acceptance of their own physiological and emotional states, whatever they are, offers them safe inner space, helps them to self-regulate and enables them to be present with the client.

If the therapist is in a mobilised state, they need to calm their ANS, and if in an immobilised state, they need to mobilise. By being mindfully aware of their body, the therapist can sense what the body would like to do for regulation (Levine, 1997) enabling them to take additional self-regulating actions. In mobilised states the therapist may further self-regulate by bringing attention to their breathing, prolonging the out-breath, and bringing awareness to the soles of their feet. In an immobilised state the therapist needs to mobilise themselves, for instance by breathing deeply (because breathing in the immobilised states slows down and becomes shallow), by moving their hands and legs, and changing body posture. Therapists might also want to use other resources to help themselves to regulate.

Without mindful awareness of the body and their physiological states, a therapist cannot be present, and cannot realise when they are dysregulated. We believe the majority of the mistakes which therapists make are the result of their dysregulated autonomic states.

Regulation of the client's hyper and hypoarousal

Nervous systems crave reciprocal interaction to be regulated and to feel safe (Porges, 2017). The therapist through their own regulated state implicitly co-regulates the client. They can also regulate the client in active ways by enhancing the client's mindful awareness and self-compassion or by other strategies.

There are various strategies for regulating the activation of a client's ANS defence system. When the client is in a *mobilised state*, in *hyperarousal*, the therapist helps the client to down-regulate the arousal. The therapist does this implicitly through calm presence, which is conveyed through a kind look, gentle voice, soft facial expression, and gestures. The therapist needs to slow down the client's pace and lead the client to mindful observation and recognition of their physiological state. Mindful awareness, decentred perspective and acceptance all contribute to regulation. If the activation of ANS is very high, we do not explore that state in detail or leave the client to stay in that state alone. The therapist helps the client to realise that they are in hyperarousal and helps them to down-regulate. Breathing rhythm with longer exhalation (Geller, 2018) and inviting the client to become mindfully aware of their hands and feet (Levine, 2018) can be useful in this regard. Different types of sound (vocalisation, music and musical instruments, including tuning forks) can be used for the regulation of hyper or hypoarousal (Erbida Golob & Žvelc, 2015). Other specific techniques, like the *calm imaginary place*, can also be used. The therapist by regulating the client, at the same time regulates themselves.

When a client is in an immobilised state, their ability to be aware of their internal sensations is severely limited (Levine, 2018). First, the therapist invites the client to become mindfully aware of their immobilised state. Here the mobilising of the client's ANS is needed. The therapist initiates this by inviting the client to move; it can be in an actual physical movement or imaginary. The therapist also guides the client into being mindfully aware of any feelings about how the body may wish to move or any sensations of strength (Levine, 2018). Vocalising the out-breath and singing can also help to activate the ventral vagal tone (Porges, 2017, Levine, 2018). The therapist should join in with the client and in this way self-regulates and also saves the client from feeling embarrassment. The therapist's soft voice usually does not help; it can even intensify feelings of danger and shame (Levine, 2018). What is needed here is a directive, encouraging, strong but respectful and not rough voice. When the client's ANS is regulated, within the window of tolerance, the therapist can start or proceed with other tasks in the therapy.

"I am not alone": Vignette from a therapy session

We will now systematically, step by step, introduce the practical use of a therapist's mindful awareness and regulation in the course of a therapy session, starting with the therapist's awareness of their own body and physiological states. We will present part of a therapy session between a female therapist and her client Tina, fully describing the following seven *therapeutic tasks* that are related to the therapist's mindful awareness and physiological regulation: (1) The therapist mindfully prepares for the session, (2) The therapist is mindfully aware of her body/physiological sensations and emotions during the session and assesses her autonomic state, (3) The therapist self-regulates, (4) The therapist attunes to the client and mentalises about the client's state, (5) The therapist mindfully observes the client, (6) The therapist promotes mindful awareness within the client, (7) The therapist regulates the client. These seven tasks are all interconnected steps in the therapy. They can be generalised to other sessions and other cases.

   With all of these tasks, the therapist uses her *metacognitive skills*. She mentalises about the meaning of the observed body sensations, physiological and emotional states, which she recognises within herself and in the client. This mentalisation and reflection accompany mindful awareness and observation in the course of therapy. The therapist wants to understand her own and her client's mental and autonomic states.

Step 1: The therapist mindfully prepares for the session

The therapist has a break, where she prepares herself for the next therapy session. The preparation consists of being present and mindfully aware. She is aware that her breathing is calm, she feels the warmth of the heater and looks through the window at the mountains that are bathed in sunshine. She loves them. She feels a sense of awe and yearning, looking at them. Then she remembers some details from the last session with the client. She feels warmth towards the client. She recalls the intention why she is here waiting for Tina, and how she is her client's fellow traveller helping her on her life journey. Being in touch with this intention deepens the therapist's spiritual awareness, which is already evoked with looking at the mountains.

Step 2: The therapist is mindfully aware of her body/physiological sensations and assesses her autonomic state

Client Tina arrives. There is a cordial greeting between them. When Tina sits down, she exhales deeply, as if here is safe and she can finally relax. She starts to talk about the things she had to do at work which were stressful, but she managed to do them very well. Tina is happy and proud of her success. The therapist while listening to and observing Tina, is at the same time mindfully aware of her own body sensations, physiological states, emotions, and thoughts. The therapist is aware that she feels happy for and proud of Tina, and that she feels ease and warmth in her body.

Later in the session, Tina begins to talk with a reasonably enthusiastic voice, but with an accelerated tempo about a meeting at work the next day, where she will meet the man she is beginning to be attracted to. While listening to Tina, the therapist is mindfully observing: "*I am aware of a painful sensation in my stomach. I am also aware of my stronger heartbeat, my breathing is …, I don't know, it is not at ease and calm, and my hands are cold and clammy.*" The therapist is aware of her physiological changes. Through mindful observation of her body, she also becomes aware of her emotions "*I sense anxiety.*"

Awareness of her own physiological state (accelerated heartbeat, irregular breathing, cool and clammy hands, painful sensation in the stomach and sensing fear) helps the therapist to assess the state of her autonomic nervous system (ANS): "*I think I am mobilising; approaching the hyperaroused state.*"

The therapist uses the word "approaching" because, despite the activation of her sympathetic system, she could nevertheless observe and tolerate her sensation and feelings; she was not flooded with them. The therapist knows that she attunes and synchronises with the client's physiology quite easily. She knows that physiological synchrony is a common process in psychotherapy. Now she wants to prevent further synchronisation with Tina's dysregulated physiology. The therapist is also aware of the important theoretical premise: for psychotherapy treatment to be effective, it is "necessary to keep the autonomic nervous system out of states of defence" (Porges, 2017, p. 24) and within the window of tolerance (Ogden et al., 2006; D. J. Siegel, 1999). Through mindful awareness, she prevents further arousal of her ANS; she grounds herself and by that regulates herself. She sees mindful awareness as taming the "wild," dysregulated processes, which have their origins in trauma. She has experience of self-regulation and regulation of clients, and that gives her confidence and security.

Step 3: The therapist self-regulates

For regulation of her mobilised state, our therapist uses mindful awareness processes: present moment awareness, acceptance, and decentred perspective. She is aware of her body and her present physiological and emotional states in an accepting way. Based on mindful awareness of the body, adaptive actions of the body arise. The therapist starts to breathe in a soothing rhythm. She is also self-compassionate, putting her hand on her stomach in a kind and loving way, and saying to herself: "*Everything is OK. The body is telling me an important story; important processes are going on right now in the therapy.*"

We can see how the therapist is from a decentred perspective observing the content of her mind. The process could be outlined: "*I observe you, the content of my mind, I am not merged with you, and I think you are important. I am safe here from my observing and loving place.*" She is not fighting against the observed processes; she is accepting them. At the same time, with the acceptance, self-compassion and decentred perspective, she is providing care, support, and a safe space for herself.

With the regulation of the therapist's autonomic state and activation of her ventral vagus, the look in her eyes, tone of her voice, facial expressions, posture, movements, and gestures are all changing. The autonomic system of the therapist provides calm and safe information to the client and may implicitly co-regulate Tina. Tina will through the processes of neuroception (Porges, 2017), latently (subconsciously) detect those changes in the therapist, and there is a high possibility that her physiology will also calm down. The impact of the therapist's autonomic states on the client also depends on client factors and we cannot be certain how the client will react to the therapist's regulated ventral vagal state. In cases of severe trauma, clients may develop faulty neuroception, which means, that they might "detect risk when there is no risk or identify cues of safety when there is risk" (Porges, 2017, p. 20).

Mindful awareness and self-regulation help the therapist to function within the window of tolerance, be socially engaged, present, and to further attune to herself and the client.

Step 4: The therapist attunes to the client and mentalises about the client's state

While the therapist is becoming aware of her sensations and is regulating herself, at the same time she also mentalises, looking for the meaning of what she perceives in her body:

> "I am feeling my stomach ache, my heart is beating faster, my breath is irregular, and my hands are sweating. I sense anxiety. How come I am beginning to feel this right now? I wonder, what is the meaning of these sensations? Does this remind me of something? If I were meeting somebody I would be excited, maybe anxious, but not with this pain and in fear … Am I resonating with something that is going on in Tina's body right now? … Maybe Tina is frightened; maybe she is hyperactivated; she might have a stomach ache. I'll check."

Because of the mutual interaction of the client's and therapist's physiology, there is a high possibility that the client is also experiencing physiological changes and is probably in the dysregulated autonomic state. Based on the therapist's awareness of her own physiological and emotional state, our therapist has a sense of the client's physiological and emotional state, which is the basis for her empathy and attunement. In other words, the therapist is becoming aware of her bodily and emotional countertransference. Based on her awareness of her body and physiological sensations, she has a hypothesis about the client's states. What the therapist feels might be similar to what the client is feeling. Alternatively, it may be a feeling that is different from the client's, but triggered by the client's state. This process can be explained by physiological synchrony, mimicry, and emotional resonance. Our therapist's internal processes, from awareness, self-regulation, and mentalisation, are quick, taking less than a minute.

Step 5: The therapist mindfully observes the client

The therapist also mindfully observes the client's state, which is revealed through the client's body. The therapist, with her open and accepting mind, follows any changes in the client's body. She observes the posture, gestures, the way the client looks, talks, the quality of the voice, features of the skin, breathing, muscle tone, and movements. She is attentive to *changes* in the client's body, as the changes in the body show changes in the client's inner world (in physiology and emotions) (Lowen, 1975/1988; Reich, 1942/1988). She is particularly attentive to her client's breathing because the internal (psychological) state is always revealed through the breath (Reich, 1942/1988). The therapist is accepting of whatever it is that she notices about her client. She knows that the client's body is telling a significant story about the client (Erskine, 2014), and she sincerely appreciates and values this. She is open to any hypothesis regarding the meaning of her client's behaviour. She is not anxious or eager about getting any particular insights; sometimes, she can't explain the observations she has, and that is fine, too. In her mindful way, she accepts what is. From this position, she can then decide on meaningful action.

The therapist mindfully observes: "*Tina is speaking in an accelerated tempo, her eyes are restless, she looks tense in her shoulders, and she is not taking time to breathe in.*" The therapist connects this observation with an observation of her own state and mentalises: "*I have this feeling like I can't feel her, connect with her any more. I was becoming hyperactivated and felt anxiety; probably she is experiencing anxiety … but it seems that she wants to avoid her sensations and feelings. She is blocking her breathing. I am going to inquire about what is happening inside of her.*"

Up until now, we have been presenting the therapist's inner processes in psychotherapy. We see that the activity of the therapist is not limited only to her outer actions – her methods and interventions in the classical sense – but also to her inner, invisible "activity" – being mindfully aware, interoception, self-regulation, co-regulation, self-compassion, emotional resonance, observation of the client, and mentalising. These processes are the *internal activity of the therapist*. We suggest they should primarily be led by a bottom-up process (Ogden et al., 2006). This means that the therapist first becomes mindfully aware of the body; other activities and interventions are then built on the therapist's contact with the body.

In the next two steps, the therapist will explicitly communicate with her client.

Step 6: The therapist promotes mindful awareness within the client

The therapist decided that she will ask Tina what she is experiencing inside of herself. With this phenomenological inquiry (Erskine et al., 1999) the therapist is raising Tina's awareness of her internal world. The therapist wants to develop and promote the client's mindful awareness *within* the therapy sessions. She starts by asking Tina what she is experiencing in her body. The therapist is starting phenomenological inquiry from the bottom-up, to ground the content of the client's story in her body awareness and experience (Fosha, 2000b; Ogden et al., 2006). Tina can come into contact with herself through the connection with her body and emotions within the safe therapeutic relationship (Fogel, 2013; Fosha, 2000b; Moursund & Erskine, 2004; Ogden et al., 2006).

172 Methods and interventions

THERAPIST: *Tina, if we now stop a little ... and we turn our attention to our bodies ...* (The therapist talks more slowly; pauses for a moment, she turns her attention to her body as well.) *What are you experiencing in your body right now?*

CLIENT: *Hm ... I don't know ... I am aware that I was not aware of my body until now. Let's see.* (stops for a few seconds) *It is quite uncomfortable. I feel tense in my body and pressure in my chest. My heart is pounding.*

If the client answered right away, with words like: "I'm OK", "nothing", "nothing special", she is probably not taking time to observe mindfully, and perhaps she is trying to protect herself by avoiding her sensations. In our case, Tina mindfully observes and becomes mindfully aware of feeling uncomfortable, of having pressure in her chest.

Because Tina was able to come into contact with her body sensations, the therapist wants to lead her further into mindful awareness of her emotions. She knows that when clients come into contact with their body and core emotions, usually the cognitive level also changes. They enter a different cognitive state of mind, where they can reach forgotten memories and get new insights, accessing deeper layers of unconscious material (Fosha, 2000b). Clients often go in circles with their stories and problems (Angus & Greenberg, 2011). Getting into contact with their bodies and emotions within the window of tolerance can help them break out of these circles.

THERAPIST: *Which emotion do you feel?*

CLIENT: *I guess anxiety ... fear ... and ... can it be ... embarrassment? A little.*

The tension in Tina's body, stronger heartbeat, feeling fear and embarrassment all point to sympathetic mobilisation.

Before the therapist asked Tina about her body state, Tina was in a dysregulated, mobilised state. When the therapist slowed down the therapy by initiating a mindful pause from "talking", Tina followed the therapist and then mindfully observed and verbalised her inner state. From these signs, the therapist knows that Tina has activated her social engagement system and is already more regulated. The therapist also feels more at ease in her own body, and her hands are warmer. Because of all these indications, the therapist decides to proceed with the inquiry. Tina's body and emotional awareness may lead to previously "unknown" thoughts and memories.

THERAPIST: *Do you have any thoughts, pictures, or memories that flip through your mind, right now?*

CLIENT: (after some seconds) *I have a thought: don't tell her. It's none of her business. You'll regret it.*

Tina is remembering something significant. Although she is struggling to share this memory with the therapist she feels safe enough to express her thoughts which is the sign of a good alliance. "Breaking the ordinary talking" about the meeting the next day and bringing mindful space into the therapy, gives the client and the therapist a chance to enter deeper levels of the therapy.

THERAPIST: (with an accepting look and gentle voice, reflects) *Mm-hm. There is something you are aware of, but you are struggling to tell me.*

The therapist acknowledges Tina's struggle and her protective mechanism. She does not fight the client's process of protection. With her look and the tone of her voice, she communicates to Tina that she is accepting her and her protective mechanisms. She also implicitly communicates that she understands, that the struggle is there for a reason. She talks to Tina's Adult self-state, to bring her back into the here and now. She wants to activate Tina's mindful observation and decentred perspective.

CLIENT: *Mm-hm.*

Silence. The therapist offers a mindful and compassionate presence.

THERAPIST: *You have a good reason for that. … For struggling to tell me or not.*

The therapist acknowledges and validates (Erskine et al., 1999) Tina's feelings and protective mechanisms. She conveys acceptance and compassion for Tina. Tina is holding her breath. The therapist spontaneously gets a picture in her mind of a small lonely girl sitting in the corner. The image is in different shades of grey. The therapist has a feeling that it is difficult to reach the girl. She feels a sense of loneliness, sadness, and pain; and also that it is somewhere far off, almost unreachable. She uses this image and with a gentle, accepting, and compassionate voice says:

THERAPIST: *It was there for a long time. You were all alone with this. Nobody knew.*

In her voice and through other nonverbal pathways there vibrates the feeling of loneliness, sadness, pain, and yearning for contact. The therapist addresses Tina's Child self-state. By the therapist's attunement to Tina, and acknowledging, accepting, and validating Tina's protective mechanisms, they paradoxically melt, and Tina speaks:

CLIENT: (slowly) *I have a picture. Of my neighbour. Touching me. I am small.*

Tina looks down, her spine and shoulders bent, and her breathing "stops".

Step 7: The therapist regulates the client

Tina turns her eyes away and flops into a powerless position. The therapist, at that moment, recognises in herself that her breath is becoming shallow and a feeling of coldness is crawling inside of her. The therapist realises that she is approaching a lighter "version" of hypoarousal, which Rothschild (2017) calls the lethargic state. The therapist assumes that Tina is also entering an immobilised state and decides that regulation is needed. The therapist opens her chest to let her breath in fully and "starts" breathing. She moves her palms and feet gently. The awareness of her own and her client's autonomic states and knowing what to do, bring energy and safety to the therapist. She comes from hypoarousal back to the ventral vagal autonomic state and asks the client:

THERAPIST: (in a kind, but determined voice) *Tina, would you mind looking at me?*

The immobilised state is the state of being shut down and cut off from connection with the outside world. The therapist is inviting Tina to come back into contact with her because she knows they have previously built a strong alliance. Her intention is not to leave Tina alone; she was alone for too long. She also knows that by having eye contact with the client, she can regulate her better. She trusts that with the help of her grounded and regulated ANS state, she can co-regulate Tina. At the same time, she is continuing to support herself and take care of herself by breathing and slightly moving her hands and feet from time to time. Movement mobilises the therapy field.

CLIENT: (looks at the therapist)

This is a good sign. Tina later said that it was as if there was a life-saving rope in the therapist's eyes, something which was bringing her back. She felt that the therapist was with her. Tina also moves her hands and feet. Then she says:

CLIENT: *I want to stand, I want to breathe, and I want to move.*

Tina initiates this progression. They both stand up, walk, breathe, stretch, and shake. With moving, they are regulating themselves, climbing the hierarchy levels of ANS, from immobilisation to safe mobilisation.

CLIENT: *I want to live!*

Immobilisation, when it is a defensive state, symbolically represents death; whereas mobilisation arising out of immobilisation, symbolically represents birth and life.

THERAPIST: (with a firm voice) *Yes!*

She feels even more energy rising in her body and that she can emotionally connect with the client's words.

THERAPIST: *Where in your body do you feel "I want to live"?*

The therapist wants to anchor Tina's experience in her body. However, it may be too soon.

CLIENT: *I think I felt it in all of my body … my arms and legs were strong … but now … as if something would like to prevent me from feeling this … Like there is an obstacle in my chest, preventing me from breathing fully.*

Tina cannot integrate her awakening desire to be fully alive; a part of her is "protecting" her from being "alive". The therapist is at first disappointed that the feeling of aliveness disappeared so quickly, and is wondering if her intervention was too early. Then she says to herself that although it is precious that Tina could feel this desire to live, according to trauma theory, we cannot expect that she will feel safe with this feeling. The therapist hypothesises that what was stopping Tina from letting herself be fully alive was her shame and guilt.

THERAPIST: (with an accepting voice) *Mm-hm, you felt "I want to live" clearly in your body, and then the feeling started to vanish. There is meaning to it.* (a few seconds later with a gentle voice) *It was not your fault … and the neighbour is the one who did wrong. He had no right to do that.*

The therapist provides the message to Tina's Child and Adult self-states that she is not guilty and responsible, and that she does not need to punish herself. Tina has as a child concluded that what happened was because of her and that it was her fault. This schema was probably activated in the session, and the therapist gives Tina new information that provides a *juxtaposition* to old emotional learning.

The therapist leans closer, puts her hand on her own chest (which promotes compassion and self-compassion) and says:

THERAPIST: *I am glad you told me …* (silence) *I appreciate you told me. I am with you.*

Tina looks at her, nods and starts to cry. It is an expression of deep pain and self-compassion, and with it comes relief. The therapist is moved, and her eyes start to water. She feels the compassion flowing from her heart. It was a precious moment of deep inner contact within the client and between the client and the therapist. Even though the therapist has not had the same experience as the client, she knows her vulnerable part; being alone, sad, and yearning for contact. She also knows the guilt and the shame … Being compassionate to the client, she was also providing compassion to herself. It was a moment of shared humanity between two human beings, two souls connected in their vulnerability, which makes them stronger, loving, and alive. It was a moment of meeting, of I–Thou relationship (Buber, 1999).

In the next session, Tina connected her feelings of anxiety and embarrassment related to the man she was attracted to, with the abuse by her neighbour. Tina gained the insight that the desire to approach the man she was attracted to was linked to the fear of abuse and humiliation and the prohibition from enjoyment. She started to understand that her wounded Child self-state activates in relationships with men. Tina then briefly described what happened with the neighbour and what happened afterwards. The therapist was mindful about their autonomic states and initiated regulation when needed. They processed the event a few months later when Tina felt ready for it.

In MCIP we want to promote mindfulness, compassion, and self-compassion in the therapists, as well as in the clients. We want to enhance our clients' resources and widen their tolerance to stay with their feelings, body sensations, and thoughts. We wish them to be present while telling their profound stories. At the same time, we, as therapists, also want to stay present while the clients are telling their stories. In that way, the memories, thoughts, emotions, and body sensations can be integrated. Then the stories become healing.

12 The transforming power of mindfulness: Mindful processing[1]

In Chapter 9, we describe methods of relational mindfulness and compassion that invite the client into present moment awareness, decentred perspective, acceptance, and self-compassion. Those methods enhance mindfulness and compassion processes through an attuned and involved therapeutic relationship. They provide a foundation for all other interventions in MCIP. In addition to those relational methods, we also use various intrapsychic methods that invite the client into mindful awareness and compassion. In these methods, the focus is on the client's relationship with themselves. The attuned therapeutic relationship is still there but as a background to the client's intrapsychic work. The role of the therapist is the role of the catalyst for the client's internal process, so that clients, from the position of the *observing self,* relate to their internal experience and various self-states. They are embracing their inner world with mindful awareness and compassion. Intrapsychic methods provide a deepening of the clients' processes, as they give the clients more time and space to be with their inner world. Both relational and intrapsychic methods are complementary and are often used interchangeably during one session.

Mindful processing and transformation of inner experience

We have previously proposed that mindfulness promotes natural healing of the organism, where change happens spontaneously by acceptance and awareness of internal experience (G. Žvelc, 2014; Žvelc & Žvelc, 2008, 2009). Mindfulness not only promotes an open and accepting relationship to the inner experience but also promotes processing and transformation of emotions, physical sensations, and cognitions. We have termed this process *mindful processing* (Žvelc & Žvelc, 2008). We proposed that with mindful awareness, clients can process and integrate disturbing experiences. When we are able to embrace our experience with acceptance, curiosity, and openness, the inner experience starts to transform. The processes of present moment awareness, decentred perspective, acceptance, and self-compassion are at the heart of this process of transformation.

Psychological problems are frequently a consequence of the tendency to avoid or escape from painful experience (S. C. Hayes, et al., 1999). We often cannot stay with and accept our experience. This is a primary mechanism behind most defence mechanisms (McWilliams, 2011). Clients who come for psychotherapy are often distanced from their experiences and are trying to control or repress difficult emotions, disturbing thoughts, and body sensations. They develop an aversive stance towards their experience, which eventually brings additional pressure, symptoms, and self-criticism. With mindful awareness, we provide a new accepting context for inner experience, which is the exact opposite of defence mechanisms, such as repression or dissociation. Inviting clients into a mindful processing mode can reverse the cycle of avoidance of inner experience.

Mindful processing may be one of the main mechanisms of change in different psychotherapies which are concerned with the processing of emotional and somatic experience. It may be one of the mechanisms behind the effectiveness of EMDR therapy. In EMDR this process is called "dual awareness", where the client maintains "a non-evaluative 'observer' stance with respect to emotion and to the flow of somatic, affective, cognitive and sensory associations" (F. Shapiro, 2018, p. 233). It enables the client to stay present while simultaneously experiencing elements of past traumatic memories. The non-evaluative observer stance refers to mindful processes of the present moment, acceptance, and decentred awareness. We proposed that mindful awareness is crucial for trauma treatment, regardless of the treatment method (Žvelc & Žvelc, 2009). It enables clients to come into contact with traumatic memories and at the same time observe them as the loving witness.

Fundamental assumptions of mindful processing method

Based on the understanding that mindful awareness can promote the processing of painful experiences, we have developed a method that is focused entirely on promoting mindful processing. This method provides a context in psychotherapy in which mindful processing can occur. In mindful processing, we are intentionally bringing mindful awareness to painful feelings, body sensations, or other experiences. We are using the power of mindful awareness for the transformation of the personal sense of self. This method was in its initial form presented for the first time at the fourth European conference on positive psychology (Žvelc & Žvelc, 2008). In the last ten years, we have further developed and refined the method. We have integrated the method with the theory of memory reconsolidation (Ecker et al., 2012), polyvagal theory (Porges, 2011, 2017), Fosha's (2000a, 2000b) concept of metatherapeutic processing and EMDR (F. Shapiro, 2018). The mindful processing method is used within the overall framework of MCIP, and it can be easily integrated within other therapeutic approaches. Relational mindfulness and compassion methods are the foundations for its use.

With mindful processing, the therapist invites the client to become aware of their moment-to-moment subjective experience with curiosity and acceptance. The client comes into contact with disturbing experiences, evoked by painful memories or dysfunctional schema. They are invited to attend to body sensations related to the disturbing experience and mindfully observe their inner world. After a few moments of mindful awareness, the client is gently invited to come into contact with the therapist and share with them their inner experience. After short moments of sharing, the client is again invited into mindful awareness of their inner world. In mindful processing, the client alternates between mindful awareness of their inner world and the relational experience of sharing that with the therapist. The client is invited to pay attention to any experience that emerges from moment-to-moment. Through such an exchange of internal and external contact, the client's experience starts to transform and process. These two aspects of mindful processing can also be described as intrapersonal and interpersonal attunement (D. J. Siegel, 2007). In intrapersonal attunement, the client attends to themselves with compassion, kindness, and acceptance. When the client shares their experience with the therapist, the interpersonal attunement of the therapist helps the client to accept and embrace their experience. Presence, acceptance, and the attunement of the therapist promote a new "relational" experience, which is an antidote to previous relationship ruptures when the client had to deny and repress their inner experience.

In mindful processing, every moment is valuable and meaningful. We invite the client to pay attention from moment-to-moment and to embrace each moment with acceptance and loving-kindness. The psychotherapist's task is to embody the qualities of mindful awareness and to encourage the client to do the same. The therapist facilitates and invites the client to become a loving witness to their inner experience. They invite the client to relate to their experience from the position of the observing self, which manifests in present moment awareness, decentred perspective, acceptance, and self-compassion.

In contrast to the relational mindfulness methods that we describe in Chapter 9, the therapist is here less active in terms of verbal interventions. The therapist gives space to the client to fully immerse into their own experience. The therapist is a guide that facilitates the client's mindful process.

Body-centred method focused on interoception

Mindful processing starts with focusing on body sensations connected to the disturbing experience. This is taken from Gendlin's (1981) focusing approach and gestalt therapy (Perls et al., 1951). In mindful processing, the primary focus is on body-felt experience from which other elements of subjective experience arise (emotions, cognitions, memories …). Attention to the body-felt sense is like an anchor, to which we regularly invite the client to return. Interoception is one of the main processes of the mindful processing method. Mindful processing integrates both bottom-up and top-down processing, as the client alternates between mindful awareness and reflection on the experience.

Importance of therapist's mindful presence and attunement

During mindful processing, the therapist should relate to themselves and the client from the position of the observing self. They have to be fully present and aware of what is happening both within themselves and what is happening with the client. The therapist offers an accepting space to all of the client's experiences that are emerging from moment-to-moment. The therapist is not trying to change the contents of the client's experience; their role is to remain curious and open and to contain the process and emotions that are arising. Only such a stance can promote mindfulness in the client. If the therapist cannot stay present with "what is", but is oriented towards achieving a goal, this will have an impact on the client. The therapist's embodiment of a mindful stance is crucial. In Chapter 11, we write about the importance of the mindful presence of the therapist that helps the client to stay within the social engagement system and helps to regulate the client's experience. The mindfulness of the therapist is, through the process of physiological synchrony, a catalyst for the mindful awareness of the client.

Trust in inner wisdom and innate capacity for processing

In mindful processing, the therapist trusts the client's inner wisdom. This is congruent with Rogers (1957), who proposed that the therapist's role is to create the right conditions in the course of therapy which will help the client to facilitate his innate tendency to actualize. Unconditional positive regard of the therapist is based on their trust in "the integrity and dependability of his client's organismic tendency to actualise" (Tudor & Worrall, 2006, p. 88). In MCIP, the client's mindful awareness creates the conditions for processing to occur. If the client can be present with their experience, the change will come spontaneously. Often this does not come in the way we expect, so the therapist remains open and curious regarding the ongoing process of the client. The therapist has to tolerate the experience of not-knowing, with no predetermined goal for the client and being empty of expectations. Their only intention is related to being a loving and compassionate witness who is concerned for the welfare for the client.

Mindful processing as relational meditation

The method of mindful processing shares similarities with mindfulness meditation. It is like meditation in a relationship, and it could be called *relational meditation*. There are two mindful people in the room, and the therapist is continually inviting the client to pay attention to the present moment with acceptance. Clients who come for therapy because of mental health problems often have difficulty accepting their inner experience. They find it hard to tolerate and stay with disturbing thoughts and emotions. Mindfulness meditation is sometimes "too hard" for them; they become lost in their experience and have great difficulty in developing a decentred perspective. In mindful processing, the therapist helps them establish a mindful stance, which involves the capacity to observe inner experience. The therapist provides *cues of safety* for the clients so that they can risk diving deep into their experience. The therapist's presence can promote a mindful stance in the client that would be difficult to achieve alone. Moreover, such a stance promotes the processing and integration of disturbing experiences.

In mindful processing, the client alternates between mindful awareness of their inner world and sharing their experience with the therapist. Contact with the therapist provides a grounding for the client in the present moment, which is similar to focusing on the breath in mindfulness meditation. In most forms of mindfulness meditation, the meditator is monitoring their attention. When it floats away from its primary focus, the meditator becomes aware of this and gently brings it back. In mindful processing, the therapist helps the client to monitor their attention and helps them to maintain mindful awareness, with frequent reminders for the client to stay aware of the present moment. When meditating alone, we can become lost in our thoughts, emotions, and sensations, especially if painful memories and emotions emerge. Because of this, we may move towards either the distant or merged pole of the triangle of relationship to experience (see Figure 3.2, Chapter 3). The therapist in our mindful processing method helps the client to stay a loving witness to inner experiences.

The mindful processing method and memory reconsolidation

We propose that the beneficial effects of mindful processing can be explained by the process of memory reconsolidation (Ecker, 2015; Ecker et al., 2012; Lane et al., 2015). The mindful processing method includes all of the phases that Ecker et al. (2012) found to be necessary for therapeutic memory reconsolidation: accessing sequence, transformative sequence, and verification.

In the accessing sequence, the emotional learning that is behind the symptoms is identified and retrieved, bringing it into explicit awareness and identifying disconfirming knowledge. In MCIP, the client and therapist together discover core dysfunctional relational schemas that are behind the symptoms and identify knowledge from past or present experience that is contrary to these schemas (see Chapter 10). In the preparation phase of mindful processing, we select the dysfunctional schema and related autobiographical memories that will be targeted in mindful processing.

The second phase refers to the transformative sequence, where old emotional learning is juxtaposed with new disconfirming knowledge (Ecker et al., 2012). This step unlocks synapses that maintain target learning, opening a time window of about five hours during which old learning can be dissolved by new learning (Ecker et al., 2012). For memory reconsolidation, repeated juxtaposition experiences that provide mismatch and experiential dissonance are needed. In the final verification phase, the aim is to ascertain whether memory reconsolidation has occurred by observation of certain markers of transformational change (Ecker et al., 2012). Both these phases are an essential part of our mindful processing method.

Mindful processing starts with the activation of dysfunctional schema and focusing on related body sensations. In order for memory reconsolidation to occur, old emotional learning has to be activated and experienced. In mindful processing, clients often spontaneously come into contact with disconfirming experiences that are in contrast to old dysfunctional memories. We usually do not specifically seek disconfirming knowledge but rather trust in the client's inherent brain capacity for processing and for transformation to come by itself through the inherent ability of the organism for processing. How does this occur? We propose four main hypotheses as to how the juxtaposition experience in mindful processing occurs.

Decentred awareness of schemas activates the brain's innate error detection system

Through mindful awareness of dysfunctional schema, there often spontaneously arise new insights and experiences that are contrary to old emotional learning. The brain can be understood as an error detecting system. As Seth (2013) describes, there is an increasing view within cognitive science and neuroscience that "prediction and error corrections provide fundamental principles for understanding brain operation" (p. 565). The predictive coding theory of brain functioning proposes that "the brain is continuously attempting to minimize the discrepancy or 'prediction error'" (Seth, 2013, p. 566).

We propose that when we become mindfully aware of dysfunctional schema, the brain automatically detects memories and knowledge that are contrary to old "truth". In this way clients through mindful processing come into contact with new experiences that are incongruent with dysfunctional schemas. In everyday life, when schemas are activated, we usually become merged with them and view our world through them. We are unaware that schemas influence our experience and behaviour. Because of this, it is less likely that we will detect information that is inconsistent with the schema.

In mindful processing, we are relating to schema activation from a decentred perspective. We observe the schema activation from the position of the loving witness, instead of looking through the glasses of the schema itself. This helps us to become spontaneously aware of the knowledge that is inconsistent with the schema. Dysfunctional schemas provide a rigid view of the world, which often reflects our childhood way of coping and experiencing the world. When we can relate to our schemas from a decentred perspective, we also begin to notice knowledge and experiences that are contrary to old schemas. We relate to our experience from a broader perspective that is no longer limited to the eyes of the dysfunctional schema. In our brain there exist memories and knowledge that are both consistent and inconsistent with dysfunctional schemas. Mindful awareness of schemas activates the brain's innate error detecting system, which brings to awareness also experiences that are contrary to old schemas.

Another important process in mindful processing is *interoception*, where the therapist regularly invites the client to focus their attention on body sensations. The predictive coding model of interoception may help us to understand how processing occurs at the level of body sensations (Farb et al., 2015; Seth, 2013; Seth et al., 2012). This model describes how "interoceptive processing regularly involves a comparison between immediate sensation and simulated past and future states" (Farb et al., 2015, p. 7). If the immediate sensation is different from previous expectations, the sensation can be changed to fit previous expectations, or prior expectations are updated to fit current body sensations. Although this process can operate automatically and unconsciously, if automatic responses fail to reduce prediction error, we may become aware of that and can actively engage in regulation (Farb et al., 2015).

In mindful processing, we are mindfully aware of body sensations related to the dysfunctional schema. Body sensations are activated in a new context of safety, acceptance, and nonjudgment that promotes their transformation. We propose that this process produces a prediction error where there is a mismatch between expected states and current body experience. Body sensations are tolerated and accepted, as opposed to the previous way of avoidance. During mindful processing, body sensations transform, and clients feel differently in their body. This may change prior expectations related to body sensations and provide emotional regulation (Farb et al., 2015).

In terms of relational schemas theory, subsymbolic elements of schemas are in this way updated and changed. This often happens automatically, even without conscious elaboration. The client, after a few cycles of mindful awareness of body sensations and sharing feels differently in their body. We speculate that in this process there is a continuous updating of subsymbolic aspects of schemas. The predictive coding model of interoception may be one explanation for this process.

Mindful processing transforms emotions and provides new emotional experiences

Through mindful awareness, painful emotions are processed and transformed. For example, the client who may have started processing with an experience of fear related to a dysfunctional schema may end up with a feeling of power and strength. New emotional experience acts as a mismatch to old emotional learning.

For emotional change to happen, the client has to feel and experience the emotion, tolerate, and accept it (Fosha, 2000b; Greenberg, 2008; Greenberg & Paivio, 1997). Our clinical experience is congruent with Fosha's (2000a, 2000b) findings that fully experiencing core affect releases adaptive action tendencies – coping responses and resources – together with liveliness and energy. Greenberg (2008, p. 53) argues that "a maladaptive emotional state can be transformed best by undoing it with another more adaptive emotion". In MCIP, mindful awareness and compassion enable the client to be fully aware and accepting of their affect and also promote a new emotional experience of compassionate and loving presence. The painful experience, for instance of anxiety, fear, powerlessness, or shame, is imbued with the energy of awareness, acceptance, and compassion, which results in the transformation of affect.

In our experience with clients, we have found that if clients can truly and mindfully observe their experience, the experience starts to transform. If the client cannot be mindful of their emotional experience, then affect regulation or other methods will be needed first.

Mindful awareness itself as a source of disconfirming knowledge

Another source of disconfirming knowledge is the mindful state itself. Relating to our experiences with openness, acceptance, and compassion is in stark contrast

```
┌─────────────────────────────┐
│      1. PREPARATION          │
└─────────────────────────────┘
               │
               ▼
┌─────────────────────────────┐
│      2. ACTIVATION OF        │
│      SCHEMA / MEMORY         │
└─────────────────────────────┘
               │
               ▼
```

3. CYCLE OF MINDFUL PROCESSING

```
┌──────────────────────┐           ┌──────────────────────┐
│  MINDFUL AWARENESS    │ ◄──────► │      SHARING          │
└──────────────────────┘           └──────────────────────┘
          ▲                                   │
          │         ╭──────────────╮          │
          │         │ NEW EXPERIENCES│         │
          │         │  LEADING TO    │         │
          │         │ JUXTAPOSITION  │         │
          │         ╰──────────────╯          │
          │      ┌──────────────────────┐     │
          └──────│  CHECKING ORIGINAL    │◄────┘
                 │       ISSUE           │
                 └──────────────────────┘
                            │
                            ▼
```

```
┌─────────────────────────────┐
│    4. PROCESSING OF          │
│    JUXTAPOSITION             │
│    EXPERIENCE                │
└─────────────────────────────┘
               │
               ▼
┌─────────────────────────────┐
│    5. METATHERAPEUTIC        │
│    PROCESSING                │
└─────────────────────────────┘
               │
               ▼
┌─────────────────────────────┐
│    6.  INTEGRATION           │
└─────────────────────────────┘
               │
               ▼
┌─────────────────────────────┐
│    7. VERIFICATION           │
└─────────────────────────────┘
```

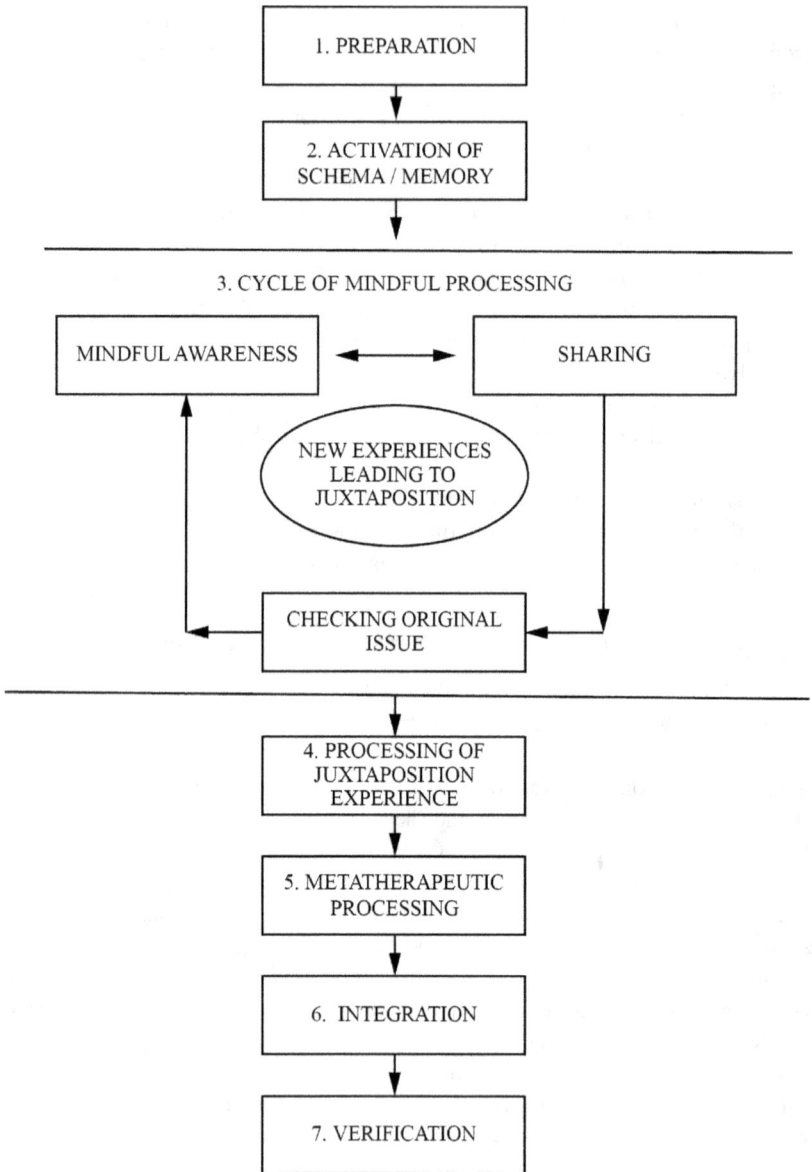

Figure 12.1 Schematic presentation of the mindful processing method

with avoidance and self-criticism. We often avoid painful experiences, and we tend to push them out of awareness. We may fear something terrible will happen if we were to experience particular memories. So activation of schemas, memories, and self-states in a new accepting context may provide a valuable mismatch experience to our old ways of relating to ourselves.

Sometimes it is the fear of painful memories that is driving the symptoms. Clients may experience anxiety as they are unconsciously afraid of contacting painful memories. Mindful processing itself may be a new experience that is contrary to an old schema that painful experiences are dangerous, and that it is better to avoid them.

Attuned psychotherapy relationship as a corrective relational experience

In mindful processing, a new corrective experience with a mindful and compassionate therapist may provide a juxtaposition experience to old relational failures. Dysfunctional schemas and traumatic memories are often related to negative relational expectations. When they are activated, clients can fear that other people, including the therapist, will hurt them, shame them, or react in other painful ways. When old traumatic memories or schemas are activated, the client's old expectations can be *juxtaposed* with an accepting and compassionate therapeutic relationship (Erskine, 2015; Erskine et al., 1999).

Phases of the mindful processing method

In this section, we describe the seven phases of mindful processing: (1) Preparation, (2) Activation of the schema/memory, (3) The cycle of mindful processing, (4) Mindful processing of the juxtaposition experiences, (5) Metatherapeutic processing, (6) Integration, (7) Verification. These seven phases should be seen more like guidelines rather than something fixed. Mindful processing can be used flexibly in psychotherapy for the experiential exploration and processing of current issues, processing of past painful experiences and for developing positive resources. We use it also in supervision for the exploration of therapists' countertransference. Figure 12.1 schematically presents these seven phases of our mindful processing method.

Phase 1: Preparation

Preparation for mindful processing includes both the therapist and the client.

Preparation of the therapist

In mindful processing, the therapist's ability to be mindful is crucial. During mindful processing, the therapist is fully present and relates to the client from the position of a loving witness. Preparation of the therapist may include brief mindfulness exercises before the session, such as brief body scan, mindful attention to breathing or exercises that promote self-compassion (such as the *loving hand*). It is important for the therapist to reaffirm their intention to be fully present and compassionate with the client. The therapist's ongoing practice of mindfulness may be beneficial in developing this capacity to be mindful with the client. In addition to mindful practice, the therapist's training, supervision, and personal therapy are essential for cultivating the therapist's ability to stay present with the client's experience.

If the therapist and the client are preparing to work on a significant traumatic experience, the therapist has to ask themselves if they are ready to accompany the client through this process. The therapist's readiness to work with trauma is often a neglected part of trauma therapy.

Preparation of the client

Mindful processing builds upon previous phases of the therapy in which the client has already developed their capacity for mindful awareness and self-compassion, and a solid therapeutic alliance has been established. The client has to feel safe with the therapist so that they can allow themselves to be fully immersed in their world and share this with the therapist.

Not all clients are ready for mindful processing. Some clients have difficulty attending to their inner experience, even for a short time. These clients typically suffer from high or low emotional arousal, related to unresolved traumatic experiences and have difficulty regulating their emotions. They have great difficulty staying within the window of tolerance and social engagement system. For these clients it is vital to assess their ability to be in a mindful state of mind before introducing mindful processing. Such clients would need a more extensive preparation phase that would focus on developing their ability to contain difficult emotions and developing their capacity for self-regulation. Methods of relational mindfulness and compassion (see Chapter 9) are beneficial in this regard, as they help clients to develop the capacity to stay present with their emotions and provide regulation of emotions. These methods are also crucial for developing a good therapeutic alliance, which is the foundation for using the mindful processing method. Trust in the therapeutic relationship is needed so that a client feels free to experience whatever they may experience.

In addition to the general preparation of the client for mindful processing, preparation also takes place in the session itself. Before the start of mindful processing, the therapist may invite the client to do a brief mindfulness exercise, such as awareness of the body, breathing, or just a simple invitation to be in the present moment. We also use mindful meditation related to the diamond model of the observing self or exercises that promote self-compassion, such as a loving hand (see Chapter 10).

> "*Be aware that you are here. Look at the room, what do you see, what do you hear. Sense your body sitting in the chair …*"

Such preparation enables the client to begin the mindful processing method from the position of a loving witness. Being in the position of a loving witness also implies that the client is within the social engagement system (Porges, 2017) and window of tolerance (Ogden et al., 2006).

Choosing the target for mindful processing

The main targets for processing need to be chosen. Mindful processing can focus on a specific traumatic memory, dysfunctional schema, or any disturbing emotions or sensation. It can also focus on positive experiences and emotions. The Self-Narrative System (see Chapter 7) may point us towards which target would be good to process in order to facilitate change in the personal sense of self. In previous phases of MCIP, the client and the therapist have already identified the main dysfunctional schemas and autobiographic memories that can be a target for mindful processing.

Description of mindful processing to the client

The therapist describes the method to the client and makes an agreement about the use of mindful processing.

> *"At the beginning, I will invite you to focus on the body sensation which you experience when you think about this painful issue. Your task is to observe what is happening inside. Gently notice what is happening. Thoughts, images, emotions, or body sensations may arise. There is no plan for what should happen. The task is to notice and be aware of your experiences. After some time, I will invite you to share with me what has occurred. You will just tell me what you noticed. After that, I will again invite you to observe and notice what is happening for you at that moment. And then again, I will invite you to share your subjective experiencing. So we will alternate between your internal process of experiencing and your sharing of that experience.*
>
> *There is no plan for what should happen. The task is just to be mindful and in contact with your inner experience. Maybe sometimes nothing new will emerge, you just report on that. If some thoughts or emotions arise that you don't want to share, you just tell me that you don't want to share them. That is completely fine. If you would like to stop this exercise, you just tell me or lift up your hand. How does that sound to you? Are you willing to proceed with this method?"*

During the periods of internal focus, the client can have their eyes either closed or looking at a certain point in the room.

> *"You observe and notice what is happening with openness and acceptance. We call this aspect of you, which observes the contents of the mind, the loving witness. During mindful processing, you can have your eyes closed or focused on something in the room. This is similar to meditation, where we often have our eyes closed or focused on a certain point in the room. Do you have any preference? During the session, you can experiment with what feels better for you."*

Some clients do not want to close their eyes as they feel they are losing control. They prefer to keep their eyes open. Sometimes we may suggest the main focus of attention based on their position on *the triangle of relationship to experience* (see Chapter 3). Some clients, who have difficulties in making contact with body sensations and emotions, find it easier to close their eyes so that they exclude the external environment and focus just on their internal process. For clients who are overwhelmed with their emotions and are experiencing high sympathetic arousal, focusing on a point in the room may be more calming and stable. Some clients can quickly get into contact with their inner world, even without closing their eyes or focusing on any particular point. They may prefer no focus at all. So it is important to be attuned to their experience.

An additional focus of attention

The main aim of mindful processing is to facilitate the client's mindful awareness during the processing phase. This can be promoted by different means. For some clients, who suffer from complex trauma, it is challenging to stay in the window of tolerance and to be present with experience. So for them, we may include an additional focus of attention to promote present moment and decentred perspective by inviting them to attend to their breath during processing. Awareness of breathing brings the client into the present moment and promotes self-regulation. Other focuses of attention may be creatively chosen together with the client, including, for instance, music on which the client focuses during processing. Certain music which includes *prosodic* vocals can promote activation of the social engagement system (Porges, 2017). For some clients, an activity like unstructured drawing can be beneficial by helping the clients to attend to their inner experience while drawing. Some clients may like tactile stimulation and may, for example, like to play with a piece of playdough. Some clients feel that their therapist is the greatest source of safety and groundedness. So for them looking at the therapist while engaging in the observation of their inner world may help them to stay inside the window of tolerance.

During the mindful processing phase, we may also integrate methods from other therapeutic approaches so that clients can remain mindful during processing. We may include bilateral stimulation, which originates in EMDR therapy (F. Shapiro, 2018). The therapist may interchangeably gently tap the client's right and left hand. In addition to bringing attention to the present moment and decentred perspective, tapping provides an additional sense of the therapist's presence. We can also use special devices that provide bilateral stimulation, such as electronic, audio, or tactile devices.

Any additional focus of attention is chosen together with the client. We may present the client with different options for focusing attention and ask the client what he feels would help most in staying present during the processing phase.

> *"During observation of your inner world, you may experience disturbing images, thoughts or emotions that may pull you out of your position as the loving witness. In order to stay*

present with your experience, we sometimes include an additional focus of attention. Some people like to focus on their breath, listen to music, draw or play with playdough. Some clients prefer to watch their therapist, who gives them a sense of safety. Some people find helpful tapping or holding in their hand devices that provide bilateral stimulation (show). What do you sense would be helpful for you?"

Based on the process of the client, we may creatively adjust the focus of attention during processing. If the client is not suffering from significant trauma and has a good ability for mindful awareness, an additional focus of attention is not necessary. However, with clients who are prone to dissociation, an additional focus of attention is often necessary to help them stay present and within the social engagement system.

Phase 2: Activation of the schema/memory

In phase 2, we invite the client to activate dysfunctional schemas, memories, or come into contact with any other experience they would like to process and mindfully explore. Usually it is the issue which the client and therapist chose as a target in the preparation phase.

Awareness of body sensation connected to the disturbing issue

The primary entry point in mindful processing is awareness of any body sensation connected to the issue.

THERAPIST: *When you think about the whole issue, what do you feel in your body now? Where do you feel it in your body now?*

Utilising the Scale of Physiological Arousal (SPA)

In order to assess the state of physiological arousal connected to the disturbing issue, we use the Scale of Physiological Arousal (SPA). We developed the SPA for measuring physiological hypoarousal and hyperarousal (see Figure 12.2).

The scale extends from −5 to +5. Hypoarousal is on a scale from −1 to −5; it covers such signs as the absence of sensations, feeling numb, feeling frozen, "empty-headed", spacing out; 0 is the optimal arousal point which manifests in feeling calm, relaxed, safe, focused, and grounded. Hyperarousal is on a scale from +1 to +5. It covers a higher intensity of emotions and physiology such as feelings of being upset, anxious, disturbed, nervous etc.

We educate the client about the theory behind the functioning of the autonomic nervous system regarding arousal zones (see Chapters 5 and 11).

> *How would you assess your arousal on a scale from -5 to +5?*
> *- 5 is the most frozen or collapsed you have ever felt,*
> *0 is optimal arousal,*
> *and +5 is the most upset and disturbed you have ever felt in your life.*
>
> **Hypoarousal**   -5 -4 -3 -2 -1 0 1 2 3 4 5   **Hyperarousal**
>
> | | | |
> |---|---|---|
> | Feeling numb | Feeling calm | Feeling upset |
> | Collapsed | Relaxed | Feeling disturbed |
> | Feeling frozen | Feeling safe | Feeling anxious |
> | "Empty-headed" | Focused | Nervous |
> | Spacing out | Grounded | Heart beating |

Figure 12.2 The Scale of Physiological Arousal (SPA)

We then ask our client how they would assess their arousal from −5 to +5 on the SPA.

THERAPIST: *When you think about the issue now, how would you assess your arousal on a scale from −5 to +5. −5 is the most frozen or collapsed you have ever felt, 0 is optimal arousal, and +5 is the most upset and disturbed you have ever felt in your life.*

Focusing on body sensation related to the issue

THERAPIST: *Focus on that body sensation and just observe what is happening.*

The therapist is attuned to the client and to their experience, observing the nonverbal signs of the client and also the client's process of experiencing. The therapist is fully aware and present, in contact with self and the client. After a few moments, the therapist asks: *"What is happening now?"* or *"What are you noticing?"*. The client shares their experience with the therapist.

Phase 3: Cycle of mindful processing

In the cycle of mindful processing, there are two main subphases: (1) The client's mindful awareness of internal processes and (2) Sharing with the therapist. The client alternates between mindful awareness of inner processes and the sharing of their experience with the therapist. The cycle of mindful processing also includes checking the original issue.

Subphase 3.1
Mindful awareness of internal processes

The client's mindful internal awareness is initiated with an invitation to be present with their experience.

"Be aware of that and notice what is happening inside you."
"Be aware of (sensation, thought, feeling)."
"Observe that (experience) with loving eyes."

In this phase, the client is centred on their internal experience. Through mindful awareness, the client becomes increasingly aware of their body sensations, emotions, thoughts, and other contents of awareness. The client relates to experiences with openness, acceptance, decentred perspective, and compassion. In this phase, clients may have their eyes open or closed, or focused on a certain point in the room. Additional focuses of attention may have been selected, as described in the preparation phase. The therapist, with their nonverbal attitude, encourages the client to experience whatever they may experience.

The therapist's primary intervention is expressed in a short invitation to awareness and acceptance of experience such as *"Just be aware of that," "Observe that," "Focus on that," "Make room for this experience."* If the client can stay witness to their experience, there is no need for the therapist to do much else verbally. The therapist is following the client and inviting them to pay attention to the present moment. However, when the client is moving away from being a loving witness to their experience, the therapist may intervene accordingly, so that the client can become mindful again. In this way, the therapist promotes regulation of the client's autonomic nervous system and helps the client to stay inside the window of tolerance.

In Chapter 9, we describe methods of relational mindfulness and compassion that can also be used flexibly in the mindful processing method. The triangle of relationship to internal experience (see Figure 3.2, Chapter 3) helps the therapist to determine when the client is losing the stance of the loving witness and is becoming merged or distanced regarding their experience. Sometimes clients are distanced from their emotions and body sensations. In this case, the therapist may gently invite the client to attend to and accept the experience. This is often done by attending to and focusing on body sensations and emotions or by validation of the client's experience.

"Just focus on that sensation/emotion."
"Make room for this sadness."
"They are important tears. Just let them come."
"Just let yourself feel this."

Sometimes the clients are so merged with their thoughts, emotions, or physiological sensations they have difficulty with decentring from their experience. In this case, the task is to develop an appropriate distance from the experience.

The therapist may promote decentring with an invitation to observe the experience:

"Just observe these thoughts."
"Make a distance between you and your emotions and observe what you are experiencing."
"Put your emotions out into the room outside of you. And just observe them."

Contact with the observing self also promotes decentring:

> "*Imagine that you are awareness, and these thoughts appear in it.*"
> "*Become aware of who or what is aware of all these emotions.*"
> "*Come into contact with a wise part of you, the part, which has wisdom and love. Just look at the experience through the eyes of wisdom.*"

If the client is critical and judgemental towards their experience, the therapist may invite the client to self-compassion and loving-kindness.

> "*If you are willing, put your hand on your heart, feel the warmth of it and embrace the sadness.*"
> "*Imagine that someone who cares for you is here with you. Just imagine that you are looking now through the eyes of that loving person …*"

Body sensations are the main anchor to which we are regularly inviting the client to return. So when we sense that the client is losing contact with self, awareness of body sensations helps the client to come back to the present moment and back into contact with themselves. This is especially important when the client starts intellectualising and becoming removed from the experience. Sometimes clients can become dysregulated because they become merged with disturbing images or thoughts. Attending to body sensations can lower the emotional arousal, as clients are no longer focused on the disturbing images or thoughts.

It is crucial to assess the client in terms of their position on the triangle of relationship to experience and to check whether the client is within the social engagement system and window of tolerance (see Chapter 11). If the client is in a dysregulated state, it is crucial to provide physiological regulation. Relational mindfulness and compassion methods may help the client to stay mindful and in the position of the loving witness. The therapist may acknowledge, validate, or normalise the client's experience and provide regulation of affect. The client through the process of *neuroception* senses the therapist's calm state of ANS, which also promotes the client's physiological regulation. Besides relational regulation, we may also use other interventions to help the client come within the social engagement system.

Subphase 3.2 Sharing with the therapist

After a few moments of mindful awareness of the present experience, connected to the disturbing issue, the therapist invites the client to share their inner experience. The therapist uses their attunement skills to know when is the right time to ask the client to make contact with the therapist.

> "*Tell me what is happening now.*"

or

> "*O.K. What do you notice?*"

In this subphase, the client is invited to find words for their inner experience and share that with the therapist. This phase promotes the symbolisation of emotions and somatic experiences. The therapist is attuned to the client and gently invites the client to accept and be aware of whatever is present. The mindful presence of the therapist invites the client to mindful awareness. If the client can stay in the window of tolerance and can be present with their experience, the therapist is just following the client and is not actively intervening. The basic idea is to stay with the client's phenomenological moment-to-moment experience and not to interfere with their process. We trust in the client's innate inner wisdom. However, if the client becomes dysregulated and starts losing the witnessing position, the therapist intervenes more actively.

Subphase 3.3 Alternating between mindful awareness and sharing

The therapist invites the client to alternate between mindful awareness and sharing the experience with the therapist. Rhythmic attunement to the client is crucial to determine the amount of time for each subphase. Usually, mindful processing alternates quite quickly between these two phases. At the beginning of mindful processing, we invite the client to attend to their inner world for about 10–20 seconds. However, each client may process differently. Some clients need a longer time to come into contact with themselves and to notice what they are experiencing. On the other hand, some clients are quickly overwhelmed, so just a few seconds of mindful awareness may be enough.

Example of the cycle of mindful processing:

THERAPIST: *When you think about the event with your boss, what do you feel in your body now?*
CLIENT: *I feel that something is emerging … like some dark feeling. I am not sure what it is.*
THERAPIST: *Allow yourself to be with it. Make space for it.* (the therapist is promoting acceptance of experience.)
CLIENT: (mindful awareness) *It is like a bullet in my stomach … Like something old and painful.*
THERAPIST: *Mm-hm. Observe and be curious …*
CLIENT: (mindful awareness) *Now came an event from childhood. When I was five years old, my father wanted me to eat up all of this disgusting vegetable soup. I resisted and then I was beaten.*
THERAPIST: *Ok, just observe it and be aware of your breathing.*
CLIENT: (mindful awareness) *I feel anger … Like the bullet was this anger, which stayed in me.*
THERAPIST: *Allow yourself to be with whatever comes.*
CLIENT: (mindful awareness) *Just now I've had a picture, that bullet came from my stomach and I throw it into my father. I feel angry. I would like to tell him what I should have told him long ago.*
THERAPIST: *Trust your intuition and go with whatever comes.*
CLIENT: *"You had no right to do it! Lots of children do not like disgusting vegetables!"* (in an angry tone)

Subphase 3.4 Checking the original issue

When, during processing, we sense that the client has experienced a significant shift in terms of new insights, changed perspective or emotional/body experiences, we may invite the client to check the original issue. This subphase is taken from EMDR (F. Shapiro, 2001). We have included it because in our experience, it promotes memory reconsolidation, as the client contrasts old emotional learning with new experiences gained during processing. In this way, the client can become simultaneously aware of old and new knowledge. As we regularly invite the client to check the original experience, the client can experience repeated juxtapositions.

We may also invite the client to check the original issue when the client's associations are becoming too distant from the original issue. In this way, the client comes back into contact with the original issue.

THERAPIST: *If you bring* (the original issue) *into your awareness, what comes up?*

If new associations are coming and the original issue is still painful, we invite the client into another cycle of processing, starting with subphase 3.1 – mindful awareness of internal processes.

If the issue is processed, the client will usually report new insights, changed perspective, positive affects, peacefulness, or strength in the body. They will experience the original issue without intense emotional and physiological arousal. We may ask the client to check the state of their arousal with the Scale of Physiological Arousal (SPA):

THERAPIST: *When you think about the original issue now, how would you assess your arousal on a scale from −5 to +5? −5 is the most frozen or collapsed you have ever felt, 0 is optimal arousal, and +5 is the most upset and disturbed you have ever felt in your life.*

Phase 4: Mindful processing of the juxtaposition experiences

During mindful processing, new insights and experiences often come spontaneously that are contrary to old dysfunctional schemas. For memory reconsolidation, repeated juxtapositions between old and new learning are necessary (Ecker et al., 2012). In this phase, we intentionally promote explicit awareness of the juxtaposition between old and new learning.

Subphase 4.1 Highlighting the new learning

We may ask the client about new emotional learning:

"*When you think about the original issue, what is new?*"
"*How do you experience now the original issue, what is different?*"

We may also highlight the new learning with a simple acknowledgement:

> *"So you discovered that not all men are mean, that some may be ok."*
> *"So you discovered that you are valuable, even if you make a mistake."*
> *"You discovered that you are worthy, even if other people criticise you or try to humiliate you."*

New learning is not necessarily always expressed in words. When processing implicit emotional memories, sometimes new learning is more in the form of a transformed body-felt sense, new emotional experience, or transcendent experiences, such as deep peace and love. We invite the client to be aware of this newness in relation to the old experience.

Subphase 4.2 Mindful processing of the juxtaposition between old and new learning

Ecker et al. (2012) describe how it is crucial for memory reconsolidation that clients are simultaneously aware of the contrast between old and new emotional learning which have to be experienced at the same time. Congruent with this, we invite the client to be mindfully aware of both old and new learning. A decentred perspective enables observation of competing truths at the same time.

THERAPIST: *Become aware of this contrast between believing that you are a bad person and the experience that you are OK even if you make a mistake. Be aware of both at the same time.*

or

THERAPIST: *Become aware of both experiences at the same time. You felt that something's wrong with you, and now you experience this deep acceptance of yourself and sense you are a normal human being.*

Cognitive awareness of a juxtaposition experience is not enough for memory reconsolidation. Juxtaposition has to be fully felt in the body, so we invite the client to focus on body sensation.

THERAPIST: *When you think about both issues together* (therapist names them), *what do you feel now in your body? Focus on that.*

After this, we initiate another cycle of mindful processing (phase 3).

Phase 5: Metatherapeutic processing

In this phase, we integrate Fosha's concept of *metatherapeutic processing*, which is the processing of the client's experience of positive affect connected to successful therapeutic work (Fosha, 2000a, 2000b; Fosha & Conceição, 2019). It involves the processing of positive, transformational emotional change and the experience of the therapeutic relationship that promoted the change (Fosha, 2000a, 2000b; Fosha & Conceição, 2019; Iwakabe & Conceicao, 2016).

THERAPIST: *What is it like for you to have this experience?* (name the positive, transformational experience the client has just had here in the therapy)

or

THERAPIST: *What is it like for you to experience this whole process with me?*

The therapist may also disclose their own experience of the client's mindful processing. Self-disclosure by the therapist may deepen the relational contact and encourage the client to share their experience of the relationship.

THERAPIST: *I feel moved by a sense of compassion that you felt today for yourself. Thank you for letting me be a witness to your experience. And what is it like for you sharing this with me?*

When the client shares their experience with the therapist, we invite them to begin a new cycle of processing (phase 3), which involves cycles of mindful experience and sharing with the therapist. Through this process, clients can experience transformational affects (Fosha, 2000a; Fosha & Conceição, 2019) such as pride, joy, mourning for the self, tears of joy, being moved, gratitude.

Mindful processing occurs in the presence of an attuned and mindful therapist. During the mindful processing, the client may experience deep contact with the therapist, which may be a significant new experience that is in contrast to old experiences of relational failures. If the client experienced such a corrective relational experience, we might also invite them to process this juxtaposition experience with the therapist. We invite the client to focus on the difference between previous relational experiences and their new experience with the therapist.

Phase 6: Integration

In this phase, the aim is to provide closure for mindful processing and integration of the new experience. The client is invited to check the original issue and to reflect on the whole experience. This provides further integration. We also tell the client that processing and memory reconsolidation may continue. Memory reconsolidation research suggests that taking a nap within a period of six hours after therapy may be helpful for memory reconsolidation (Lane et al., 2015).

Repeated juxtaposition experiences may also occur between sessions. We invite the client to remain mindfully aware during the week of the contrast between old dysfunctional schemas and the new learning, which came through mindful processing. One option, which Ecker and colleagues (2012) suggest is that the therapist together with the client writes down on a card both the old emotional learning and the new learning gained through mindful processing. The client is then invited to remain aware while at home of both aspects. We combine this instruction with a suggestion for mindfulness practice focused on the juxtaposition experience:

"You can do a short mindfulness exercise, such as attending to your breath. And then you take your card and focus on what we've written down, both the old and the new learning. And become aware of what is happening inside you. You become aware of your body sensation, emotions, thoughts. And after that, you again turn your attention to your breath."

Phase 7: Verification

At the next session, we re-evaluate the client's processing and verify whether memory reconsolidation has occurred by observing markers of transformational change (Ecker et al., 2012). Successful memory reconsolidation shows in non-reactivation, symptom cessation, and effortless performance (Ecker et al., 2012). Successful processing shows in lowered emotional and physiological arousal and a new perspective and insight towards the original issue. We also check how the client coped during the week in connection with the usual triggers of schemas. If memory reconsolidation did not occur, and the client is still aroused regarding the issue, we can continue with mindful processing.

Note

1 The chapter includes some material adapted from "Mindful processing in psychotherapy: Facilitating natural healing process within attuned therapeutic relationship" by G. Žvelc, 2012, *International Journal of Integrative Psychotherapy*, *3*(1), 42–58 (www.integrative-journal.com/index.php/ijip/article/view/54). CC BY. Adapted with permission of the author.

13 Self-compassion: The road to a loving and healing inner relationship

Our children's grandfather once said to our sons when you start to love yourself that is the beginning of a long-lasting loving relationship. In every moment of our life, no matter what the circumstances, no matter if we are succeeding or failing, we can be friends with ourselves, we can always be by our side, wishing us well. This is accessible to all of us, at any time, anywhere. We can lean on this aspect of ourselves, which loves us and supports us. There is a "deep well of compassion" inside each of us (Desmond, 2016, p. 91).

Every person has a specific relationship with themselves. This relationship can be loving, warm, supporting, and friendly or violent, cold, rejecting, and pushing. The aspect of ourselves which immanently holds love and compassion is our *observing/transcendent self*. MCIP helps the client to rebuild the bond with that compassionate aspect of us and create a loving inner relationship. While being self-compassionate, we relate in a profoundly different way to ourselves and promote transformation and change. Self-compassion leads to regulation and widens the window of tolerance. Self-compassion provides safety, which is the essential prerequisite for human balance, well-being, and satisfying social interactions. It is a relational state (Neff, 2011). Through self-compassion, a person relates to themselves, and at the same time feels a connection to other people. They may also feel a connection to life and the world.

Working with self-compassion in psychotherapy consists of motivating the client and contracting for self-compassion work, assisting the client in finding and enhancing self-compassion, working with obstacles, and leading the client to bring self-compassion to the vulnerable or protecting parts of themselves (self-compassion processing). We describe the first three therapeutic tasks in Chapter 10. In this chapter, we focus on self-compassion processing.

Transforming power of self-compassion: Self-compassion processing

Self-compassion processing is a processing of unresolved and painful issues with the help of self-compassion. It represents the third phase of MCIP (see Chapter 8). If strategies for enhancing self-compassion, described in Chapter 10, successfully invoke self-compassion within the client, we can then use this self-compassion for processing unresolved and painful issues. Metaphorically speaking, by learning how to sail in pretty calm waters with a favourable wind, we can then use the strategies for promoting self-compassion also in a stormy sea and strong wind.

Self-compassion processing is indicated when clients are upset about some disturbing event, when they are self-critical, self-punishing, or self-pushing. We first awake self-compassion within the client and then we invite the client, in their imagination, to go from their place of self-compassion, into a specific stressful scene. We ask the client to be mindfully aware of what they are now noticing. Connecting the state of suffering (in the stressful scene) with the self-compassionate state, spontaneously transforms, in a more functional way, how the client sees the scene, how they feel and think about themselves and the problem. Receiving compassion (from ourselves or others) while feeling pain provides transformation (Desmond, 2016). "Compassion transforms and integrates the mind" (P. Gilbert, 2010, p. 175). We suggest that connecting the states of suffering to mindful awareness and self-compassion enables memory reconsolidation (Ecker et al., 2012; Ecker & Vaz, 2019) and with that comes the change of relational schemas (G. Žvelc, 2009b). Figure 13.1 illustrates how mindful awareness and compassion directed to our suffering leads to transformation and integration of the personal sense of self.

There are two fundamental steps in self-compassion processing:

1   Mindful awareness of one's own suffering and pain.
2   Bringing self-compassion to one's own suffering.

Mindful awareness of own suffering and pain

In the first step, it is crucial that the client recognises and becomes mindfully aware of their suffering (Neff, 2011). By suffering, we mean physical or psychological pain, like feeling anxiety, shame, guilt, powerlessness, unworthiness, or emptiness. It is essential that the client comes in contact with their pain (Desmond, 2016). The client can be in touch with pain if they can tolerate it. This means that they are not overwhelmed by it and not avoiding it, but are the loving witness to it. To be able to do this, the client needs to have developed mindful capacity in the earlier phases of therapy.

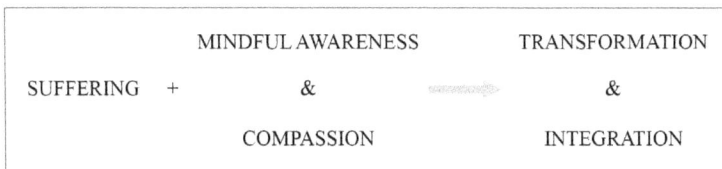

		MINDFUL AWARENESS		TRANSFORMATION
SUFFERING	+	&		&
		COMPASSION		INTEGRATION

Figure 13.1 The transforming effect of mindful awareness and compassion

We lead the client into taking a decentred perspective and accepting awareness of their pain. We ask the client to describe the event that evoked suffering and within this event to concretely define what was most painful for them. The therapist might say:

> *"Go to the situation when you criticised yourself the most. What do you see?* (therapist waits for the answer) *Where are you? .... What are you doing? ... How do you look? ... What body posture do you have?"*

Asking tangible things enables the client to recognise the moment of suffering and to feel the pain. Realising and seeing themselves suffering (usually triggered by viewing the "surrendered" body posture of themselves), often naturally evokes self-compassion.

Bringing self-compassion to own suffering

When a client comes mindfully into contact with their suffering and pain, then we lead them to evoke and bring self-compassion to their pain. They embrace their suffering "with open acceptance and love" (Desmond, 2016, p. 115). Usually, we do this in two ways that are often combined within a single therapy session: (a) Promoting the real or imagined compassionate touch of the client on themselves within a situation of suffering and (b) Invoking a self-compassionate inner dialogue within the situation of suffering.

Promoting the real or imagined compassionate touch of the client on themselves

The therapist promotes the real or imagined compassionate touch of the client on themselves in the situation of suffering. The therapist may say:

> *"I suggest, if you agree, ... put your hand on your heart in a kind and loving and way."*

The therapist saying this in a gentle, kind, soft voice also puts their hand on their own chest, aware of both their own and the client's breathing.

After a short while, the therapist says gently:

> *"What are you noticing?"*

If the client feels warmth and kindness to themselves, which also provide physiological regulation, the therapist proceeds:

> *"Go to a situation where you felt that pain ..."* (and repeats some features of the painful situation that they have previously explored.)
> *"Imagine that you are there now. Look at yourself with kind and loving eyes and be aware of the pain ...* (stops a little) *What is happening?* or *What do you notice?"*

If the client feels self-compassion towards themselves in the situation of suffering, the therapist can further propose the imagined touch within the imagined "critical" situation:

> *"Come closer to yourself … and, if you feel comfortable with that, in your imagination, gently put your hand on your shoulder."*

The therapist may raise their hand (in reality), and in their own imagination, put their hand on the client's shoulder in the imagined scene. After a short while, the therapist asks: *"What do you notice?"* or *"What is happening?"*

Invoking self-compassionate inner dialogue

When the therapist sees that the self-compassion process is starting to take effect, they initiate a self-compassionate inner dialogue within the situation of the client's suffering. The therapist can ask:

> *"Look at yourself in this situation with loving eyes and be aware of the pain that you feel. What could you say to yourself (from the compassionate part of you)? What kind words of support and love could you tell? Remember that feeling pain is what we all share."*

The therapist may then ask:

> *"How is it for you (or part of you) hearing these words of compassion? How do you feel? What do you feel in your body?"*

We promote self-compassion also in other ways. Clients can imagine their *wise and compassionate self* from the future who visits their "current" self. Clients can also look at themselves through the eyes of a beloved or imagined compassionate person or an animal. Spiritual resources can also be used. Clients can be invited to look at themselves from the position of a figure from their spiritual or religious tradition (like an angel, God, or a saint). The therapist does not force the client to feel self-compassion. They acknowledge and validate whether the client currently cannot bring compassion to themselves while remaining compassionate towards the client.

Memory reconsolidation, transformation, and grieving

When we bring compassion to the suffering self or self-state, profound transformation and integration may happen (Desmond, 2016; P. Gilbert, 2010). If we awaken self-compassion when an unresolved painful or traumatic memory is activated, we are bringing new information to the psychological system. Connecting new bodily and emotional felt information with the activation of old memory enables memory reconsolidation (Ecker, 2018; Ecker et al., 2012; Ecker & Vaz, 2019; Lane et al., 2015). Through memory reconsolidation, transformation of relational schemas happens and the integration of a personal sense of self. A client feels the situation and "sees" themselves and others in a profoundly different way.

Receiving compassion or self-compassion may also trigger the grieving process (P. Gilbert, 2010). The contrast between what was needed then and a new compassionate internal relationship provides the experience of juxtaposition and may start the grieving process. It is the grieving related to witnessing the pain of what happened to us and also what did not happen; what we needed and missed. It is the mourning for the lost part of our life, which could have been different, better. The grieving process is profoundly transforming if it is embraced by self-compassion.

Markers for initiating self-compassion processing

The markers indicating when to initiate self-compassion strategies within the client include inner self-critique and shame, inner pressure to work hard, illness, or suffering in any other way (being anxious, guilty, feeling unworthy, powerless, etc.).

Inner critique

The *inner critique* comes from the critical self-state and is directed to the criticised, vulnerable self-state. The style and content of self-critique vary from person to person and also within the person. There are different levels and intensity of inner critique that are reflected in words ranging from: "You didn't do well. You messed up; why didn't you …" to "You are incapable, you suck, you are an idiot, I hate you, you don't deserve to live." The consequences of inner critique can be feeling shame, feeling inadequate, powerlessness, hopelessness etc. The body also feels pressure from the self-critique; it is as if something is pulling you down and taking your strength. People can physically bend their arms and spines, lower their head, breathe more shallowly, feel a lack of energy etc. Self-compassion is a significant antidote for self-critique and shame (Sedighimornani et al., 2019).

Inner pressure to work hard

The self-state which pressures the client to work hard can be connected with self-criticism, but also carries some specific features. It provides the voice in our heads and the pressure in our bodies which force us to work hard and usually to hurry. By submitting to this self-state, we lose sight of our needs and our values. We do not rest when it is needed, because the work has to be done. There is no time today, and there will be no time tomorrow. You have to hurry; you have to work hard. There is no time to eat and drink properly, no time for your own interests, your own soulful activities; no time for your friends; not even for sex. Gradually by neglecting your needs, you do not feel the need for them anymore. By continuously living under inner pressure, a person can develop anxiety, or depressive symptoms, burnout syndrome or illness.

When we work with self-criticism and self-pressuring, it is important that we understand the function of self-states that are critical and self-pressuring. These are protective self-states that were developed as an adaptation to painful and often traumatic circumstances. We work with such self-states according to the phases of relational mindfulness and compassion (see Chapter 9). We validate and normalise the important function they serve. In this process, protective self-states transform and become more internally supportive together with the integration of vulnerable self-states.

Self-compassion brings a person creative regret and love from which they may wish to take care of and nurture themselves. A client may come to recognise their values, realise what things are worth for them, how life is worth living. From these insights, which are thought and felt, there come motivation and decision for new behaviour.

In the following sections, we will share two vignettes which illustrate self-compassion processing. Self-compassion processing can be done by connecting self-compassion either to the client's present painful issues or to the client's past unresolved issues and dissociated self-states.

Bringing self-compassion to clients' present painful issues

We can promote self-compassion in our clients when they are dealing with the external or internal stressors in their life, without necessarily touching memories from the distant past. However, present painful issues are often related to activation of dysfunctional schemas that are generalisations of past experiences.

Therapy vignette: Bringing self-compassion to internal criticism

During one therapy session, the client Anna is talking:

CLIENT: *Maybe you remember I was invited to do a lecture about a theme, connected to my work. I was not keen on driving to the other side of the country. You know that I like my work, but I am anxious about doing presentations … and the participants were a group who can be tough and demanding. But since I was invited and would like to spread the ideas we are developing with my colleagues, I decided to go.* (Client's pace is accelerated.)

THERAPIST: *Yes, I remember you were telling me you would go.*

CLIENT: *So, last weekend I was there. Oh, and it was a disaster.* (Client's shoulders slump, and she looks down.)

THERAPIST: (interested, leans forward) *Tell me, what happened?*

CLIENT: (looks at the therapist) *I was giving my lecture, I remember at some parts I was satisfied with myself, thought I was doing well … But you know* (with upset voice) *after the break, some participants left! And in the second part, when I tried to engage them, they were very passive, unresponsive; and* (the client is talking faster and faster and doesn't breathe) *at the end, I've got vague feedbacks, that they didn't understand some things and that I was not practical enough.*

The therapist is aware that her body is restless, and she is mindful of her urge to take a deep breath. The therapist, detecting the client's hyperarousal (her hurrying, not taking a proper breath) and her own body reaction, decides to initiate the mindful awareness process within the client and the process of regulation.

THERAPIST: *Anna, would you mind turning your attention to your body and see how your body is reacting.*

The therapist is promoting within the client mindful awareness of her body.

CLIENT: *I am agitated. I am shaking. It was so shameful!*
THERAPIST: *You have a thought: it was shameful.* (the therapist is promoting a decentred perspective within the client) *What other thoughts do you have, Anna?*
CLIENT: *You were no good. You are no good. You are stupid. And useless. You shouldn't give lectures anymore! Ever!*
THERAPIST: *This is very tough.*

The therapist is acknowledging the intensity of the client's inner critique. Identifying self-critique is one of the markers for self-compassionate work in therapy.

CLIENT: *Yes. It is. From one part of myself, I know it was not so bad and that I don't deserve such a strong critic and punishment. But I don't feel like that. I just feel like a big bunch of shit. I felt almost that I don't deserve to live.*

From knowing Anna's history, the therapist thinks that past self-states are being activated. Anna's introjected self-state has become very apparent. She is relating to herself in the same way she perceived her mother related to her in the past when she made a mistake: *"You are no good! You are stupid! And useless!"* There is also an introjected part from her peers in childhood humiliating her. Her archaic Child self-state is also activating; she feels and thinks like she used to feel and think when she was a child, being attacked and humiliated by her mother or peers: *"I am afraid. I feel shame. I feel worthless. I don't deserve to live."* The therapist decides she will not today directly work with past self-states, but instead, she would like to activate a resourceful self-compassionate state within Anna and help Anna to bring it to her present issue.

The therapist initiating the self-compassion process puts her hand on her chest, feels compassionate towards Anna, and says:

THERAPIST: *Anna, are you willing to do something with me? Please put your hand on your chest in a gentle way and breathe.*

Client Anna starts visibly to breathe again and gently puts her hand on her chest. Anna's ANS activation is calming down from hyperarousal. The therapist's look, voice, and words, the client's gentle hand on her chest, attention to her breathing, all these help Anna to regulate.

THERAPIST: *If you agree, go with your mind back to the hall where you gave your lecture.* (pause) *Are you there now?*
CLIENT: (nods) *Yes.*

The client imagines the hall with her eyes open. The therapist wants her to stay present in the here and now, in contact with the therapist. Closing her eyes may have led her quickly back to hyperarousal. Open eyes, in this case, enables Anna to be dually aware, to be safer and within the window of tolerance and to keep a mindful stance during the process.

THERAPIST: *Which moment from the lecture is the worst for you?*
CLIENT: *The feedback part. I especially see one woman with a strict, somehow deformed face: "I didn't get what I expected."* (The client imitates her in a somewhat teasing way.)
THERAPIST: *Let's look at yourself at that moment … in that hall, in front of all the participants, in front of that woman, like you would look from a bird's perspective … Let's look at yourself with loving eyes* (soft and gentle voice of the therapist). *What do you see?*
CLIENT: *I see myself so exposed. My shoulders are unprotected.* (Client speaks softly and starts crying.)
THERAPIST: (her voice touched by the clients suffering) *Mm-hm, mm-hm.*
CLIENT: *I want to touch my shoulders; I want to pat them …*
THERAPIST: *Yes, let's do that.*

The therapist raises her hand and pats the client's imaginary shoulder (with her hand in the air), while her other hand stays on her heart. The client does the same; lifts one hand, and pats her imagined shoulder while the other hand stays on her chest. The pace is slow, and the therapy room is quiet, somehow solemn, almost sacred. The therapist has a feeling that Anna is "blessed" at this moment in her state of suffering. Compassion opens a way to spiritual experience. When compassion arises, it is often felt like spiritual love or a presence of "blessing".

CLIENT: (still crying, in a soft way; very touched by the process and says with a gentle smile) *I give her a kiss on the top of her head.*
THERAPIST: (responding to the client's words with nodding and a gentle smile) *Is there anything you would like to say to yourself?*

The loving inner relationship started when the client put her hand on her chest and then went on to pat herself on the shoulder and gave herself a kiss. Now the therapist invites her into a self-compassionate dialogue with words.

CLIENT: (speaking slowly) *You went all that way with a good intention to deliver your knowledge. Some of them understood you and liked your talk and did acknowledge that, and some of them just didn't. You remember – there is a story: "You can never please all people." It is an impossible task. (silence) You did it well. Everything's fine. I love you …. Now I hug her (looks at the therapist).*

For memory reconsolidation and transformation of dysfunctional schema, we should become simultaneously aware of dysfunctional schema together with new contradictive information (Ecker, 2018; Ecker et al., 2012). In this vignette, the client's dysfunctional schema *"I am bad, incompetent, I don't deserve to exist"* was activated. Anna was becoming mindful of her inner critic and started to bring self-compassion to herself. She was gentle, supporting, and loving to herself. This was shown in her feelings, words, and deeds. This new attitude was brought together with the self-state, activated by the old dysfunctional schema. By developing and activating a different, loving relationship towards herself, the old schema started to transform.

To consolidate new neural learning, the therapist decides to activate the client's old schema again and lead the client to bring a self-compassionate state to it.

THERAPIST: *This is a very touching process, also for me.* (The therapist discloses her experience.) *Anna, can we go a step further?*

CLIENT: *Yes?*

THERAPIST: *Can you now activate the state when you were highly critical of yourself; when you were saying you are a bunch of shit; you don't deserve to live.* (The therapist is imitating the critical voice; she invites Anna to activate this state. She extends her left arm with the palm up – as if the critical state were on her left hand.) *You have it? Ok. And now activate your compassionate state, when you pet and kiss yourself, tell yourself you are ok, everything is fine, I love you* (she says this in a compassionate voice, extending now her right arm also with her hand palm up). *You have it? Ok. So now: be aware of both states; the critical one* (lifting slightly her left hand) *and the compassionate one* (lifting slightly her right hand). (short silence) … *What happens?… What do you get?*

CLIENT: (Repeats the hand movements. She is silent for a while. It seems a lot is going on.) *Wow, it is like … like going from one universe to another … amazing … when I look and feel, both of them.* (Silence)

THERAPIST: (present, nodding)

CLIENT: *I feel sorry for myself* (a tear in her eye). (Silence) … *I didn't deserve that … I didn't deserve that …*

The client starts the grieving process, realising how cruel she was in the way she was acting towards herself.

CLIENT: *I want to stay faithful to myself … when I am being so critical, I am not faithful to myself. This is not genuine care. Even if I have something to improve, it is impossible to improve from this critical part …* (more tears) … *I want to be able to stay with myself. To be faithful, to be truthful …*

THERAPIST: (present) *Mm-hm, mm-hm, yes, let's breathe.*

CLIENT: *Now I feel peace. I feel myself. The energy. It is pleasant and somehow quiet.* (silence) *And now, looking at you; I am getting tears again, thank you … to be with me … to support me, to lead me through this process.*

THERAPIST: (gets teary eyes, too)

The therapist is deeply touched. It felt for her as a meeting of souls. She knows the suffering the client was going through; she is moved by the client's compassionate process and touched by the client's gratitude.

THERAPIST: *Anna, I'm very glad that we are going through this process together.*

In the next session the therapist asks Anna how the last session was for her; what feelings and thoughts she had after the meeting. Anna says that she felt very good, at peace with herself and the world. It felt like a spiritual experience. When she came back home, she made love with her husband; it was a great feeling. She also noticed she was very present with her children and had pleasure with them and the activities she did. The therapist is attuned to her; sharing her gentle joy with Anna.

THERAPIST: *Do you agree to go back to the topic which you brought last time?… When you think about your lecture at that place, what do you get now?*

CLIENT: *It doesn't upset me anymore. My body stays calm. I did what I did; I can think what I may do differently next time … but I feel I am OK and a competent person. And now I see the people who praised me after that lecture. Now they stand out from the rest.* (She smiles.)

We can see how transformation and integration has occurred: the scene has changed, the old schema transformed, the client, faced by the challenging situation, is able to remain grounded, feeling worthy, competent, and safe.

THERAPIST: *Ok. It is interesting how your feelings and images have changed. I am glad. … And now if you imagine that you are going to deliver your next lecture, what happens?*

The therapist wants to consolidate this new memory in different ways; to connect and integrate it into the client's anticipation of future events, which is also the activation of implicit memory.

CLIENT: *Who says that I will be going to a next lecture?* (smiles) *I am joking … (pause) yes, I feel some anxiety. But I will deliver speeches. I want to do it. When I look at myself making an imagined future speech, I feel it makes sense; it is meaningful to me.*

Bringing self-compassion to clients' past issues and archaic Child self-states

There are many unresolved issues stemming from the past. Children, often based on their magical and egocentric thinking (Piaget & Inhelder, 1966/1986), conclude that they created events or influenced them. If the circumstances were terrible or tragic, they often conclude that they were responsible and guilty. In adolescence and adulthood, if traumatic or painful events happen, we may re-experience archaic Child self-states and can attribute guilt to ourselves, that we somehow caused or influenced the circumstances and we blame ourselves for that. We can also feel guilty for some genuine reason from our Adult self-mode when we indeed did something wrong (for instance, driving drunk and causing a car accident injuring our partner). Whatever it was, we deserve to receive compassion and be self-compassionate regarding traumatic, tragic, and other stressful events we went through or are going through. It is important to note that being compassionate does not mean excusing us or someone else for bad deeds.

When facing overwhelmingly stressful and traumatic events, we create or reinforce dysfunctional schemas (like "I am bad", "I am not safe", "I am powerless", etc.). These schemas influence how we interpret the present and predict the future (D. J. Siegel, 1999; G. Žvelc, 2009b). Being compassionate to our past self-states that are related to activation of dysfunctional schemas can help us to transform the schemas.

During any traumatic event which was unbearable, where we were not strong enough to fight, and we had no means of escape, we "escaped" into ourselves (Kalsched, 1996). Physiologically speaking we froze or collapsed. On the psychological level, we split the self; we created a part which was untouchable from the outside world. Afterwards, we seek refuge there when we feel hurt; but on the other hand, we avoid this part and would like to get rid of it, because it reminds us of the traumatic event. It reminds us of being weak, unworthy, and unsafe. One client described such split off part: "*I see a girl sitting in a dark room, in a dark corner, I hardly see her. She is so distant.*" Others see a wall and feel that somebody is behind the wall. If clients can't get rid of such parts, they reject them; they are cold to them, ignoring or criticising them. On other occasions, they are merged with them and feel like a victim, hopeless and helpless.

The goal of therapy is to re-discover and integrate split parts of the clients, to bring them "home" (Erskine et al., 1999). Through the therapist's compassion and the client's self-compassion to these self-states, gradually they transform and integrate into the Adult self-mode. From our clinical experience, we think that for work with self-compassion connected to past issues and dissociated self-states, it is important that the client is able to be self-compassionate. Without self-compassion, there may not be enough resources within the client for trauma work.

Therapy vignette: Trauma processing by bringing self-compassion to Child self-state

In this vignette, we present an example of connecting with and bringing self-compassion to an archaic Child self-state.

In the therapy session, the client Julia is talking about how it is difficult for her to allow herself to be seen; this also touches upon her belief "I am not important". She feels anxiety, a lump in her throat and stiffness in her body.

THERAPIST: (gently) *Julia, I would like to invite you to direct your attention to the anxiety, the lump in your throat and the thought: what I say is not important … If you go back to your childhood, when did this feeling first appear?*

CLIENT: (short silence) *I see myself in a living room … I am alone.*

THERAPIST: *You are alone in a living room. What do you see? What does the room look like?*

CLIENT: *It is pretty dark in the room. There is a couch … I sit on the floor … there's a door to the kitchen.*

THERAPIST: (gently and kind) *How old are you?*

CLIENT: (pause) *I am small. Maybe five.*

THERAPIST: *How do you look?*

CLIENT: *I am in a lovely dress. I have long hair … I am cute … you would like me.* (She smiles.)

THERAPIST: *Yes, I am sure I would like you.* (gently smiling, too) *What did they call you when you were a child?*

CLIENT: *Julie.*

THERAPIST: *Julie, what is it that is hardest for you?*

CLIENT: *That there is nobody around.*

THERAPIST: *Who do you miss?*

CLIENT: *Mommy …*

THERAPIST: *Mm-hm, mommy. How do you explain to yourself that Julie is alone, that there is no mommy?*

CLIENT: *It is not important what I feel …*

The therapy is going at a slow pace. The client is speaking in short sentences. It seems she is restricting herself. The therapist decides to inquire how she is feeling. At the same time, this is a response to the client's belief "it is not important what I feel".

THERAPIST: *What do you feel now, Julia?*

CLIENT: *There is such loneliness.*

The client reveals loneliness from the third-person perspective: "there is …" It seems she is not in full contact with feeling loneliness. The therapist decides to continue with the phenomenological inquiry into body sensations which might lead the client into deeper contact with herself on an emotional level.

THERAPIST: *What do you feel in your body now?*
CLIENT: *It's like I have a heavy weight on myself.*
THERAPIST: *I have a sense that you have tears wanting to be wept.*

The therapist acknowledges her client's tendency to cry.

CLIENT: *Yes, there is sadness all the time.*

The pace is still slow. It seems the client is in slight hypoarousal; detached from her sadness, the fear, the pain. She is talking about feelings in the third person. The therapist is aware that she has a good reason for that.

THERAPIST: *Where is mommy?*
CLIENT: (with the "adult" voice) *She was depressed.*
THERAPIST: *How did little Julie explain to herself that there is no mommy around?*

The therapist is exploring the child's meaning of the situation.

CLIENT: (Silence. She tightens her lips and becomes restless.) *Papa said because I am naughty* (with the voice of a young girl) *... and I believed it ... I thought I am bad.*
THERAPIST: (The energy returns to the therapy field, the therapist feels sadness and pressure in her throat, a sensation like just before crying). *Mm-hm, mm-hm, let yourself feel this. It hurts.*
CLIENT: (starts to cry)

The therapist is present and compassionate. The client comes into touch with her deep pain. It is an appropriate moment for encouraging self-compassion.

THERAPIST: *Julia, shall we explore ways together that will give you more support ... If you agree let's go now to little Julie in the living room. Let me first ask you, what do you see now?*
CLIENT: *She sits on the floor, and she is sad.*
THERAPIST: (speaking gently but firmly) *I am with you. Can you go to this room, now, as an adult, and approach her?* (pauses) *What happens if you approach her? Does she let you approach her?*

The therapist feels that adult Julia needs support, and that is why she says that she is with her. It is important that the client is simultaneously staying in the Adult self-mode and within the window of tolerance when visiting the Child self-state.

CLIENT: *Yes, she lets me. I sit next to her. I feel tenderness towards her ... The room is lighter now ... She looks at me. She still has a sad look.*

THERAPIST: *She is sad because there is no mommy, and papa told her it's because she was naughty. She thinks that it is her fault ... that mommy feels bad and is not here with her. Shall we tell her the truth?*

CLIENT: (nodding, silence) *... I don't know how to start. Help me.*

THERAPIST: *Julia, may I sit closer to you?*

The therapist wants to give support to Julia with body vicinity. Later Julia said that the therapist coming closer to her was a crucial turning point in the session.

THERAPIST: (to little Julie) *Dear Julie, mommy is not here, because she is ill. It is not your fault.*

CLIENT: *My dear Julie, mommy is not feeling well, she is ill, but it is not because of you; people get ill, that's how it is. It was not your fault.* (pause) *I love you.*

THERAPIST: (present, touched) *Mm-hm, mm-hm.*

CLIENT: (silence; then she turns to the therapist) *She needed touch; she needed hugs.*

THERAPIST: (compassionate, normalising the child's need) *Yes, she needed touch; she needed hugs ... I am sorry that nobody noticed that ...*

Client gently cries. She is going through her grieving process for the parents' loving presence and touch she missed in her childhood.

CLIENT: *Now I feel her very much. I want to hug her ... Do you have a cushion?*

Julia warmly hugs the cushion in her lap, gently rocking it. She feels deep compassion for the wounded part of herself. There is a gentle smile on her face. She closes her eyes, and when she opens them, there are sparkles in her eyes. She is hugging little Julie in her imagination. The therapist feels tenderness and compassion towards the little Julie and the adult Julia. It is a precious and touching moment.

CLIENT: (holding and rocking the cushion) *It feels so good.*

THERAPIST: (present, touched)

A little later in the session:

CLIENT: *You are mine ... mine ... And it is not true that she didn't want to see you because you were terrible. Just she was ill ... you are a precious little girl. I love you.*

A little later:

THERAPIST: *Julia, can you feel Julie inside of you? As part of you?*

CLIENT: *Yes ... yes ...* (deep sigh) *... All this is difficult to accept.*

THERAPIST: (Looking at the client, who looks on the one hand like someone reborn, on the other hand, also tired.) *What do you mean when you say "all"?*

212 Methods and interventions

CLIENT: *The little girl said to me: how many years I have been waiting that you will come to see me. That you will stop blaming me.*

These are very touching words; on the one hand, they evoke sadness and regret; on the other, hope. The "girl" found her voice, found the words; got the strength! From being in Adult Julia's hug, she experienced acceptance and safety. From this safe haven, strength and assertiveness began to rise. Julia started the session with talking about difficulties in allowing herself to be seen and believing that she is not important. And then, the right to be heard and the strength and braveness to be seen were unlocked.

The little girl, with words "*I have been waiting that you will stop blaming me*" is being assertive and probably talking to some critical part of Julia, too. Here we can see that further work with the introjected critical self-state and possible other self-states who were criticising and pushing away the vulnerable part, is needed (for this session it is enough, it would be too much to work with them as well). An alliance between all these different self-states is needed, so that the changes which have happened in the session can integrate and consolidate, and that her personal sense of self becomes harmonious. The therapist continues encouraging the connection between little Julia and the Adult self-mode.

THERAPIST: *Julie spoke very significant words to you. What would you like to tell her?*
CLIENT: (speaking gently, tears in her eyes) *I hear you ... I hear you ... I am here. I am sorry. I won't let you go ... ever. I am here.*
THERAPIST: *What do you feel now, Julia?*
CLIENT: *I am touched. I feel more whole. I am also sad to see how it was hard for me when I was small ... And pretty tired, too.*
THERAPIST: *You went through an in-depth process ... Being open to compassion is beautiful and at the same time, painful. Grieving is part of that ... I am touched by the work you did, and I am glad I could be with you in this process.*

The therapist and the client started closing the session. Julia said that she had a feeling that something literally changed in her brain.

Julia within the therapeutic process touched a deep, denied pain, and conveyed compassion to her inner Child self-state, who carried that pain. Up until then, the little girl Julie was living alone in a room. Part of herself was split off from the Adult self-mode, symbolised by a dark room in a flat. The vital part of the flat, the living room, was in the dark. The little girl was left alone, not just from significant others, also by Julia herself. In the session, Julia recognised and embraced the pain of the wounded girl and built an affectionate bond with her. By accepting the pain and reconnecting with a vital part of herself, the locked energy, dignity, feelings of importance, strength, and worthiness were released and became accessible to Julia. She was becoming more whole.

Afterword

We have come to the end of our book, and we ask ourselves, what now? Where does this journey of integration lead? Integration is a process that never ends, and we are aware that there are many themes we have left unexplored that will be important in the future.

We are fascinated by *how much we don't know* about what is happening between people who are involved in the psychotherapeutic process. In this book, we have written about an invisible bond between us – the physiological intersubjective field – which is attracting increasing scientific research. But we think there is even more to it. We believe that people are deeply interconnected, but the nature of such interconnection has not yet been sufficiently scientifically explored. We hope that in the future we will be able to understand more about the subtle energetic exchanges happening between people, and that we will understand the bond of interconnection in psychotherapy more profoundly.

An important topic, which is often overlooked in western psychotherapy, is the importance of spirituality. Mindfulness and compassion were historically part of wisdom traditions, where the primary goal was not an enhancement of our personal sense of self, but spiritual growth. One of the central concepts in MCIP is the observing/transcendent self, which is related to the spiritual dimension. We write about two states of consciousness related to the observing/transcendent self: the mindful state of consciousness and nondual awareness. While our book is mostly about the importance of mindful awareness and compassion, we have in many chapters touched upon the subject of nondual awareness, which is in western psychology still mostly unexplored. Becoming aware of the transcendent self has the potential to spark the dawn of nondual awareness that manifests in experiences of oneness, inner peace, and interconnection. We have also proposed a potential phase of psychotherapy focused on spiritual development. We think that in the future, mindfulness- and compassion-oriented approaches have to build on their roots in wisdom traditions and further explore the importance of spiritual development for human beings.

We started the book with Maša's dream of interconnection, and we will finish with another dream. It is our shared dream that our book will challenge your mind, touch your hearts, and inspire you in your work with your clients.

Appendix

Online supplements

Online resources for readers of *Integrative Psychotherapy: A Mindfulness- and Compassion- Oriented Approach* are available at: www.mcip.eu

Supplements include scales for researchers and clinicians: Relational Needs Satisfaction Scale (RNSS), Test of Object Relations (TOR), and Pictorial Test of Separation and Individuation (PTSI); case presentation resources; Glossary of this book; and other related materials.

References

Ainsworth, M. D. S., Blehar, M. C., Waters, E., & Wall, S. (1978). *Patterns of attachment: A psychological study of the strange situation.* Erlbaum.

Albahari, M. (2006). *Analytical Buddhism: The two-tiered illusion of self.* Palgrave Macmillan.

Albahari, M. (2014). Insight knowledge of no self in Buddhism: An epistemic analysis. *Philosopher's Imprint, 14*(21), 1–30.

Alexander, F., & French, T. M. (1980). *Psychoanalytic therapy: Principles and application.* University of Nebraska Press. (Original work published 1946)

Andrews, J. D. W. (1993). The active self model. In G. Stricker & J. R. Gold (Eds.), *Comprehensive handbook of psychotherapy integration* (pp. 165–183). Springer. https://doi.org/10.1007/978-1-4757-9782-4_13

Angus, L. E., & Greenberg, L. S. (2011). *Working with narrative in emotion-focused therapy.* American Psychological Association.

Aron, L. (1996). *A meeting of minds: Mutuality in psychoanalysis.* Analytic Press.

Aron, L. (2000). Self-reflexivity and the therapeutic action of psychoanalysis. *Psychoanalytic Psychology, 17*(4), 667–689.

Assagioli, R. (1993). *Psychosynthesis: The definitive guide to the principles and techniques of psychosynthesis* (3rd ed.). Thorsons. (Original work published 1965)

Baldwin, M. W. (1992). Relational schemas and the processing of social information. *Psychological Bulletin, 112*, 461–484.

Baldwin, M. W., Granzberg, A., Pippus, L., & Pritchard, E. T. (2003). Cued activation of relational schemas: Self-evaluation and gender effects. *Canadian Journal of Behavioural Science, 35*(2), 153–163. https://doi.org/10.1037/h0087197

Bar-Kalifa, E., Prinz, J. N., Atzil-Slonim, D., Rubel, J. A., Lutz, W., & Rafaeli, E. (2019). Physiological synchrony and therapeutic alliance in an imagery-based treatment. *Journal of Counseling Psychology, 66*(4), 508–517. https://doi.org/10.1037/cou0000358

Barber, J. P., Muran, J. C., McCarthy, K. S., & Keefe, J. R. (2013). Research on dynamic therapies. In M. J. Lambert (Ed.), *Bergin and Garfield's handbook of psychotherapy and behavioral change* (6th ed., pp. 443–495). John Wiley & Sons.

Beisser, A. (1971). The paradoxical theory of change. In F. J. & I. L. Shepherd (Eds.), *Gestalt therapy now: Theory, techniques, applications* (pp. 77–80). Harper & Row.

Benjamin, J. (1995). *Like subjects, love objects: Essays on recognition and sexual difference.* Yale University Press.

Benoit, D., & Parker, K. C. H. (1994). Stability and transmission of attachment across three generations. *Child Development, 65*, 1444–1456.

Berne, E. (1961). *Transactional analysis in psychotherapy: A systematic individual and social psychiatry.* Grove Press.

Berne, E. (1966). *Principles of group treatment.* Grove Press.

Berne, E. (1967). *The games people play: The psychology of human relationship.* Grove Press.

Berne, E. (1972). *What do you say after you say hello?* Grove Press.

Bishop, S. R., Lau, M., Shapiro, S., Carlson, L., Anderson, N. D., Carmody, J., Segal, Z. V., Abbey, S., Speca, M., Velting, D., & Devins, G. (2004). Mindfulness: A proposed operational definition. *Clinical Psychology: Science and Practice, 11*(3), 230–241. https://doi. org/10.1093/clipsy/bph077

Bluck, S., & Habermas, T. (2000). The life story schema. *Motivation and Emotion, 24*(2), 121–147. https://doi.org/10.1023/A:1005615331901

Bollas, C. (1987). *The shadow of the object: Psychoanalysis of the unthought known.* Free Association Books.

Bordin, E. S. (1979). The generalizability of the psychoanalytic concept of the working alliance. *Psychotherapy: Theory, Research and Practice, 16*, 252–260.

Bowlby, J. (1969). *Attachment and loss: Vol. 1 Attachment.* Penguin Books.

Brach, T. (2012). Mindful presence: A foundation for compassion and wisdom. In C. K. Germer & R. D. Siegel (Eds.), *Wisdom and compassion in psychotherapy: Deepening mindfulness in clinical practice* (pp. 35–47). Guilford Press.

Bromberg, P. M. (1996). Standing in the spaces: The multiplicity of self and the psycho-analytic relationship. *Contemporary Psychoanalysis, 32*(4), 509–535. https://doi.org/10. 1080/00107530.1996.10746334

Brown, K. W., & Ryan, R. M. (2003). The benefits of being present: Mindfulness and its role in psychological well-being. *Journal of Personality and Social Psychology, 84*(4), 822–848.

Bruce, N. G., Manber, R., Shapiro, S. L., & Constantino, M. J. (2010). Psychotherapist mindfulness and the psychotherapy process. *Psychotherapy, 47*(1), 83–97. https://doi.org/ 10.1037/a0018842

Buber, M. (1999). *Princip dialoga [The dialogic principle]* (J. Zupet, Trans.). Društvo izdajateljev časnika 2000.

Bucci, W. (1997). *Psychoanalysis and cognitive science: A multiple code theory.* Guilford Press.

Buzzell, L., & Chalquist, C. (2009). *Ecotherapy: Healing with nature in mind.* Sierra Club Books.

Cardaciotto, L., Herbert, J. D., Forman, E. M., Moitra, E., & Farrow, V. (2008). The assessment of present-moment awareness and acceptance: The Philadelphia Mindfulness Scale. *Assessment, 15*(2), 204–223. https://doi.org/10.1177/1073191107311467

Cassibba, R., Coppola, G., Sette, G., Curci, A., & Costantini, A. (2017). The transmission of attachment across three generations: A study in adulthood. *Developmental Psychology, 53* (2), 396–405. https://doi.org/10.1037/dev0000242

Castonguay, L. G., Eubanks, C. F., Goldfried, M. R., Muran, J. C., & Lutz, W. (2015). Research on psychotherapy integration: Building on the past, looking to the future. *Psychotherapy Research, 25*(3), 365–382. https://doi.org/10.1080/10503307.2015.1014010

Castonguay, L. G., & Hill, C. E. (2007). Introduction: Examining insight in psychotherapy. In L. G. Castonguay & C. E. Hill (Eds.), *Insight in psychotherapy* (pp. 3–5). American Psychological Association.

Cavicchioli, M., Movalli, M., & Maffei, C. (2018). The clinical efficacy of mindfulness-based treatments for alcohol and drugs use disorders: A meta-analytic review of rando-mized and nonrandomized controlled trials. *European Addiction Research, 24*(3), 137–162. https://doi.org/10.1159/000490762

Choi-Kain, L. W., & Gunderson, J. G. (2008). Mentalization: Ontogeny, assessment, and application in the treatment of borderline personality disorder. *American Journal of Psychiatry, 165*(9), 1127–1135. https://doi.org/10.1176/appi.ajp.2008.07081360

Chopik, W. J., Edelstein, R. S., & Grimm, K. J. (2019). Longitudinal changes in attachment orientation over a 59-year period. *Journal of Personality and Social Psychology, 116*(4), 598–611. https://doi.org/10.1037/pspp0000167

Cooper, M. (2019). *Integrating counselling & psychotherapy: Directionality, synergy and social change.* Sage.

Cooper, M., & McLeod, J. (2007). A pluralistic framework for counselling and psychotherapy: Implications for research. *Counselling and Psychotherapy Research, 7*(3), 135–143. https://doi.org/10.1080/14733140701566282

Cozolino, L. (2002). *The neuroscience of psychotherapy: Building and rebuilding the human brain.* W. W. Norton & Company.

Crits-Christoph, P., Gibbons, M. B. C., & Mukherjee, D. (2013). Psychotherapy process-outcome research. In M. J. Lambert (Ed.), *Bergin and Garfield's handbook of psychotherapy and behavioral change* (pp. 298–341). John Wiley & Sons.

Černetič, M. (2005). Biti tukaj in zdaj: Čuječnost, njena uporabnost in mehanizmi delovanja [Being here and now: Mindfulness, its use and mechanisms of work]. *Psihološka Obzorja/Horizons of Psychology, 14*(2), 73–92.

Černetič, M. (2017). Struktura konstrukta čuječnosti: Zavedanje doživljanja in sprejemanje doživljanja [The structure of the mindfulness construct: Awareness and acceptance of experience]. *Psihološka Obzorja/Horizons of Psychology, 26*, 41–51. https://doi.org/10.20419/2017.26.465

Černigoj, M. (2007). *JAZ in MI: Raziskovanje temeljev socialne psihologije* [I and WE: Researching fundamentals of social psychology]. IPSA, Inštitut za integrativno psihoterapijo in svetovanje.

Dana, D. (2018). *The polyvagal theory in therapy: Engaging the rhythm of regulation.* W.W. Norton & Company.

De Meulemeester, C., Vansteelandt, K., Luyten, P., & Lowyck, B. (2018). Mentalizing as a mechanism of change in the treatment of patients with borderline personality disorder: A parallel process growth modeling approach. *Personality Disorders: Theory, Research, and Treatment, 9*(1), 22–29. https://doi.org/10.1037/per0000256

Deikman, A. J. (1982). *The observing self: Mysticism and psychotherapy.* Beacon Press.

Deikman, A. J. (1996). I = Awareness. *Journal of Consciousness Studies, 3*(4), 250–357. http://deikman.com/awareness.html

Desmond, T. (2016). *Self-compassion in psychotherapy: Mindfulness-based practices for healing and transformation.* W.W. Norton & Company.

Dimaggio, G., Montano, A., Popolo, R., & Salvatore, G. (2015). *Metacognitive interpersonal therapy for personality disorders: A treatment manual.* Routledge.

Dimberg, U., Thunberg, M., & Elmehed, K. (2000). Unconscious facial reactions to emotional facial expressions. *Psychological Science, 11*(1), 86–89. https://doi.org/10.1111/1467-9280.00221

di Pellegrino, G., Fadiga, L., Fogassi, L., Gallese, V., & Rizzolatti, G. (1992). Understanding motor events: A neurophysiological study. *Experimental Brain Research, 91*(1), 176–180. https://doi.org/10.1007/BF00230027

Dunn, R., Callahan, J. L., & Swift, J. K. (2013). Mindfulness as a transtheoretical clinical process. *Psychotherapy: Theory, Research, Practice, Training, 50*(3), 312–315. https://doi.org/10.1037/a0032153

Ecker, B. (2015). Memory reconsolidation understood and misunderstood. *International Journal of Neuropsychotherapy, 3*, 2–46. https://doi.org/10.12744/ijnpt.2015.0002-0046

Ecker, B. (2018). Clinical translation of memory reconsolidation research: Therapeutic methodology for transformational change by erasing implicit emotional learnings driving symptom production. *International Journal of Neuropsychotherapy, 6*(1), 1–92. https://doi.org/10.12744/ijnpt.2018.0001-0092

Ecker, B., Robin, T., & Hulley, L. (2012). *Unlocking the emotional brain: Eliminating symptoms at their roots using memory reconsolidation.* Routledge.

Ecker, B., & Vaz, A. (2019, June 6–8). *Beyond common and specific factors: Memory reconsolidation as a transtheoretical mechanism of change and unifying framework in psychotherapy* [Conference session]. SEPI XXXV Annual Meeting, Lisbon, Portugal.

Elliott, R., Bohart, A. C., Watson, J. C., & Murphy, D. (2018). Therapist empathy and client outcome: An updated meta-analysis. *Psychotherapy, 55*(4), 399–410. https://doi.org/10.1037/pst0000175

Elliott, R., Bohart, A., Watson, J. C., & Greenberg, L. S. (2011). Empathy. In J. C. Norcross (Ed.), *Psychotherapeutic relationships that works (Vol. 1): Evidence-based therapist contributions* (pp. 132–152). Oxford University Press.

Elliott, R., Greenberg, L. S., Watson, J., Timulak, L., & Freire, E. (2013). Research on humanistic-experiential psychotherapies. In M. J. Lambert (Ed.), *Bergin and Garfield's handbook of psychotherapy and behavioral change.* (6th ed., pp. 495–539). John Wiley & Sons.

Elliott, R., Slatick, E., & Urman, M. (2001). Qualitative change process research on psychotherapy: Alternative strategies. In J. Frommer & D. L. Rennie (Eds.), *Qualitative psychotherapy research: Methods and methodology* (pp. 69–111). Pabst Science.

Engler, J., & Fulton, P. R. (2012). Self and no-self in psychotherapy. In C. K. Germer & R. D. Siegel (Eds.), *Wisdom and compassion in psychotherapy: Deepening mindfulness in clinical practice* (pp. 176–189). Guilford Press.

Erbida Golob, M., & Žvelc, M. (2015). Uporaba zvenečih vilic kot intervencija v psihoterapiji: Preliminarna raziskava [The use of tuning forks as intervention in psychotherapy]. *Kairos, Slovenian Journal of Psychotherapy, 9*(3), 25–42.

Erskine, R. G. (1988). Ego structure, intrapsychic function, and defense mechanisms: A commentary on Eric Berne's original theoretical concepts. *Transactional Analysis Journal, 18*(1), 15–19. https://doi.org/10.1177/036215378801800104

Erskine, R. G. (1991). Transference and transactions: Critique from an intrapsychic and integrative perspective. *Transactional Analysis Journal, 21*(2), 63–76. https://doi.org/10.1177/036215379102100202

Erskine, R. G. (1993). Inquiry, attunement, and involvement in the psychotherapy of dissociation. *Transactional Analysis Journal, 23*(4), 184–190. https://doi.org/10.1177/036215379302300402

Erskine, R. G. (1997). The therapeutic relationship: Integrating motivation and personality theories. In R. G. Erskine (Ed.), *Theories and methods of an integrative transactional analysis* (pp. 7–19). TA Press.

Erskine, R. G. (2001). The psychotherapist' s myths, dreams and realities. *International Journal of Psychotherapy, 6*(2), 133–140. https://doi.org/10.1080/13569080120085796

Erskine, R. G. (2009). Life scripts and attachment patterns: Theoretical integration and therapeutic involvement. *Transactional Analysis Journal, 39*(3), 207–218. https://doi.org/10.1177/036215370903900304

Erskine, R. G. (2010). Life scripts: Unconscious relational patterns and psychotherapeutic involvement. In R. G. Erskine (Ed.), *Life scripts: A transactional analysis of unconscious relational patterns* (pp. 1–29). Karnac Books.

Erskine, R. G. (2014). Nonverbal stories: The body in psychotherapy. *International Journal of Integrative Psychotherapy, 5*(1), 21–33.

Erskine, R. G. (2015). *Relational patterns, therapeutic presence: Concepts and practice of integrative psychotherapy.* Karnac Books.

Erskine, R. G. (2016). A transactional analysis of obsession: Integrating diverse concepts and methods. In R. G. Erskine (Ed.), *Transactional analysis in contemporary psychotherapy* (pp. 1–27). Routledge.

Erskine, R. G. (2019a). Developmentally based, relationally focused integrative psychotherapy: Eight essential points. *International Journal of Integrative Psychotherapy, 10*, 1–10.

Erskine, R. G. (2019b). Child development in integrative psychotherapy: Erik Erikson's first three stages. *International Journal of Integrative Psychotherapy, 10*, 11–34.

Erskine, R. G. (2019c, November 15–17). *Compassion, hope, and forgiveness in the therapeutic dialogue* [Conference presentation]. Manchester Institute for Psychotherapy Conference, Manchester, UK.

Erskine, R. G., & Moursund, J. P. (1988). *Integrative psychotherapy in action.* Sage.

Erskine, R. G., Moursund, J. P., & Trautmann, R. L. (1999). *Beyond empathy: A therapy of contact-in-relationship.* Brunner/Mazel.

Erskine, R. G., & Trautmann, R. L. (1996). Methods of an integrative psychotherapy. *Transactional Analysis Journal, 26*(4), 316–328. https://doi.org/10.1177/036215379602600410

Erskine, R. G., & Trautmann, R. L. (1997). The process of integrative psychotherapy. In *Theories and methods of an integrative transactional analysis: A volume of selected articles* (pp. 79–95). TA Press. (Original work published 1993)

Erskine, R. G., & Trautmann, R. L. (2003). Resolving intrapsychic conflict: Psychotherapy of Parent ego states. In C. Sills & H. Hargdane (Eds.), *Ego states (Key concepts in transactional analysis: Contemporary views)* (pp. 109–135). Worth Publishing.

Erskine, R. G., & Zalcman, M. J. (1979). The racket system: A model for racket analysis. *Transactional Analysis Journal, 9*, 51–59.

Ettema, E. J., Derksen, L. D., & van Leuwen, E. (2010). Existential loneliness and end-of-life care : A systematic review. *Theoretical Medicine and Bioethics, 31*, 141–169. https://doi.org/10.1007/s11017-010-9141-1

Eubanks, C. F., & Goldfried, M. R. (2019). A principle-based approach to psychotherapy integration. In J. C. Norcross & M. R. Goldfried (Eds.), *Handbook of psychotherapy integration.* (3rd ed., pp. 88–105). Oxford University Press.

Eubanks, C. F., Muran, J. C., & Safran, J. D. (2018). Alliance rupture repair: A meta-analysis. *Psychotherapy, 55*(4), 508–519. https://doi.org/10.1037/pst0000185

Evans, K. R., & Gilbert, M. C. (2005). *An introduction to integrative psychotherapy.* Palgrave Macmillan.

Fairbairn, W. D. (1986). A revised psychopathology of the psychoses and psychoneuroses. In P. Buckley (Ed.), *Essential papers on object relations* (pp. 71–101). New York University Press. (Original work published 1941)

Fairbairn, W. R. D. (1986). The repression and the return of bad objects (with special reference to the 'war neuroses'). In P. Buckley (Ed.), *Essential papers on object relations* (pp. 102–126). New York University Press. (Original work published 1943)

Falb, M. D., & Pargament, K. I. (2012). Relational mindfulness, spirituality, and the therapeutic bond. *Asian Journal of Psychiatry, 5*(4), 351–354. https://doi.org/10.1016/j.ajp.2012.07.008

Farb, N. A. S., Anderson, A. K., & Segal, Z. V. (2012). The mindful brain and emotion regulation in mood disorders. *Canadian Journal of Psychiatry, 57*(2), 70–77. https://doi.org/10.1177/070674371205700203

Farb, N. A. S., Segal, Z. V., Mayberg, H., Bean, J., Mckeon, D., Fatima, Z., & Anderson, A. K. (2007). Attending to the present: Mindfulness meditation reveals distinct neural modes of self-reference. *Social Cognitive and Affective Neuroscience, 2*(4), 313–322. https://doi.org/10.1093/scan/nsm030

Farb, N., Daubenmier, J., Price, C. J., Gard, T., Kerr, C., Dunn, B. D., Klein, A. C., Paulus, M. P., & Mehling, W. E. (2015). Interoception, contemplative practice, and health. *Frontiers in Psychology, 6*, 1–26. https://doi.org/10.3389/fpsyg.2015.00763

Fernández-Alvarez, H., Consoli, A. J., & Gómez, B. (2016). Integration in psychotherapy: Reasons and challenges. *American Psychologist, 71*(8), 820–830. https://doi.org/10.1037/amp0000100

Ferrari, M., Hunt, C., Harrysunker, A., Abbott, M. J., Beath, A. P., & Einstein, D. A. (2019). Self-compassion interventions and psychosocial outcomes: A meta-analysis of RCTs. *Mindfulness*. https://doi.org/10.1007/s12671-019-01134-6

Ferrari, P. F., & Gallese, V. (2007). Mirror neurons and intersubjectivity. In S. Bråten (Ed.), *On being moved: From mirror neurons to empathy* (Vol. 1, pp. 73–88). John Benjamins. https://doi.org/10.1075/aicr.68.08fer

Finlay, L. (2016). *Relational integrative psychotherapy: Engaging process and theory in practice*. Wiley Blackwell.

Flückiger, C., Del, A. C., Wampold, B. E., & Horvath, A. O. (2018). The alliance in adult psychotherapy: A meta-analytic synthesis. *Psychotherapy, 55*(4), 316–340. https://doi.org/10.1037/pst0000172

Fogel, A. (2013). *Body sense: The science and practice of embodied self-awareness*. W.W. Norton & Company.

Fonagy, P., Gergely, G., Jurist, E. L., & Target, M. (2004). *Affect regulation, mentalization, and the development of the self*. Karnac Books.

Fonagy, P., Steele, H., & Steele, M. (1991). Maternal representations of attachment during pregnancy predict the organisation of infant–mother attachment at one year of age. *Child Development, 62*, 891–905.

Fonagy, P., & Target, M. (2006). The mentalization-focused approach to self pathology. *Journal of Personality Disorders, 20*(6), 544–576. https://doi.org/10.1521/pedi.2006.20.6.544

Ford, B. Q., Lam, P., John, O. P., & Mauss, I. B. (2018). The psychological health benefits of accepting negative emotions and thoughts: Laboratory, diary, and longitudinal evidence. *Journal of Personality and Social Psychology, 115*(6), 1075–1092. https://doi.org/10.1037/pspp0000157

Fosha, D. (2000a). Meta-therapeutic processes and the affects of transformation: Affirmation and the healing affects. *Journal of Psychotherapy Integration, 10*(1), 71–97. https://doi.org/10.1023/A:1009422511959

Fosha, D. (2000b). *The transforming power of affect: A model for accelerated change*. Basic Books.

Fosha, D., & Conceição, N. (2019, June 6–8). *How to be a transformational therapist and integrate transformational work into your clinical practice: Insights from the clinical practice of and research into AEDP* [Conference session]. SEPI 35th Annual Meeting, Lisbon, Portugal.

Frankl, V. E. (1992). *Kljub vsemu rečem življenju da* [Yes to life: In spite of everything] (J. Bohak, J. Stabej, Trans.). Mohorjeva družba. (Original work published 1946)

Frankl, V. E. (1994). *Volja do smisla. Osnove in raba logoterapije* [The will to meaning: Foundations and applications of logotherapy] (J. Stabej, Trans.). Mohorjeva družba. (Original work published 1969)

Fraser, J. S. (2018). *Unifying effective psychotherapies: Tracing the process of change*. American Psychological Association.

Freud, S. (2013). The psychotherapy of hysteria. In J. Breuer & S. Freud (Eds.), *Studies in Hysteria* (A. A. Brill, Trans.) (pp. 141–168). Digireads.com Publishing. (Original work published 1895)

Fromm, E. (1976). *To have or to be*. Bloomsbury Academic.

Fucci, E., Abdoun, O., Caclin, A., Francis, A., Dunne, J. D., Ricard, M., Davidson, R. J., & Lutz, A. (2018). Differential effects of nondual and focused attention meditations on the formation of automatic perceptual habits in expert practitioners. *Neuropsychologia, 119*, 92–100. https://doi.org/10.1016/j.neuropsychologia.2018.07.025

Ganesan, V. (2017). *Direct teaching of Bhagavan Ramana: Self-attention expounded in his own words of wisdom*. Sri Ramanasramam.

Geller, S. M. (2018). Therapeutic presence and polyvagal theory: Principles and practices for cultivating effective therapeutic relationships. In S. W. Porges & D. Dana (Eds.), *Clinical applications of the Polyvagal theory: The emergence of polyvagal-informed therapies*. (pp. 106–126). W.W. Norton & Company.

Geller, S. M., & Greenberg, L. S. (2012). *Therapeutic presence: A mindful approach to effective therapy*. American Psychological Association.

Geller, S. M., Greenberg, L. S., & Watson, J. C. (2010). Therapist and client perceptions of therapeutic presence: The development of a measure. *Psychotherapy Research, 20*(5), 599–610. https://doi.org/10.1080/10503307.2010.495957

Geller, S. M., & Porges, S. W. (2014). Therapeutic presence: Neurophysiological mechanisms mediating feeling safe in therapeutic relationships. *Journal of Psychotherapy Integration, 24*(3), 178–192. https://doi.org/10.1037/a0037511

Gendlin, E. (1981). *Focusing*. Bantam Books.

Gerhardt, S. (2004). *Why love matters: How affection shapes a baby's brain*. Routledge.

Germer, C. K. (2005). Mindfulness: What is it? What does it matter? In C. K. Germer, R. D. Siegel, & P. R. Fulton (Eds.), *Mindfulness and psychotherapy* (pp. 3–28). Guilford Press.

Germer, C. K. (2012). Cultivating compassion in psychotherapy. In C. K. Germer & R. D. Siegel (Eds.), *Wisdom and compassion in psychotherapy: Deepening mindfulness in clinical practice* (pp. 93–110). Guilford Press.

Germer, C., & Neff, K. (2013). The mindful self-compassion training program. In T. Singer, & M. Bolz (Eds.), *Compassion: Bridging practice and science* (pp. 364–396). Max-Planck Institute.

Gibbons, M. B. C., Crits-Christoph, P., Barber, J. P., & Schamberger, M. (2007). Insight in psychotherapy: A review of empirical literature. In L. G. Castonguay & C. E. Hill (Eds.), *Insight in psychotherapy* (pp. 143–167). American Psychological Association.

Gilbert, M., & Orlans, M. (2011). *Integrative therapy: 100 key points and techniques*. Routledge.

Gilbert, P. (2009). *The compassionate mind: A new approach to life's challenges*. New Harbinger Publications.

Gilbert, P. (2010). *Compassion focused therapy: Distinctive features*. Routledge.

Goldberg, S. B., Tucker, R. P., Greene, P. A., Davidson, R. J., Kearney, D. J., & Simpson, T. L. (2019). Mindfulness-based cognitive therapy for the treatment of current depressive symptoms: A meta-analysis. *Cognitive Behaviour Therapy, 6073*. https://doi.org/10.1080/16506073.2018.1556330

Goldberg, S. B., Tucker, R. P., Greene, P. A., Davidson, R. J., Wampold, B. E., Kearney, D. J., & Simpson, T. L. (2018). Mindfulness-based interventions for psychiatric disorders: A systematic review and meta-analysis. *Clinical Psychology Review, 59*, 52–60. https://doi.org/10.1016/j.cpr.2017.10.011

Goldfried, M. R. (1980). Toward the delineation of therapeutic change principles. *American Psychologist, 35*(11), 991–999. https://doi.org/10.1016/j.appsy.2009.10.015

Goldfried, M. R., Pachankis, J. E., & Goodwin, B. J. (2019). A history of psychotherapy integration. In J. C. Norcross & M. R. Goldfried (Eds.), *Handbook of psychotherapy integration.* (3rd ed., pp. 28–63). Oxford University Press.

Goldfried, M. R., & Padawer, W. (1982). Current status and future directions in psychotherapy. In M. R. Goldfried (Ed.), *Converging themes in psychotherapy* (pp. 3–49). Springer.

Goldin, P. R., & Gross, J. J. (2010). Effects of Mindfulness-based stress reduction (MBSR) on emotion regulation in social anxiety disorder. *Emotion, 10*(1), 83–91. https://doi.org/10.1037/a0018441

Gómez, B., Iwakabe, S., & Vaz, A. (2019). International themes in psychotherapy integration. In J. C. Norcross & M. R. Goldfried (Eds.), *Handbook of psychotherapy integration.* (3rd ed., pp. 448–485). Oxford University Press.

Greenberg, L. (2008). Emotion and cognition in psychotherapy: The transforming power of affect. *Canadian Psychology, 49*(1), 49–59. https://doi.org/10.1037/0708-5591.49.1.49

Greenberg, L. S., Auszra, L., & Herrmann, I. R. (2007). The relationship among emotional productivity, emotional arousal and outcome in experiential therapy of depression. *Psychotherapy Research, 17*(4), 482–493. https://doi.org/10.1080/10503300600977800

Greenberg, L. S., & Paivio, S. C. (1997). *Working with emotions in psychotherapy.* Guilford Press.

Greenberg, L. S., Rice, L. N., & Elliot, R. (1993). *Facilitating emotional change: The moment-by-moment process.* Guilford Press.

Greenberg, L. S., & Watson, J. C. (2006). *Emotion-focused therapy for depression.* American Psychological Association.

Grof, S. (1988). *The adventure of self-discovery: Dimensions of consciousness and new perspectives in psychotherapy and inner exploration.* State University of New York Press.

Guistolise, P. G. (1996). Failures in the therapeutic relationship: Inevitable and necessary? *Transactional Analysis Journal, 26*(4), 284–288. https://doi.org/10.1177/036215379602600403

Guntrip, H. (1993). *Schizoid phenomena, object relations and the self.* Karnac Books. (Original work published 1968)

Hanh, T. N. (1998). *The heart of the Buddha's teaching.* Harmony Books.

Hanley, A. W., Nakamura, Y., & Garland, E. L. (2018). The Nondual Awareness Dimensional Assessment (NADA): New tools to assess nondual traits and states of consciousness occurring within and beyond the context of meditation. *Psychological Assessment.* https://doi.org/10.1037/pas0000615

Hargaden, H., & Sills, C. (2002). *Transactional analysis: A relational perspective.* Brunner/Routledge.

Harris, R. (2007). *The happiness trap: How to stop struggling and start living.* Trumpeter Books.

Hatfield, E., Bensman, L., Thornton, P. D., & Rapson, R. L. (2014). New perspectives on emotional contagion: A review of classic and recent research on facial mimicry and contagion. *Interpersona: An International Journal on Personal Relationships, 8*(2), 159–179. https://doi.org/10.5964/ijpr.v8i2.162

Hautamäki, A., Hautamäki, L., Neuvonen, L., & Maliniemi-Piispanen, S. (2010). Transmission of attachment across three generations: Continuity and reversal. *Clinical Child Psychology and Psychiatry, 15*(3), 347–354. https://doi.org/10.1177/1359104510365451

Hayes, A. M., & Feldman, G. (2004). Clarifying the construct of mindfulness in the context of emotion regulation and the process of change in therapy. *Clinical Psychology: Science and Practice, 11*(3), 255–262. https://doi.org/10.1093/clipsy/bph080

Hayes, S. C. (1984). Making sense of spirituality. *Behaviorism, 12*, 99–110. https://contextua lscience.org/files/Hayes%201984.pdf

Hayes, S. C. (2019). *A liberated mind: How to pivot toward what matters.* Penguin/Avery.

Hayes, S. C., & Hofmann, S. G. (2018). Introduction. In S. C. Hayes & S. G. Hofmann (Eds.), *Process-based CBT: The science and core clinical competencies of cognitive behavioral therapy* (pp. 1–7). Context Press: An Imprint of New Harbinger Publications.

Hayes, S. C., Law, S., Malady, M., Zhu, Z., & Bai, X. (2019). The centrality of sense of self in psychological flexibility processes: What the neurobiological and psychological correlates of psychedelics suggest. *Journal of Contextual Behavioral Science, 15*, 30–38. https://doi.org/10.1016/j.jcbs.2019.11.005

Hayes, S. C., & Spencer, S. (2005). *Get out of your mind & into your life: The new acceptance and commitment therapy.* New Harbinger Publications.

Hayes, S. C., Strosahl, K. D., & Wilson, K. G. (1999). *Acceptance and commitment therapy: An experiential approach to behavior change.* Guilford Press.

Hayes, S. C., Strosahl, K. D., & Wilson, K. G. (2012). *Acceptance and commitment therapy: The process and practice of mindful change* (2nd ed.). Guilford Press.

Helm, J. L., Sbarra, D. A., & Ferrer, E. (2014). Coregulation of respiratory sinus arrhythmia in adult romantic partners. *Emotion, 14*(3), 522–531. https://doi.org/10.1037/a0035960

Hilton, L., Hempel, S., Ewing, B. A., Apaydin, E., Xenakis, L., Newberry, S., Colaiaco, B., Maher, A. R., Shanman, R. M., Sorbero, M. E., & Maglione, M. A. (2017). Mindfulness meditation for chronic pain: Systematic review and meta-analysis. *Annals of Behavioral Medicine, 51*(2), 199–213. https://doi.org/10.1007/s12160-016-9844-2

Hofmann, S. G., & Hayes, S. C. (2018). The history and current status of CBT as an evidence based therapy. In S. C. Hayes & S. G. Hofmann (Eds.), *The process-based CBT: The science and core clinical competencies of cognitive behavioral therapy* (pp. 7–22). Context Press: An Imprint of New Harbinger Publications.

Hofmann, S. G., & Hayes, S. C. (2019). The future of intervention science: Process-based therapy. *Clinical Psychological Science, 7*(1), 37–50. https://doi.org/10.1177/2167702618772296

Hofmann, S. G., Sawyer, A. T., Witt, A. A., & Oh, D. (2010). The effect of mindfulness-based therapy on anxiety and depression: A meta-analytic review. *Journal Consulting Clinical Psychology, 78*(2), 169–183. https://doi.org/10.1037/a0018555

Høglend, P., & Hagtvet, K. (2019). Change mechanisms in psychotherapy: Both improved insight and improved affective awareness are necessary. *Journal of Consulting and Clinical Psychology, 87*(4), 332–344. https://doi.org/10.1037/ccp0000381

Hölzel, B. K., Lazar, S. W., Gard, T., Schuman-Olivier, Vago, D. R., & Ott, U. (2011). How does mindfulness meditation work. *Perspectives on Psychological Science, 6*(6), 537–559. https://doi.org/10.1177/1745691611419671

Horowitz, M. J. (1998). *Cognitive psychodynamics: From conflict to character.* John Wiley & Sons.

Horst, K., Newsom, K., & Stith, S. (2013). Client and therapist initial experience of using mindfulness in therapy. *Psychotherapy Research, 23*(4), 369–380. https://doi.org/10.1080/10503307.2013.784420

Howell, E. F. (2011). *Dissociative identity disorder.* Routledge.

Iacoboni, M. (2009). Imitation, empathy, and mirror neurons. *Annual Review of Psychology, 60*(1), 653–670. https://doi.org/10.1146/annurev.psych.60.110707.163604

International Integrative Psychotherapy Association. (2020). *Definition.* https://integrativea ssociation.com/the-association/

Iwakabe, S., & Conceicao, N. (2016). Metatherapeutic processing as a change-based therapeutic immediacy task: Building an initial process model using a task-analytic research strategy. *Journal of Psychotherapy Integration, 26*(3), 230–247. https://doi.org/10.1037/int0000016

Jain, S., Shapiro, S. L., Swanick, S., Roesch, S. C., Mills, P. J., Bell, I., & Schwartz, G. E. R. (2007). A randomized controlled trial of mindfulness meditation versus relaxation training: Effects on distress, positive states of mind, rumination, and distraction. *Annals of Behavioral Medicine, 33*(1), 11–21.

James, M., & Jongeward, D. (1996). *Born to win: Transactional analysis with gestalt experiments.* Addison-Wesley. (Original work published 1971).

James, W. (2007). *The principles of psychology* (Vol. 1). Cosimo. (Original work published 1890)

Josipovic, Z. (2010). Duality and nonduality in meditation research. *Consciousness and Cognition, 19*(4), 1119–1121. https://doi.org/10.1016/j.concog.2010.03.016

Josipovic, Z. (2014). Neural correlates of nondual awareness in meditation. *Annals of the New York Academy of Sciences, 1307*(1), 9–18. https://doi.org/10.1111/nyas.12261

Josipovic, Z. (2016). Love and compassion meditation: A nondual perspective. *Annals of the New York Academy of Sciences, 1373*(1), 65–71. https://doi.org/10.1111/nyas.13078

Josipovic, Z. (2019). Nondual awareness: Consciousness-as-such as non-representational reflexivity. In N. Srinivasan (Ed.), *Progress in brain research: Meditation* (Vol. 244, pp. 273–298). Netherlands: Elsevier. https://doi.org/10.1016/bs.pbr.2018.10.021

Jung, C. G. (2010). *AION* (D. Flis, T. Drev, Trans.). Celjska Mohorjeva družba. (Original work published 1951)

Kabat-Zinn, J. (1990). *Full catastrophe living: How to cope with stress, pain and illness using mindfulness meditation.* Piatkos.

Kabat-Zinn, J. (1994). *Wherever you go, there you are: Mindfulness meditation in everyday life.* Hyperion.

Kalsched, D. (1996). *The inner world of trauma: Archetypal defenses of the personal spirit.* Routledge.

Kappen, G., Karremans, J. C., Burk, W. J., & Buyukcan-Tetik, A. (2018). On the association between mindfulness and romantic relationship satisfaction: The role of partner acceptance. *Mindfulness, 9*(5), 1543–1556. https://doi.org/10.1007/s12671-018-0902-7

Karvonen, A., Kykyri, V. L., Kaartinen, J., Penttonen, M., & Seikkula, J. (2016). Sympathetic nervous system synchrony in couple therapy. *Journal of Marital and Family Therapy, 42*(3), 383–395. https://doi.org/10.1111/jmft.12152

Kernberg, O. F. (1976). *Object-relations theory and clinical psychoanalysis.* Jason Aronson.

Khoury, B., Lecomte, T., Fortin, G., Masse, M., Therien, P., Bouchard, V., Chapleau, M. A., Paquin, K., & Hofmann, S. G. (2013). Mindfulness-based therapy: A comprehensive meta-analysis. *Clinical Psychology Review, 33*(6), 763–771. https://doi.org/10.1016/j.cpr.2013.05.005

Kleinbub, J. R. (2017). State of the art of interpersonal physiology in psychotherapy: A systematic review. *Frontiers in Psychology, 8*, 2053. https://doi.org/10.3389/fpsyg.2017.02053

Klimecki, O., & Singer, T. (2012). Empathic distress fatigue rather than compassion fatigue? Integrating findings from empathy research in psychology and social neuroscience. In B. Oakley, A. Knafo, G. Madhavan, & D. S. Wilson (Eds.), *Pathological altruism* (pp. 368–383). Oxford University Press. https://doi.org/10.1093/acprof

Knox, S., Hess, S. A., Hill, C. E., Burkard, A. W., & Crook-Lyon, R. E. (2012). Corrective relational experiences: Client perspectives. In L. G. Castonguay & C. E. Hill (Eds.),

Transformation in psychotherapy. Corrective experiences across cognitive behavioral, humanistic, and psychodynamic approaches (pp. 191–213). American Psychological Association.

Kohut, H. (1977). *The restoration of the self.* International Universities Press.

Kohut, H. (1984). *How does analysis cure?* University of Chicago Press.

Krägeloh, C. (2018). Phenomenological research fails to capture the experience of nondual awareness. *Mindfulness, 10*, 15–25. https://doi.org/10.1007/s12671-018-0995-z

Kuyken, W., Warren, F. C., Taylor, R. S., Whalley, B., Crane, C., Bondolfi, G., Hayes, R., Huijbers, M., Ma, H., Schweizer, S., Segal, Z., Speckens, A., Teasdale, J. D., Van Heeringen, K., Williams, M., Byford, S., Byng, R., & Dalgleish, T. (2016). Efficacy of mindfulness-based cognitive therapy in prevention of depressive relapse an individual patient data meta-analysis from randomized trials. *JAMA Psychiatry, 73*(6), 565–574. https://doi.org/10.1001/jamapsychiatry.2016.0076

Lane, R. D., Lee, R., Nadel, L., & Greenberg, L. (2015). Memory reconsolidation, emotional arousal, and the process of change in psychotherapy: New insights from brain science. *Behavioral and Brain Sciences, 38*, 1–64. https://doi.org/10.1017/S0140525X14000041

Lanius, R. A. (2015). Trauma-related dissociation and altered states of consciousness: A call for clinical, treatment, and neuroscience research. *European Journal of Psychotraumatology, 6*, 1–9. https://doi.org/10.3402/ejpt.v6.27905

Levenson, R. W., & Gottman, J. M. (1983). Marital interaction: Physiological linkage and affective exchange. *Journal of Personality and Social Psychology, 45*(3), 587–597. https://doi.org/10.1037/0022-3514.45.3.587

Levine, P. A. (1997). *Waking the tiger: Healing trauma.* North Atlantic Books.

Levine, P. A. (2018). Polyvagal theory and trauma. In S. W. Porges & D. Dana (Eds.), *Clinical applications of the polyvagal theory: The emergence of polyvagal-informed therapies* (pp. 3–26). W.W. Norton & Company.

Lichtenberg, J. D. (2017). Narrative and meaning: Our story begins. In J. D. Lichtenberg, F. M. Lachmann, & J. L. Fosshage (Eds.), *Narrative and meaning: The foundation of mind, creativity and the psychoanalytic dialogue* (pp. 1–51). Routledge.

Little, R. (2006). Ego state relational units and resistance to change. *Transactional Analysis Journal, 36*(1), 7–19. https://doi.org/10.1177/036215370603600103

Lomas, T., Medina, J. C., Ivtzan, I., Rupprecht, S., & Eiroa-Orosa, F. J. (2019). A systematic review and meta-analysis of the impact of mindfulness-based interventions on the well-being of healthcare professionals. *Mindfulness, 10*(7), 1193–1216. https://doi.org/10.1007/s12671-018-1062-5

Lowen, A. (1988). *Bioenergija: Revolucionarno zdravljenje duševnih in telesnih motenj s pomočjo govorice telesa* [Bioenergetics: The revolutionary therapy that uses the language of the body to heal the problems of the mind]. Cankarjeva založba. (Original work published 1975)

Luborsky, L., Singer, B., & Luborsky, L. (1975). Comparative studies of psychotherapies: Is it true that "Everyone has won and all must have prizes"? *Archives of General Psychiatry, 32*(8), 995–1008. https://doi.org/10.1001/archpsyc.1975.01760260059004

Luoma, J. B., Hayes, S. C., & Walser, R. D. (2007). *Learning ACT: An acceptance & commitment therapy skills-training manual for therapists.* New Harbinger Publications.

Lutz, A., Dunne, J. D., & Davidson, R. J. (2006). Meditation and the neuroscience of consciousness: An introduction. In P. Zelazo, M. Moscovitch, & E. Thompson (Eds.), *The Cambridge Handbook of Consciousness (Cambridge Handbooks in Psychology).* Cambridge University Press. https://doi.org/10.1017/CBO9780511816789.020

MacBeth, A., & Gumley, A. (2012). Exploring compassion: A meta-analysis of the association between self-compassion and psychopathology. *Clinical Psychology Review, 32*(6), 545–552. https://doi.org/10.1016/j.cpr.2012.06.003

Mahler, M. S., Pine, F., & Bergman, A. (1975). *The psychological birth of the human infant.* Hutchinson.

Main, M., & Solomon, J. (1990). Procedures for identifying infants as disorganised/disoriented during the Ainsworth Strange Situation. In M. T. Greenberg, D. Cicchetti, & E. M. Cummings (Eds.), *Attachment in the preschool years: Theory, research, and intervention* (pp. 121–160). University of Chicago Press.

Malachi, T. (2004). *The gnostic gospel of St. Thomas: Meditations on the mystical teachings.* Llewellyn Publications.

Malachi, T. (2005). *Living gnosis: A practical guide to gnostic Christianity.* Llewellyn Publications.

Marci, C. D., Ham, J., Moran, E., & Orr, S. P. (2007). Physiologic correlates of perceived therapist empathy and social-emotional process during psychotherapy. *Journal of Nervous and Mental Disease, 195*(2), 103–111. https://doi.org/10.1097/01.nmd.0000253731.71025.fc

Marci, C. D., & Orr, S. P. (2006). The effect of emotional distance on psychophysiologic concordance and perceived empathy between patient and interviewer. *Applied Psychophysiology Biofeedback, 31*(2), 115–128. https://doi.org/10.1007/s10484-006-9008-4

Martin, J. R. (1997). Mindfulness: A proposed common factor. *Journal of Psychotherapy Integration, 7*(4), 291–312.

McAdams, D. P. (2001). The psychology of life stories. *Review of General Psychology, 5*(2), 100–122. https://doi.org/10.1037//I089-2680.5.2.100

McAdams, D. P., & McLean, K. C. (2013). Narrative identity. *Current Directions in Psychological Science, 22*(3), 233–238. https://doi.org/10.1177/0963721413475622

McAleavey, A. A., Xiao, H., Bernecker, S. L., Brunet, H., Morrison, N. R., Stein, M., Youn, S. J., Castonguay, L. G., Constantino, M. J., & Beutler, L. E. (2019). An updated list of principles of change that work. In L. G. Castonguay, M. J. Constantino, & L. E. Beutler (Eds.), *Principles of change: How psychotherapists implement research in practice* (pp. 13–37). Oxford University Press.

McGill, J., Adler-Baeder, F., & Rodriguez, P. (2016). Mindfully in love: A meta-analysis of the association between mindfulness and relationship satisfaction. *Journal of Human Sciences and Extension, 4*(1), 89–101.

McHughs, L., & Stewart, I. (2012). *The self and perspective taking: Contributions and applications from modern behavioral science.* Oaklands, CA: New Harbinger Publications.

McHughs, L., Stewart, I., & Almada, P. (2019). *A contextual behavioral guide to the self: Theory and practice.* New Harbinger Publications.

McNeel, J. R. (1976). The parent interview. *Transactional Analysis Journal, 6*(1), 61–68.

McWilliams, N. (2011). *Psychoanalytic diagnosis: Understanding personality structure in the clinical process* (2nd ed.). Guilford Press.

Messer, S. B. (2013). Three mechanisms of change in psychodynamic therapy: Insight, affect, and alliance. *Psychotherapy, 50*(3), 408–412. https://doi.org/10.1037/a0032414

Messina, I., Palmieri, A., Sambin, M., Kleinbub, J. R., Voci, A., & Calvo, V. (2013). Somatic underpinnings of perceived empathy: The importance of psychotherapy training. *Psychotherapy Research, 23*(2), 169–177. https://doi.org/10.1080/10503307.2012.748940

Mills, P. J., Peterson, C. T., Pung, M. A., Patel, S., Weiss, L., Wilson, K. L., Doraiswamy, P. M., Martin, J. A., Tanzi, R. E., & Chopra, D. (2018). Change in sense of nondual awareness and spiritual awakening in response to a multidimensional well-being program. *The Journal of Alternative and Complementary Medicine, 24*(4), 343–351. https://doi.org/10.1089/acm.2017.0160

Mitchell, S. A. (2012). *Can love last? The fate of romance over time.* W.W. Norton & Company.

Modic, K. U. (2019). *Učinkovitost in spremembe v procesu integrativne psihoterapije* [Effectiveness and changes in the process of integrative psychotherapy][Unpublished doctoral dissertation]. University of Ljubljana.

Modic, K. U., & Žvelc, G. (2015). Helpful aspects of the therapeutic relationship in integrative psychotherapy. *International Journal of Integrative Psychotherapy, 6,* 1–25. http://www.integrative-journal.com/index.php/ijip/article/view/103

Moursund, J. P., & Erskine, R. G. (2004). *Integrative psychotherapy: The art and science of relationship.* Thomson: Brooks/Cole.

Neff, K. D. (2003a). The development and validation of a scale to measure self-compassion. *Self and Identity, 2,* 223–250. https://doi.org/10.1080/15298860390209035

Neff, K. D. (2003b). Self-Compassion: An alternative conceptualization of a healthy attitude toward oneself. *Self and Identity, 2,* 85–101. https://doi.org/10.1080/15298860309032

Neff, K. D. (2011). *Self compassion: Stop beating yourself up and leave insecurity behind.* Hodder & Stoughton.

Neff, K. D., & Beretvas, S. N. (2013). The role of self-compassion in romantic relationships. *Self and Identity, 12*(1), 78–98. https://doi.org/10.1080/15298868.2011.639548

Neff, K. D., & Germer, C. K. (2013). A pilot study and randomized controlled trial of the mindful self-compassion program. *Journal of Clinical Psychology, 69*(1), 28–44. https://doi.org/10.1002/jclp.21923

Norcross, J. C. (2010). The therapeutic relationship. In B. L. Duncan, S. C. Miller, B. E. Wampold, & M. A. Hubble (Eds.), *The heart and soul of change* (2nd ed., pp. 113–142). American Psychological Association.

Norcross, J. C., & Alexander, E. F. (2019). A primer on psychotherapy integration. In J. C. Norcross & M. R. Goldfried (Eds.), *Handbook of psychotherapy integration* (3rd ed., pp. 3–27). Oxford University Press.

Norcross, J. C., & Lambert, M. J. (2018). Psychotherapy relationships that work III. *Psychotherapy, 55*(4), 303–315. https://doi.org/10.1037/pst0000193

Norcross, J. C., & Wampold, B. E. (2018). A new therapy for each patient: Evidence-based relationships and responsiveness. *Journal of Clinical Psychology, 74,* 1889–1906. https://doi.org/10.1002/jclp.22678

Norris, C. J., Creem, D., Hendler, R., & Kober, H. (2018). Brief mindfulness meditation improves attention in novices: Evidence from ERPs and moderation by neuroticism. *Frontiers in Human Neuroscience, 12,* 1–20. https://doi.org/10.3389/fnhum.2018.00315

O'Reilly-Knapp, M., & Erskine, R. G. (2003). Core concepts of an integrative transactional analysis. *Transactional Analysis Journal, 33*(2), 168–177. https://doi.org/10.1177/036215370303300208

Ogden, P. (2018). Polyvagal theory and sensorimotor psychotherapy. In S. W. Porges & D. Dana (Eds.), *Clinical applications of the polyvagal theory: The emergence of polyvagal-informed therapies* (pp. 34–49). W.W. Norton & Company.

Ogden, P., Minton, K., & Pain, C. (2006). *Trauma and the body: A sensorimotor approach to psychotherapy.* W.W. Norton & Company.

Päivinen, H., Holma, J., Karvonen, A., Kykyri, V. L., Tsatsishvili, V., Kaartinen, J., Penttonen, M., & Seikkula, J. (2016). Affective arousal during blaming in couple therapy:

Combining analyses of verbal discourse and physiological responses in two case studies. *Contemporary Family Therapy, 38*(4), 373–384. https://doi.org/10.1007/s10591-016-9393-7

Palmieri, A., Kleinbub, J. R., Calvo, V., Benelli, E., Messina, I., Sambin, M., & Voci, A. (2018). Attachment-security prime effect on skin-conductance synchronization in psychotherapists: An empirical study. *Journal of Counseling Psychology, 65*(4), 490–499. https://doi.org/10.1037/cou0000273

Palumbo, R. V., Marraccini, M. E., Weyandt, L. L., Wilder-Smith, O., McGee, H. A., Liu, S., & Goodwin, M. S. (2017). Interpersonal autonomic physiology: A systematic review of the literature. *Personality and Social Psychology Review, 21*(2), 99–141. https://doi.org/10.1177/1088868316628405

Perls, F., Hefferline, R. F., & Goodman, P. (1951). *Gestalt therapy: Excitement and growth in the human personality*. Souvenir Press.

Petzold, H. G. (2002). *Integrative therapie*. [Integrative therapy] Junfermann.

Piaget, J., & Inhelder, B. (1986). *Intelektualni razvoj deteta: Izabrani radovi* [Intellectual development of the child: Collected works]. ZUNS. (Original work published 1966)

Piaget, J., & Inhelder, B. (1990). *Psihologija deteta* [The psychology of the child] (T. Ilić, Trans.). Izdavačka knjižarnica Zorana Stojanovića. (Original work published 1966)

Porges, S. W. (2011). *The polyvagal theory: Neurophysiological foundations of emotions, attachment, communication and self-regulation*. W.W. Norton & Company.

Porges, S. W. (2017). *The pocket guide to the polyvagal theory: The transformative power of feeling safe*. W.W. Norton & Company.

Porges, S. W. (2018). Polyvagal theory: A primer. In S. W. Porges & D. Dana (Eds.), *Clinical applications of the polyvagal theory: The emergence of polyvagal-informed therapies* (pp. 50–69). W.W. Norton & Company.

Pourová, M., Řiháček, T., & Žvelc, G. (2020). Validation of the Czech version of the Relational Needs Satisfaction Scale. *Frontiers in Psychology, 11*, 359, 1–11. https://doi.org/10.3389/fpsyg.2020.00359

Price, C. J., & Hooven, C. (2018). Interoceptive awareness skills for emotion regulation: Theory and approach of mindful awareness in body-oriented therapy (MABT). *Frontiers in Psychology, 9*, 1–12. https://doi.org/10.3389/fpsyg.2018.00798

Prochaska, J. O., & Diclemente, C. C. (2019). The transtheoretical approach. In J. C. Norcross & M. R. Goldfried (Eds.), *Handbook of psychotherapy integration* (3rd ed., pp. 161–183). Oxford University Press.

Prochazkova, E., & Kret, M. E. (2017). Connecting minds and sharing emotions through mimicry: A neurocognitive model of emotional contagion. *Neuroscience and Biobehavioral Reviews, 80*, 99–114. https://doi.org/10.1016/j.neubiorev.2017.05.013

Rasmussen, P. D., Storebø, O. J., Løkkeholt, T., Voss, L. G., Shmueli-Goetz, Y., Bojesen, A. B., Simonsen, E., & Bilenberg, N. (2019). Attachment as a core feature of resilience: A systematic review and meta-analysis. *Psychological Reports, 122*(4), 1259–1296. https://doi.org/10.1177/0033294118785577

Reeck, C., Ames, D. R., & Ochsner, K. N. (2016). The social regulation of emotion: An integrative, cross-disciplinary model. *Trends in Cognitive Sciences, 20*(1), 47–63. https://doi.org/10.1016/j.tics.2015.09.003

Reich, W. (1988). *Funkcija orgazma* [The function of the orgasm]. A-Š Delo. (Original work published 1942)

Rizzolatti, G., Fadiga, L., Fogassi, L., & Gallese, V. (1999). Resonance behaviors and mirror neurons. *Archives Italiennes de Biologie, 137*(2–3),85–100. https://doi.org/10.4449/aib.v137i2.575

Robinson, J. W., Herman, A., & Kaplan, B. J. (1982). Autonomic responses correlate with counselor–client empathy. *Journal of Counseling Psychology, 29*(2), 195–198. https://doi.org/10.1037/0022-0167.29.2.195

Rogers, C. R. (1957). The necessary and sufficient conditions of therapeutic personality change. *Journal of Consulting Psychology, 21*(2), 95–103. https://doi.org/10.1037/h0045357

Rothschild, B. (2000). *The body remembers: The psychophysiology of trauma and trauma treatment.* W. W. Norton & Company.

Rothschild, B. (2006). *Help for the helper: The psychophysiology of compassion fatigue and vicarious trauma.* W.W. Norton & Company.

Rothschild, B. (2017). *Body remembers: Revolutionizing trauma treatment* (Vol. 2). W.W. Norton & Company.

Rust, M. (2008). Climate on the couch: Unconscious processes in relation to our environmental crisis. *Psychotherapy and Politics International, 6*(3), 157–170. https://doi.org/10.1002/ppi

Safran, J. D. (1990). Towards a refinement of cognitive therapy in light of interpersonal theory: II. Practice. *Clinical Psychology Review, 10*(1), 107–121. https://doi.org/10.1016/0272-7358(90)90109-N

Safran, J. D., & Kraus, J. (2014). Alliance ruptures, impasses, and enactments: A relational perspective. *Psychotherapy, 51*(3), 381–387. https://doi.org/10.1037/a0036815

Safran, J. D., & Muran, J. C. (2000). *Negotiating the therapeutic alliance: A relational treatment guide.* Guilford Press.

Safran, J. D., & Segal, Z. V. (1990). *Interpersonal process in cognitive therapy.* Jason Aronson.

Salvador, M. C. (2019). *Beyond the self: Healing emotional trauma and brainspotting.* Editorial Eleftheria.

Saxbe, D. E., Margolin, G., Spies Shapiro, L., Ramos, M., Rodriguez, A., & Iturralde, E. (2014). Relative influences: Patterns of HPA axis concordance during triadic family interaction. *Health Psychology, 33*(3), 273–281. https://doi.org/10.1037/a0033509

Saxbe, D., & Repetti, R. L. (2010). For better or worse? Coregulation of couples' cortisol levels and mood states. *Journal of Personality and Social Psychology, 98*(1), 92–103. https://doi.org/10.1037/a0016959

Sayers, W. M., Creswell, J. D., & Taren, A. (2015). The emerging neurobiology of mindfulness and emotion processing. In B. D. Ostafin, M. D. Robinson, & B. P. Meier (Eds.), *Handbook of Mindfulness and Self-Regulation* (pp. 9–22). Springer. https://doi.org/10.1007/978-1-4939-2263-5_2

Schore, A. N. (1994). *Affect regulation and the origin of the self.* Erlbaum.

Schore, A. N. (2001). The effects of early relational trauma on right brain development, affect regulation, and infant mental health. *Infant Mental Health Journal, 22*, 201–269.

Schore, A. N. (2003). *Affect dysregulation & disorders of the self.* W.W. Norton & Company.

Schore, A. N. (2019). *Right brain psychotherapy.* W.W. Norton & Company.

Schuman, M. (2017). *Mindfulness-informed relational psychotherapy and psychoanalysis: Inquiring deeply.* Routledge.

Schutte, N. S., & Malouff, J. M. (2018). Mindfulness and connectedness to nature: A meta-analytic investigation. *Personality and Individual Differences, 127*, 10–14. https://doi.org/10.1016/j.paid.2018.01.034

Schwartz, R. C. (1995). *Internal family systems therapy.* Guilford Press.

Sedighimornani, N., Rimes, K. A., & Verplanken, B. (2019). Exploring the relationships between mindfulness, self-compassion, and shame. *SAGE Open, 9*(3). https://doi.org/10.1177/2158244019866294

Segal, Z. V., Williams, J. M. G., & Teasdale, J. D. (2002). *Mindfulness-based cognitive therapy for depression: A new approach to preventing relapse.* Guilford Press.

Seth, A. K. (2013). Interoceptive inference, emotion, and the embodied self. *Trends in Cognitive Sciences, 17*(11), 565–573. https://doi.org/10.1016/j.tics.2013.09.007

Seth, A. K., Suzuki, K., Critchley, H. D., Frith, C., & Trust, W. (2012). An interoceptive predictive coding model of conscious presence. *Frontiers in Psychology, 2*, 1–16. https://doi.org/10.3389/fpsyg.2011.00395

Shallcross, A. J., Troy, A. S., Boland, M., & Mauss, I. B. (2010). Let it be: Accepting negative emotional experiences predicts decreased negative affect and depressive symptoms. *Behavioral Research and Therapy, 48*(9), 921–929. https://doi.org/doi:10.1016/j.brat.2010.05.025

Shapiro, F. (2001). *Eye movement desensitization and reprocessing: Basic principles, protocols and procedures* (2nd ed.). Guilford Press.

Shapiro, F. (2018). *Eye movement desensitization and reprocessing (EMDR) therapy: Basic principles, protocols, and procedures* (3rd ed.). Guilford Press.

Shapiro, S. L., Carlson, L. E., Astin, J. A., & Freedman, B. (2006). Mechanisms of mindfulness. *Journal of Clinical Psychology, 62*(3), 373–386. https://doi.org/10.1002/jclp.20237

Siegel, D. J. (1999). *The developing mind: Toward a neurobiology of interpersonal experience.* Guilford Press.

Siegel, D. J. (2007). *The mindful brain: Reflection and attunement in the cultivation of well being.* W. W. Norton & Company.

Siegel, D. J. (2012). *The developing mind: How relationships and the brain interact to shape who we are* (2nd ed.). Guilford Press.

Siegel, D. J. (2018). *Aware: The science and practice of presence. A complete guide to the groundbreaking Wheel of Awareness meditation practice.* Scribe Publications.

Siegel, R. D., & Germer, C. K. (2012). Wisdom and compassion: Two wings of a bird. In Christopher K.Germer & D. J. Siegel (Eds.), *Wisdom and compassion in psychotherapy: Deepening mindfulness in clinical practice* (pp. 7–34). Guilford Press.

Simpson, R., Simpson, S., Ramparsad, N., Lawrence, M., Booth, J., & Mercer, S. W. (2019). Mindfulness-based interventions for mental well-being among people with multiple sclerosis: A systematic review and meta-analysis of randomised controlled trials. *Journal of Neurology, Neurosurgery and Psychiatry*, 1051–1058. https://doi.org/10.1136/jnnp-2018-320165

Spinelli, C., Wisener, M., & Khoury, B. (2019). Mindfulness training for healthcare professionals and trainees: A meta-analysis of randomized controlled trials. *Journal of Psychosomatic Research, 120*, 29–38. https://doi.org/10.1016/j.jpsychores.2019.03.003

Stern, D. N. (1995). *The motherhood constellation: A unified view of parent–infant psychotherapy.* Basic Books.

Stern, D. N. (2004). *The present moment in psychotherapy and everyday life.* W.W. Norton & Company.

Stern, D. N. (2018). *The interpersonal world of the infant: A view from psychoanalysis and developmental psychology* (Paperback edition). Routledge. (Original work published 1998)

Stewart, I., & Joines, V. (2012). *TA today: A new introduction to transactional analysis.* Lifespace Publishing.

Stolorow, R. D. (1994). The intersubjective context of intrapsychic experience. In R. D. Stolorow, G. E. Atwood, & B. Brandschaft (Eds.), *The intersubjective perspective* (pp. 3–15). Jason Aronson.

Strauß, B., Altmann, U., Manes, S., Tholl, A., Koranyi, S., Nolte, T., Beutel, M. E., Wiltink, J., Herpertz, S., Hiller, W., Hoyer, J., Joraschky, P., Nolting, B., Ritter, V.,

Stangier, U., Willutzki, U., Salzer, S., Leibing, E., Leichsenring, F., & Kirchmann, H. (2018). Changes of attachment characteristics during psychotherapy of patients with social anxiety disorder: Results from the SOPHO-Net trial. *PLoS ONE, 13*(3), Article e0192802. https://doi.org/10.1371/journal.pone.0192802

Summers, G., & Tudor, K. (2014a). Response to "Co-creative contributions". In K. Tudor & G. Summer (Eds.), *Co-creative transactional analysis: Papers, responses, dialogues, and developments* (pp. 183–200). Karnac Books.

Summers, G., & Tudor, K. (2014b). Response to "The neopsyche: The integrating Adult ego state", and rejoinder. In K. Tudor & G. Summers (Eds.), *Co-creative transactional analysis: Papers, responses, dialogues, and developments* (pp. 69–88). Karnac Books.

Surrey, J. L. (2005). Relational psychotherapy, relational mindfulness. In C. K. Germer, R. D. Siegel, & P. R. Fulton (Eds.), *Mindfulness and psychotherapy* (pp. 91–113). Guilford Press.

Suveg, C., Shaffer, A., & Davis, M. (2016). Family stress moderates relations between physiological and behavioral synchrony and child self-regulation in mother–preschooler dyads. *Developmental Psychobiology, 58*(1), 83–97. https://doi.org/10.1002/dev.21358

Šumiga, D. (2019). Fromm's understanding of the Buddhist philosophical theory and psychoanalysis: From the phenomenal ego to the authentic being. *International Forum of Psychoanalysis,* 1–12. https://doi.org/10.1080/0803706X.2018.1521006

Taren, A. A., Creswell, J. D., & Gianaros, P. J. (2013). Dispositional mindfulness co-varies with smaller amygdala and caudate volumes in community adults. *PLoS ONE, 8*(5), 1–7. https://doi.org/10.1371/journal.pone.0064574

Taylor, P., Rietzschel, J., Danquah, A., & Berry, K. (2015). Changes in attachment representations during psychological therapy. *Psychotherapy Research, 25*(2), 222–238. https://doi.org/10.1080/10503307.2014.886791

Teper, R., & Inzlicht, M. (2013). Meditation, mindfulness and executive control: The importance of emotional acceptance and brain-based performance monitoring. *Social Cognitive and Affective Neuroscience, 8*(1), 85–92. https://doi.org/10.1093/scan/nss045

Teper, R., Segal, Z. V., & Inzlicht, M. (2013). Inside the mindful mind: How mindfulness enhances emotion regulation through improvements in executive control. *Current Directions in Psychological Science, 22*(6), 449–454. https://doi.org/10.1177/0963721413495869

Tirch, D., Schoendorff, B., & Silberstein, L. R. (2014). *The ACT practitioner's guide to the science of compassion*. New Harbinger Publications.

Totton, N. (2011). *Wild therapy: Undomesticating inner and outer worlds*. Pccs Books.

Trautmann, R. L., & Erskine, R. G. (1981). Ego state analysis: A comparative view. *Transactional Analysis Journal, 11*(2), 178–185. https://doi.org/10.1177/036215378101100218

Tschacher, W., & Meier, D. (2019). Physiological synchrony in psychotherapy sessions. *Psychotherapy Research,* 1–16. https://doi.org/10.1080/10503307.2019.1612114

Tudor, K. (2003). The neopsyche: The integrating Adult ego state. In C. Sills & H. Hargaden (Eds.), *Ego states* (pp. 201–231). Worth Publishing.

Tudor, K., & Worral, M. (2006). *Person-centred therapy: A clinical philosophy*. Routledge.

Vago, D. R., & Silbersweig, D. A. (2012). Self-awareness, self-regulation, and self-transcendence (S-ART): A framework for understanding the neurobiological mechanisms of mindfulness. *Frontiers in Human Neuroscience, 6,* 1–30. https://doi.org/10.3389/fnhum.2012.00296

Van Den Bergh, B. R. H., Van Calster, B., Smits, T., Van Huffel, S., & Lagae, L. (2008). Antenatal maternal anxiety is related to HPA-axis dysregulation and self-reported depressive symptoms in adolescence: A prospective study on the fetal origins of depressed mood. *Neuropsychopharmacology, 33*(3), 536–545. https://doi.org/10.1038/sj.npp.1301450

van der Brink, E., & Koster, F. (2015). *Mindfulness-based compassionate living.* Routledge.

van der Hart, O., Nijenhuis, E. R. S., & Solomon, R. (2010). Dissociation of the personality in complex trauma-related disorders and EMDR: Theoretical considerations. *Journal of EMDR Practice and Research, 4*(2), 76–92. https://doi.org/10.1891/1933-3196.4.2.76

van der Hart, O., Nijenhuis, E. R. S., & Steele, K. (2006). *The haunted self: Structural dissociation and the treatment of chronic traumatization.* W.W. Norton & Company.

Vieten, C. I., Wahbeh, H., Rael Cahn, B., MacLean, K., Estrada, M., Mills, P., Murphy, M., Shapiro, S., Radin, D., Josipovic, Z., Presti, D. E., Sapiro, M., Chozen Bays, J., Russell, P., VagoID, D., Travis, F., Walsh, R., & Delorme, A. (2018). Future directions in meditation research: Recommendations for expanding the field of contemplative science. *PLoS ONE, 13*(11). https://doi.org/10.1371/journal.pone.0205740

Villate, M., Villate, J., & Hayes, S. C. (2012). A naturalistic approach to transcendence: Deictic framing, spirituality, and prosociality. In L. McHugh & I. Steward (Eds.), *The self and perspective taking: Contributions and applications from modern behavioral science* (pp. 199–217). New Harbinger Publications.

Wachtel, P. L. (2008). *Relational theory and the practice of psychotherapy.* Guilford Press.

Wachtel, P. L., & Gagnon, G. J. (2019). Cyclical psychodynamics and integrative relational psychotherapy. In J. C. Norcross & M. R. Goldfried (Eds.), *Handbook of psychotherapy integration* (3rd ed., pp. 184–203). Oxford University Press.

Walder, E. H. (1993). Supervision and instruction in postgraduate psychotherapy integration. In G. Stricker & J. D. Gold (Eds.), *Comprehensive handbook of psychotherapy integration* (pp. 499–512). Springer Science & Business Media.

Wallin, D. J. (2007). *Attachment in psychotherapy.* Guilford Press.

Wampold, B. E., & Imel, Z. E. (2015). *The great psychotherapy debate: The evidence for what makes psychotherapy work.* (2nd ed.). Routledge.

Watkins, J. G. (1971). The affect bridge: A hypnoanalytic technique. *International Journal of Clinical and Experimental Hypnosis, 19*(1), 21–27. https://doi.org/10.1080/00207147108407148

Weinstock, M. (2005). The potential influence of maternal stress hormones on development and mental health of the offspring. *Brain, Behavior, and Immunity, 19*(4), 296–308. https://doi.org/10.1016/j.bbi.2004.09.006

Whitehead, R., Bates, G., Elphinstone, B., Yang, Y., & Murray, G. (2018). Letting go of self: The creation of the nonattachment to self scale. *Frontiers in Psychology, 9, 2544,* 1–12. https://doi.org/10.3389/fpsyg.2018.02544

Winnicot, D. W. (1986). The theory of the parent-infant relationship. In P. Buckley (Ed.), *Essential papers on object relations* (pp. 233–254). New York University Press. (Original work published 1960)

Winnicot, D. W. (1986). Transitional objects and transitional phenomena. In P. Buckley (Ed.), *Essential papers on object relations* (pp. 254–272). New York University Press. (Original work published 1953)

Xiao, Q., Yue, C., He, W., & Yu, J. Y. (2017). The mindful self: A mindfulness-enlightened self-view. *Frontiers in Psychology, 8,* 1752. https://doi.org/10.3389/fpsyg.2017.01752

Yalom, I. D. (2001). *The gift of therapy: Reflections on being a therapist.* Patkus Books.

Zaletel, M., Potočnik, J., & Jalen, A. (2012). Psychotherapy with the Parent ego state. *International Journal of Integrative Psychotherapy, 3*(1), 15–41.

Zessin, U., Dickhäuser, O., & Garbade, S. (2015). The relationship between self-compassion and well-being: A meta-analysis. *Applied Psychology: Health and Well-Being, 7*(3), 340–364. https://doi.org/10.1111/aphw.12051

Žvelc, G. (2009a, April, 16–19). *Present moment in integrative psychotherapy* [Conference presentation]. 4th International Integrative Psychotherapy Conference, Bled, Slovenia.

Žvelc, G. (2009b). Between self and others: Relational schemas as an integrating construct in psychotherapy. *Transactional Analysis Journal, 39*(1), 22–38. https://doi.org/10.1177/036215370903900104

Žvelc, G. (2010a). Object and subject relations in adulthood: Towards an integrative model of interpersonal relationships. *Psychiatria Danubina, 22*(4), 498–508.

Žvelc, G. (2010b). Object relations and attachment styles in adulthood [Objektni odnosi in stili navezanosti v odraslosti]. *Horizons of Psychology, 19*(2), 5–18.

Žvelc, G. (2010c). Relational schemas theory and transactional analysis. *Transactional Analysis Journal, 40*(1), 8–22. https://doi.org/10.1177/036215371004000103

Žvelc, G. (2011). *Razvojne teorije v psihoterapiji: Integrativni model medosebnih odnosov* [Developmental theories in psychotherapy: Integrative model of interpersonal relationships]. IPSA, Inštitut za integrativno psihoterapijo in svetovanje.

Žvelc, G. (2012). Mindful processing in psychotherapy: Facilitating natural healing process within attuned therapeutic relationship. *International Journal of Integrative Psychotherapy, 3*(1), 42–58.

Žvelc, G. (2014). Two aware minds are more powerful than only one: Mindfulness, relational schemas, and integrating Adult. In K. Tudor & G. Summers (Eds.), *Co-creative transactional analysis: Papers, responses, dialogues, and developments* (pp. 165–170). Karnac Books.

Žvelc, G., Černetič, M., & Košak, M. (2011). Mindfulness-based transactional analysis. *Transactional Analysis Journal, 41*(3), 241–254. https://doi.org/10.1177/036215371104100306

Žvelc, G., Jovanoska, K., & Žvelc, M. (2020). Development and validation of the Relational Needs Satisfaction Scale. *Frontiers in Psychology, 11*, 901, 1–15. https://doi.org/10.3389/fpsyg.2020.00901

Žvelc, G., & Žvelc, M. (2008, July 1–4). *The power of present moment: Mindful processing in psychotherapy and counseling* [Conference session]. Conference on Positive Psychology, Opatija, Croatia.

Žvelc, G., & Žvelc, M. (2009, April 16–19). *Loss and regain of 'now': Transforming trauma through mindful processing* [Conference session]. 4th International Integrative Psychotherapy Conference, Bled, Slovenia.

Žvelc, G., & Žvelc, M. (2011). Integrativna psihoterapija [Integrative psychotherapy]. In M. Žvelc, M. Možina, & J. Bohak (Eds.), *Psihoterapija* (pp. 565–591). IPSA, Inštitut za integrativno psihoterapijo in svetovanje.

Žvelc, M. (2008). Working with mistakes in psychotherapy: A relational model. *European Journal for Qualitative Research in Psychotherapy, 3*, 1–9.

Žvelc, M. (2011). I have feelings, too: The journey from avoidant to secure attachment. *International Journal of Integrative Psychotherapy, 2*(1), 22–44. http://integrative-journal.com/index.php/ijip/article/view/40

Žvelc, M., & Žvelc, G. (2006). Stili navezanosti v odraslosti [Attachment styles in adulthood]. *Psihološka Obzorja/Horizons of Psychology, 15*(3), 51–64.

Index

Please note that page references to Figures are followed by the letter 'f, and references to Tables the letter 't'

For Product Safety Concerns and Information please contact our EU
representative GPSR@taylorandfrancis.com
Taylor & Francis Verlag GmbH, Kaufingerstraße 24, 80331 München, Germany

www.ingramcontent.com/pod-product-compliance
Lightning Source LLC
Chambersburg PA
CBHW070356270326
41926CB00014B/2571

* 9 7 8 0 3 6 7 2 5 9 0 8 2 *